KU-246-119

Progress in
Cancer Research and Therapy
Volume 9

Endocrine Control in Neoplasia

Edited by

Rameshwar K. Sharma, Ph.D.
Associate Professor of Biochemistry
Chairman, Metabolic Regulation and Experimental Therapeutics
Basic Sciences, Memphis Regional Cancer Center
University of Tennessee Center for the Health Sciences
Memphis, Tennessee 38163

Wayne E. Criss, Ph.D.
Director of Cancer Research
Department of Biochemistry
and Howard University Comprehensive Cancer Center
Howard University College of Medicine
Washington, D.C. 20059

Raven Press ■ New York

Raven Press, 1140 Avenue of the Americas, New York, New York 10036

© 1978 by Raven Press Books, Ltd. All rights reserved. This book is protected by copyright. No part of it may be reproduced, stored in a retrieval system, or transmitted, in any form or by any means, electronic, mechanical, photocopying, recording, or otherwise, without the prior written permission of the publisher.

Made in the United States of America

Library of Congress Cataloging in Publication Data

Main entry under title:

Endocrine control in neoplasia.

(Progress in cancer research and therapy; v. 9)
Includes bibliographies and index.
1. Cancer. 2. Hormones. 3. Hormone receptors.
4. Metabolic regulation. I. Sharma, Rameshwar K.
II. Criss, Wayne E. III. Series. [DNLM: 1. Cell
transformation, Neoplastic—Congresses. 2. Hormones—
Physiology. 3. Neoplasms—Physiopathology. W1 PR667M
v. 9 / WK102.3 E561
RC262.E56 616.9′94 77–72623
ISBN 0–89004–244–6

Preface

Changes in cellular genetic information are believed by many to be involved in the process of carcinogenesis, and the mechanism by which these changes can occur is under investigation in a number of leading laboratories. Others argue that such changes may not be genetic but rather a consequence of alterations comparable to the process of cellular differentiation seen during the embryonic development of organs and tissues.

While both genetic and nongenetic changes in the cell could account for tumor development, hormones undoubtedly play a crucial role in these processes. This volume focuses on the mode of action of hormones and also on their biosynthesis, secretion, and the complex regulation of these processes. Thirty-five prominent oncologists review from basic and clinical viewpoints recent studies of hormonal responsiveness in over a dozen tumor types. These studies include levels of circulating hormones, membrane and intracellular hormone receptors, mechanisms of hormone-receptor action, cyclic nucleotide systems, intracellular biological responses to the hormones, and cellular growth responses that result from the overall action of hormones or cyclic nucleotides.

This volume will be of interest to those involved in biochemistry, cell biology, endocrinology, and clinical chemistry as they relate to the control of cellular function, as well as to clinicians who deal with the treatment of hormone-dependent tumors.

Contents

Contributors

Winston A. Anderson
Department of Zoology and Howard University Cancer Research Center
Howard University College of Medicine
Washington, D.C. 20059

Albert Castro
Department of Pathology
University of Miami School of Medicine
Miami, Florida 33152

Yoon Sang Cho-Chung
Laboratory of Pathophysiology
National Cancer Institute
National Institutes of Health
Bethesda, Maryland 20014

L. C. Costello
Department of Physiology and Biophysics
College of Medicine
Howard University
Washington, D.C. 20059

Mark E. Costlow
Department of Biochemistry
St. Jude Children's Research Hospital
332 North Lauderdale
Memphis, Tennessee 38101

Alice Dazord
Unité de Recherches sur le Controle Hormonal des Activités Cellulaires,
INSERM, U. 162
Hŏpital Debrouse
69322 Lyon Cedex 1, France

E. J. Diamond
Research Institute for Skeletomuscular Diseases
Hospital for the Joint Diseases and Medical Center
New York, New York 10035

Dennis M. Disorbo
Fels Research Institute and Department of Biochemistry
Temple University School of Medicine
Philadelphia, Pennsylvania 19140

R. B. Franklin
Department of Physiology and Biophysics
College of Medicine
Howard University
Washington, D.C. 20059

Joan T. Harmon
Diabetes Branch
National Institute of Arthritis, Metabolic and Digestive Diseases
National Institutes of Health
Bethesda, Maryland 20014

J. C. Heuson
Service de Médecine et Laboratoire d'Investigation Clinique H. J. Tagnon
Institut Jules Bordet
1000 Bruxelles, Belgium

Russel Hilf
Biochemistry Department and University of Rochester Cancer Center
University of Rochester School of Medicine and Dentistry
Rochester, New York 14642

Vincent P. Hollander
Research Institute for Skeletomuscular Diseases
Hospital for the Joint Diseases and Medical Center
New York, New York 10035

Charles Huggins
Ben May Laboratory for Cancer Research
University of Chicago Medical School
Chicago, Illinois 60637

N. Legros
Service de Médecine et Laboratoire d'Investigation Clinique H. J. Tagnon
Institut Jules Bordet
1000 Bruxelles, Belgium

Marc E. Lippman
Medicine Branch
National Institutes of Health
Bethesda, Maryland 20014

G. K. Littleton
Department of Physiology and Biophysics
College of Medicine
Howard University
Washington, D.C. 20059

Gerald Litwack
Fels Research Institute
and Department of Biochemistry
Temple University School of Medicine
Philadelphia, Pennsylvania 19140

Keishi Matsumoto
Institute for Cancer Research
Osaka University Medical School
Osaka 530, Japan

William L. McGuire
Department of Medicine
University of Texas
Health Science Center at San Antonio
San Antonio, Texas 78284

Joseph Meites
Department of Physiology
Michigan State University
East Lansing, Michigan 48824

Suresh Mohla
Department of Oncology
and Howard University Cancer Research Center
Howard University College of Medicine
Washington, D.C. 20059

Marie Monaco
Medicine Branch
National Institutes of Health
Bethesda, Maryland 20014

José M. Saez
Unité de Recherches sur le Controle Hormonal des Activités Cellulaires
INSERM, U. 162
Hǒpital Debrouse
69322 Lyon Cedex 1, France

Thomas J. Schmidt
Biochemistry of Gene Expression Section
Laboratory of Biochemistry
National Institutes of Health
Bethesda, Maryland 20014

Souei Sekiya
Department of Obstetrics and Gynecology
Chiba University School of Medicine
Chiba 280, Japan

Samir M. Shaife
Biochemistry Department
and University of Rochester Cancer Center
University of Rochester School of Medicine and Dentistry
Rochester, New York 14642

Rameshwar K. Sharma
Department of Biochemistry
and Memphis Regional Cancer Center,
University of Tennessee Center for the Health Sciences
Memphis, Tennessee 38163

Haruo Sugano
Cancer Institute
Japanese Foundation for Cancer Research
Tokyo 170, Japan

Hiroyoshi Takamizawa
Department of Obstetrics and Gynecology
Chiba University School of Medicine
Chiba 280, Japan

Guy P. Tell
Unité de Recherches sur le Controle Hormonal des Activités Cellulaires
INSERM, U. 162
Hǒpital Debrouse
69322 Lyon Cedex 1, France

E. Brad Thompson
Biochemistry of Gene Expression Section
Laboratory of Biochemistry
National Institutes of Health
Bethesda, Maryland 20014

Walter Voigt
Department of Pathology
University of Miami School of Medicine
Miami, Florida 33152

Clifford W. Welsh
Department of Anatomy
Michigan State University
East Lansing, Michigan 48824

Barnett Zumoff
Clinical Research Center
Albert Einstein College of Medicine
Montefieore Hospital and Medical Center
Bronx, New York 10467

Introduction

Claude Bernard was among the first scientists to proclaim that there must be controlling elements within the composition of fluids that bathe the cells of a multicellular organism. He proposed that the stability of this internal environment, which he called *milieu organique intérieur,* gave the organism a certain degree of functional freedom from the external environment, which he called *milieu cosmique ambiant.* It has now become evident that such stability is achieved by the coordinated activities of the endocrine and autonomic (exocrine) nervous systems.

As originally defined by Bernard, the *milieu intérieur* consists of plasma and extracellular fluids which bathe all the cells of an animal. Even though it is likely that cellular life developed from the pre-Cambrian sea which was rich in potassium and magnesium, elements more common to the intracellular environment *(milieu de la vie),* it has become obvious that multicellular organisms have evolved with a complex set of homeostatic controls which allows efficient and rapid coordination between the *milieu intérieur* and the *milieu de la vie.*

The endocrine system plays a major role in this coordination. The controlling molecules in the *milieu intérieur* include three basic types of chemicals: steroids, proteins, and catecholamines. These three classes of hormones coordinate the functioning of specific cells in a multicellular organism via a unique series of feedback control systems. Negative and positive feedback controls of the *milieu intérieur's* endocrine system regulate the oscillatory behavior observed in most organisms. This regulation may be simple or complex and directly depends upon the level of the hormones in the *milieu intérieur* and the ability of the target cell population to respond to these hormones.

A simple endocrine control system is one in which the hormone directly acts on certain target cells and directly promotes a change in the target cells (e.g. insulin–plasma glucose, parathormone–plasma calcium, aldosterone–plasma sodium). A complex endocrine control system is one in which several hormones (also possibly neural elements) and more than one set of target cells are involved. The latter system may have positive and/or negative feedback regulatory controls. An example would be the FSH-ovarian follicle-estrogen-LH-ovarian corpora lutea-progesterone cycle. By these systems, cell-to-cell coordination in a multicellular organism is promoted at a high level of efficiency. The growth and differentiation of each cell is carefully controlled to guarantee homeostasis of the *milieu de la vie.*

Unfortunately, populations of "maverick" cells sometimes occur in a multicellular organism. These maverick cells may be cancer cells. Many cancer cells appear to have lost some of their communications with the "normal" cells of the organism. However, this loss of communication is highly variable and led Charles Huggins to postulate his now widely accepted principles of cancer regulation: 1) "Cancer is not necessarily an autonomous and intrinsically self-perpetuating process," and 2) "Cancer can be sustained and even propagated by hormonal function which is not necessarily abnormal in type or exaggerated in rate, but which is operating at normal or even subnormal levels." Huggins' identification of the effective therapeutic benefits of anti-androgen treatment of human prostatic cancer and his establishment of the hormonally dependent DMBA rat mammary tumor model system has formed the rational scientific basis for the development of hormonal treatment of disease in general and of cancer specifically.

In recent years, we have begun to develop a much clearer picture of the hormonal controlling process or processes. It has become widely accepted that all hormones of the endocrine system exert their mode of action via specific hormone receptors. Specificity of hormone action resides in the presence or absence of specific hormone receptors in the target cell population, whether the target cells are normal or malignant. Two general types of hormone receptors have been identified: membrane and cytoplasmic.

Polypeptide and catecholamine hormones bind to specific receptors on the external cellular membrane surface. They exert their regulatory influences by activating specific membrane-bound enzymes (adenylate and guanylate cyclases) which produce cyclic AMP and cyclic GMP in the *milieu de la vie.* These two cyclic nucleotides coordinate intracellular processes so as to influence cellular growth and/or cellular differentiation.

Steroid hormones enter the target cell population and directly bind to cytoplasmic receptors in the *milieu de la vie.* The hormone-receptor complex enters the nucleus and interacts with the genetic material of the cell. In this way, steroid hormones influence cellular growth and/or cellular differentiation.

This book examines and summarizes our current knowledge about these hormonal receptors and their mode of regulation in cancer tissues. It illustrates how to determine or evaluate hormonal responsiveness in a variety of cancers, and how to utilize such knowledge to initiate cancer therapies. It allows us to begin to understand and extend that simple concept which Huggins put forth many years ago: "Cancers may be independent or dependent upon hormones for growth."

The Editors

Endocrine Control in Neoplasia, edited by
R. K. Sharma and W. E. Criss.
Raven Press, New York © 1978.

Two Principles in Endocrine Therapy of Cancers: Hormone Deprival and Hormone Interference*†

Charles Huggins

The Ben May Laboratory for Cancer Research, University of Chicago Medical School, Chicago, Illinois 60637

Hormones, or synthetic substances exerting physiologic effects similar thereto, are of crucial significance for growth of 7 hormone-dependent cancers of man and the animals. Two opposite sorts of change of the hormonal status can induce regression of such cancers: *(a)* deprivation of essential hormones; *(b)* hormone interference with large amounts of critical compounds.

The earliest indication that regression of advanced cancer in living creatures can be effected was derived from removal of normal organs, namely, the ovaries of women (2). This empiric therapeutic procedure was remarkable insofar as it was made before there was any concept of endocrine action. Following this discovery, Lathrop and Loeb (32) found that removal of ovaries prevented onset of mammary cancer in a considerable number of mice. Lacassagne (30) was the first to show that a correlation exists between development of cancer and hormones, since a steroid with estrogenic activity incited formation of mammary cancer; in a famous experiment weekly injections of 30 μg of estrone benzoate evoked cancer of the breast in each of 3 male mice in 5 to 6 months.

The proof that modification of hormonal status can cause regression of cancer came from a study of tumors of canine prostate (15): injection of stilbestrol resulted in a profound decrease in size of benign and malignant prostatic tumors, even those of huge size, in the dog. The hormonal control of cancer applied to far advanced carcinoma of the prostate in man (21). It was found that testoster-

* This investigation was supported by grants from the American Cancer Society and the Jane Coffin Childs Memorial Fund for Medical Research.

† This article originally appeared in *Cancer Research,* Vol. 25, August 1965, pp. 1163–1167; it appears here by permission of the original publisher. In this article, Professor Huggins clearly established the two principles of hormone deprival and hormone interference in anticancer therapy. These principles provided the working foundation for the numerous studies reported in this volume.

There is absolutely no doubt that cancer cells can regress from too little hormone or too much hormone. The major purpose of this volume is to provide for the reader an overview of the intracellular and molecular mechanisms of hormone action in cancer. These are mechanisms that have been elucidated because many excellent scientists and physicians have vigorously followed the two beautifully simple principles set out by Professor Huggins in 1965.

one accelerated the growth of human prostatic cancer, whereas, in contrast, orchiectomy or the injection of estradiol benzoate or of stilbestrol caused in most patients a dramatic and long-lasting regression of their cancers. Stilbestrol was the first synthetic substance found to be an anti-cancer drug.

There are two principles in the destruction of cancer cells in living creatures by modifications of endocrine status: *(a)* hormone deprival; *(b)* hormone interference in the cancer cell. Malignant cells can regress from too little or too much hormone. Hormone interference causes severe damage or death of cancer through *toxicity in the cancer cell* while normal cells are relatively undamaged. Not all cancers that regress from hormone deprival also regress from excessive amounts of the same hormones.

The experience with prostatic tumors led to the concept of hormone dependence and independence. This terminology (24) was first used in 1945. There is a fundamental difference between a normal hormonal target cell and its hormone-responsive malignant derivative. In a normal cell of origin supporting hormones act as catalysts of growth and metabolism, but these compounds are not essential for life of the cell. In contrast, a hormone-dependent cancer cell dies when supporting hormones are withheld or their source is removed. In consequence, a cancer cell cannot participate in growth cycles (13) characteristic of the normal cell of origin created by alternately administering and withholding supporting hormone. In hormone-dependent cancers of all sorts, prostatic and others, the supporting hormones are of cardinal importance in maintaining the life of the malignant cell. This is the principle of cancer control by hormone deprival.

Cancers can also be controlled by supplying large amounts of hormones; this is the novel principle (22) of hormone interference, a pharmacologic concept. Two cases where hormone interference kills cancer cells will be cited.

1. Heilman and Kendall (10) administered large amounts of cortisone to mice bearing a transplanted lymphosarcoma: "Although dramatic and apparently complete cures are produced, they are only temporary in a majority of the animals." Only lymphomas of adult male mice failed to be resorbed when cortisone was given, and the combined administration of cortisone *plus* estradiol-17β caused rapid regression of the tumors in these males. Whereas corticosteroids exerted lethal effects, adrenalectomy does not cause regression of lymphomas in mice.

Pearson et al. (38,39) observed that ACTH[1] or cortisone resulted in temporary regression in human lymphatic leukemia and Hodgkin's disease.

2. Huggins et al. (22,25) induced mammary carcinoma in rats, which were then treated for a limited time with large amounts of estradiol-17β *plus* progesterone. This combination of hormones excited such exuberant growth of normal mammary cells that the breast resembled that of rats late in pregnancy.

---

[1] The following abbreviations are used: ACTH, adrenocorticotropin; S-D, Sprague-Dawley strain of rats; 3-MC, 3-methylcholanthrene; 2-AAF, 2-acetaminofluorene; and 7,12-DMBA, 7,12-dimethylbenz *(a)* anthracene.

Nevertheless, many of the mammary cancers were completely extinguished (25), and 52% of the rats were free from cancer 6 months after steroids were discontinued. Landau et al. (31) found that "a combination of 50 mg of progesterone and 5 mg of estradiol benzoate injected intramuscularly and daily, induced measurable and clinically worth-while improvement in 9 of 15 patients, including 1 man, with disseminated mammary cancer. Benefit was usually obtained in patients in whom other forms of endocrine therapy such as adrenalectomy and oophorectomy had previously promoted tumor regression." Mammary cancer can regress from either hormone deprival or hormone interference from excess of hormones.

At the present time seven sorts of cancer are known to be responsive to hormonal modifications of the *milieu intérieur* since shrinkage of cancer and betterment of its host follow changes in his hormonal status. Cancers of this sort are of the breast, prostate, thyroid (1), endometrium (27), kidney (4,29), and seminal vesicle (26), and also include lymphoma and leukemia.

In a great many clinical patients, men and women, mammary cancer regresses after any of a considerable number of hormonal modifications. The regression so induced can be profound and long lasting (6,11), and, accordingly, the treatment is of value to the patient. With a single exception (22), all of the procedures found to be beneficial for human cancer of the breast were found directly at the bedside through clinical investigation. The vast amount of work in the laboratory on mammary cancer has yielded little that has been applied as therapy for women with cancer of the breast.

Hormone-dependent experimental mammary cancer. Spontaneous mammary cancer is common in the dog and mouse as well as in man. In the dog mammary cancers did not shrink after ovariectomy or adrenalectomy (23). In various strains of mice possessing the milk agent, spontaneous mammary cancers of palpable size did not regress following ovariectomy, hypophysectomy, or administration of testosterone (35). In this regard the tumors of the dog and mouse differ from many human mammary cancers. It was necessary to find a hormone-dependent experimental mammary cancer.

The key to the solution of this problem was recognition of a species with hormone-responsive cancers (14). So far as is known, the rat is unique among the species available for research on breast cancer, since only in this species are mammary cancers hormone-dependent. Hormone-dependent mammary cancer now can be produced invariably and in potentially unlimited supply with methods of extreme simplicity.

There are three methods for induction of mammary cancer in rats: exposure to (a) estrogens, (b) ionizing radiation, and (c) aromatics. Aromatics are the most efficient, since they give the highest yield of mammary carcinomas in the largest percentage of rats.

Mammary carcinoma induced by estrogens. The continued exposure to critical doses of estrogens leads to mammary cancer. The method is slow and inefficient, since many months elapse before the tumors appear and many of the animals never develop breast cancer (37). Noble and Collip (36) found that the implantation of estrone pellets into random-bred hooded rats was followed by the development of adenocarcinoma in 28 of 49 rats, the first tumor appearing after 226 days. Maisin et al. (34) implanted pellets of stilbestrol in rats that were observed for more than 300 days; no mammary cancers arose. We injected 50 μg of estradiol-17β daily for 400 days in 15 female Sprague-Dawley rats beginning at age 66 days, the rats earlier having been subjected to ovariectomy-hysterectomy. One rat developed mammary carcinoma, which was detected after 358 days; 14 rats remained free from breast cancer.

Mammary carcinoma induced by ionizing radiation. The selective induction of mammary cancer in the rat by irradiation was discovered by Hamilton (9). A single dose of radioactive isotopes, X-rays, or γ-irradiation elicits mammary tumors, which arise rather quickly, but in no series have all irradiated rats developed mammary cancer.

Hamilton et al. (9) observed a 40% incidence of mammary cancer in female S-D rats, aged 55 days, after a single injection of ^{211}At. Maisin et al. (34) found that some young female rats (strain unspecified) developed mammary cancer after total-body irradiation with X-rays. In S-D female rats, aged 52 days, given single total-body X-irradiation (400 r) and observed for 6 months, mammary carcinomas had the following characteristics (17): incidence in 29.7% of the rats; detection of 92% of the cancers within 79 days; multiple carcinomas in 18% of the rats. In experiments of Cronkite et al. (5) 79% of S-D female rats developed mammary tumors, benign and malignant, within 10 months after exposure to a single dose of total-body X-irradiation (400 r), and the first tumor was detected 41 days after the exposure. Shellabarger et al. (43) found that 56% of female S-D rats, aged 40 days, developed mammary tumors after a single total-body γ-irradiation with a ^{60}Co irradiator at age 40 days.

Mammary carcinoma induced by aromatics. Maisin and Coolen (33) painted the skin of mice repeatedly with a solution of 3-MC and found, in addition to skin cancer, that carcinoma of the mammary gland arose in 18% of the mice after 7 months. Wilson et al. (47) discovered that incorporation of an aromatic (2-AAF) in the diet of rats induced cancer in various tissues; mammary cancer arose in a small number of the animals. Shay et al. (42) observed that the daily intragastric instillation of 3-MC, 2 mg, for many months induced mammary cancer in a large percentage of Wistar rats; the tumors were detected after 129 to 383 days.

We found out (14,18) that a single large but tolerable dose of any of a considerable number of aromatics in the rat consistently induces mammary cancer selectively and rapidly. Although the conditions for induction are highly restricted, they are easily satisfied. Eight parameters have been identified in induction of mammary cancer. These are (a) the nature and (b) dose of the aromatic, (c) species, (d) strain (44), (e) age (16), and (f) the hormonal status of the rat; additionally, (g) the animals must remain free from infectious disease and (h) have no contact with cancer-protective substances (20).

In capsule, mammary cancer has always developed in our laboratory in 1,500 consecutive female rats of S-D strain, aged 50 days, given a single i.v. injection of a lipid emulsion, 1 ml, containing 7,12-dimethylbenz*(a)*anthracene, 5 mg; the animals were kept in metal cages in an air-conditioned room at 25° ± 1°C. A single feeding by gastric instillation of a solution of vegetable oil, 1 ml, containing 7,12-DMBA, 20 mg, can substitute for the lipid emulsion. The earliest mammary cancer induced by this technic was detected by palpation 20 days after 7,12-DMBA was given. In 90 consecutive rats (12) mammary cancer was detected in 28 to 92 days, mean 42.8 ± 11 days.

The mammary gland of the young adult S-D female rat stands in the forefront of cells of living creatures in its susceptibility to induction of cancer. It is equaled only by cells of certain chickens when they are inoculated with a single agent, Rous sarcoma virus I. In a famous experiment of Rous (41), cell-free filtrate of a sarcoma injected into other fowls evoked tumors of palpable size after 10 to 21 days.

Dao et al. (8) fed female rats a single dose of 7,12-DMBA and after 4 hr transplanted their mammary glands to other rats; mammary cancer arose in the homologous recipients of the grafts.

Many aromatics share in common the ability to induce mammary cancer in the rat after a single dose. In this regard, from a molecular standpoint, 4-aminodiphenyl, consisting of two rings, has the simplest strucure of the aromatic amines. The least complex of polynuclear aromatic hydrocarbons, a monomethylbenz*(a)*anthracene (7-methyl- or 12-methyl-), consists of four rings. But in efficiency of dosage, 7,12-DMBA exceeds all other aromatics by an order of magnitude.

Nature of aromatic-induced tumors in the rat. A single feeding of 7,12-DMBA, 20 mg, to 38 female S-D rats, aged 50 days, and observed for 180 days thereafter evoked tumors (25) as follows: mammary cancer, 38 rats; mammary fibroadenoma, 34 rats; ear duct carcinoma, 2 rats; leukemia, 1 rat. Tumors of other structures are less common. The tumors occur in two discontinuous series: mammary carcinoma manifests itself early, and other tumors, after 3 months.

All of the mammary cancers evoked by aromatic hydrocarbons are rather similar in cytologic appearance, and all possess the cellular pattern of papillary adenocarcinoma; mitoses are abundant. Often in some of the tumors islands of squamous carcinoma are present (50). The mammary cancers rarely metastasize but kill the host by invading muscle and skin, with consequent hemorrhage and ulceration. The respiration values (40) are similar to those of the normal lactating mammary gland; the high rate of glycolysis, which Warburg (46) found to be distinctive of the metabolism of cancer, prevailed in the induced carcinomas.

Young and Cowan (49) found that a number of the induced mammary carcinomas of the rat undergo spontaneous regression. Such tumors have these characteristics: mammary epithelium remains cubical or columnar; many mitotic figures are present; stroma of the tumor becomes heavily infiltrated with lymphocytes and other mononucleated cells. In our laboratory, we have not observed spontaneous regression of all of the cancers in any rat bearing multiple mammary cancers. It would appear that spontaneous regression is dependent on the quality of the individual tumor and is not a function of the host's immunologic status.

Hormonal prerequisites for induction of mammary cancer in the rat. The physiologic state of the mammary tree, determined by endocrine effects, is of critical significance in induction of mammary cancer. Repeated feeding of 3-MC to groups of rats evoked mammary cancer in all intact females and in no hypophysectomized mate (19). Young (48) fed 3-MC to hypophysectomized rats treated with estradiol-17β, progesterone, and bovine growth hormone; mammary carcinoma arose in 5 rats in a group of 9.

Hormonal influence on mammary cancer of the rat. Changes in hormonal status have little or no influence on hormone-independent mammary cancers. But the majority of mammary carcinomas in the rat are profoundly influenced by endocrine factors, and after appropriate changes in hormone status their growth can be accelerated or retarded, and indeed many of the growths can be extinguished.

Acceleration of growth of the mammary cancers occurs in pregnancy (7,22), in pseudopregnancy (7), and following administration of progesterone or 9α-bromo-11-ketoprogesterone (19).

Retardation of growth of mammary cancers and, at times, tumor extinction occur after ovariectomy (14) or hypophysectomy (19,28); the relative effectiveness of these two ablative procedures is shown in Fig. 1. Moreover, a severely

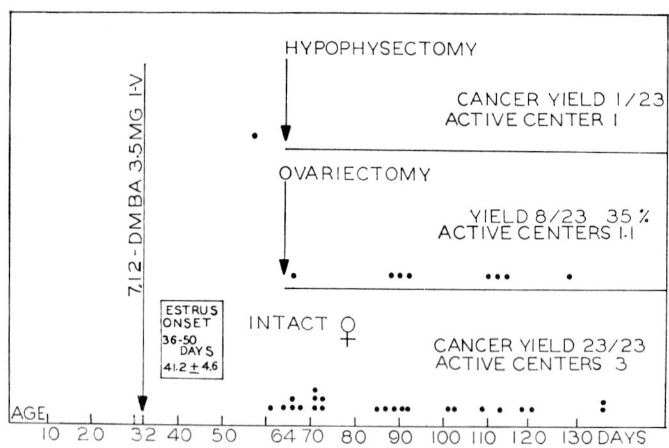

FIG. 1. The relative effectiveness of hypophysectomy and ovariectomy in extinction of mammary cancer. The age of individual rats at the time of the detection of mammary cancers, which were subsequently found at autopsy, is indicated by black dots. Mammary cancer found at autopsy is designated an active center. At the age of 32 days, just before the onset of estrus, a lipid emulsion of 7,12-dimethylbenz*(a)*anthracene (7,12-DMBA), 36 mg/kg, was injected i.v. in Sprague-Dawley female rats. At the age of 64 days, two groups of 23 rats were subjected to hypophysectomy or ovariectomy. A group of 23 rats was maintained intact. Autopsy was performed at the age of 136 days.

deleterious effect on mammary cancer follows administration of testosterone (14), estradiol-17β with progesterone (25), or equine gonadotropin (19).

Bielschowsky (3) found that mammary cancer of the rat frequently regressed during lactation, whereas ovariectomy had no effect on growth of the tumors.

The mammary cancers that diminish in size after removal of the pituitary or ovaries have a distinctive cytologic appearance. Many of the carcinoma cells are destroyed. In the remaining tumor acini the many layers of plump epithelial cells are replaced by a single layer of flat cells (14); the most obvious and consistent changes are flattening of the epithelium and an increase in size of the acinar lumina (50). Tumors unaffected by hormonal modification retain many layers of epithelial cells.

The inhibitory effect of ovariectomy on the development of mammary cancer in the rat was overcome by a daily injection of small amounts of estradiol-17β (14). It has been reported (45) that injection of growth hormone with prolactin elicited growth of tumors in rats with mammary tumors treated earlier with ovariectomy.

In the experiments of Kim and Furth (28) the growth of aromatic-induced mammary carcinoma was inhibited by ovariectomy (72%) and by hypophysectomy (87%). In their hypophysectomy series, tumors could not be identified at autopsy in 37% of the animals. Grafts of functioning pituitary tumors into hypophysectomized rats whose tumors had undergone considerable regression caused the resumption of progressive tumor growth with the reappearance of many new mammary tumors.

From the evidence that has been presented it would appear that both steroids and protein hormones are of significance in the maintenance of mammary carcinoma.

REFERENCES

1. Balme, H. W. (1954): Metastatic carcinoma of the thyroid successfully treated with thyroxine. *Lancet,* 1:812–813.
2. Beatson, G. T. (1896): On the treatment of inoperable cases of carcinoma of the mamma: Suggestions for a new method of treatment, with illustrative cases. *Lancet,* 2:104–107, 162–165.
3. Bielschowsky, F. (1947): The carcinogenic action of 2-acetylaminofluorene and related compounds. *Br. Med. Bull.,* 4:382–385.
4. Bloom, H. J. G., Dukes, C. E., and Mitchley, B. C. V. (1963): Hormone-dependent tumours of the kidney. I. The oestrogen-induced renal tumour of the Syrian hamster. Hormone treatment and possible relationship to carcinoma of the kidney in man. *Br. J. Cancer,* 17:611–645.
5. Cronkite, E. P., Shellabarger, C. J., Bond, V. P., and Lippincott, S. W. (1960): Studies on radiation-induced mammary gland neoplasia in the rat. I. The role of the ovary in the neoplastic response of the breast tissue to total- or partial-body irradiation. *Radiat. Res.,* 12:81–93.
6. Dao, T. L., and Huggins. C. (1957): Metastatic cancer of the breast treated by adrenalectomy. Evaluation and the five-year results. *J.A.M.A.,* 165:1793–1797.
7. Dao, T. L., and Sunderland, H. (1959): Mammary carcinogenesis by 3-methylcholanthrene. I. Hormonal aspects in tumor induction and growth. *J. Natl. Cancer Inst.,* 23:567–585.
8. Dao, T. L., Tanaka, Y., and Gawlak, D. (1964): Tumor induction in transplanted mammary glands in rats. *J. Natl. Cancer Inst.,* 32:1259–1275.
9. Hamilton, J. G., Durbin, P. W., and Parrott, M. (1954): The accumulation and destructive

action of astatine[211] (EKA-iodine) in the thyroid gland of rats and monkeys. *J. Clin. Endocrinol. Metab.*, 17:1161–1178.
10. Heilman, F. R., and Kendall, E. C. (1944): The influence of 11-dehydro-17-hydroxy-corticosterone (compound E) on the growth of a malignant tumor in the mouse. *Endocrinology,* 34:416–420.
11. Huggins, C. (1956): Control of cancers of man by endocrinologic methods. A review. *Cancer Res.,* 16:825–830.
12. Huggins, C. (1962): Cancer and necrosis induced selectively by hydrocarbons. In: *Horizons in Biochemistry,* edited by B. Pullman and M. Kasha, p. 497. Academic Press, New York.
13. Huggins, C. (1963): The hormone-dependent cancers. *J.A.M.A.,* 186:481–483.
14. Huggins, C., Briziarelli, G., and Sutton, H. (1959): Rapid induction of mammary carcinoma in the rat and the influence of hormones on the tumors. *J. Exp. Med.,* 109:25–42.
15. Huggins, C., and Clark, P. J. (1940): Quantitative studies of prostatic secretion. II. The effect of castration and of estrogen injection on the normal and on the hyperplastic prostate glands of dogs. *J. Exp. Med.,* 72:747–762.
16. Huggins, C., and Fukunishi, R. (1963): Mammary and peritoneal tumors induced by intraperitoneal administration of 7,12-dimethylbenz *(a)*anthracene in newborn and adult rats. *Cancer Res.* 23:785–789.
17. Huggins, C., and Fukunishi, R. (1963): Cancer in the rat after single exposure to irradiation or hydrocarbons. Age and strain factors. Hormone dependence of the mammary cancers. *Radiat. Res.,* 20:493–503.
18. Huggins, C., Grand, L. C., and Brillantes, F. P. (1961) Mammary cancer induced by a single feeding of polynuclear hydrocarbons and its suppression. *Nature,* 189:204–207.
19. Huggins, C., Grand, L. C., and Brillantes, F. P. (1959): Critical significance of breast structure in the induction of mammary cancer in the rat. *Proc. Natl. Acad. Sci. U.S.A.,* 45:1294–1300.
20. Huggins, C., Grand, L., and Fukunishi, R. (1964): Aromatic influences on the yields of mammary cancers following administration of 7,12-dimethylbenz*(a)*anthracene. *Proc. Natl. Acad. Sci. U.S.A.,* 51:737–742.
21. Huggins, C., and Hodges, C. V. (1941): Studies on prostatic cancer. I. The effect of castration, of estrogen and of androgen injection on serum phosphatases in metastatic carcinoma of the prostate. *Cancer Res.,* 1:293–297.
22. Huggins, C., Moon, R. C., and Morii, S. (1962): Extinction of experimental mammary cancer. I. Estradiol-17β and progesterone. *Proc. Natl. Acad. Sci. U.S.A.,* 48:379–386.
23. Huggins, C., and Moulder, P. V. (1944): Studies on the mammary tumors of dogs. I. Lactation and the influence of ovariectomy and suprarenalectomy thereon. *J. Exp. Med.,* 80:441–454.
24. Huggins, C., and Scott, W. W. (1945): Bilateral adrenalectomy in prostatic cancer. Clinical features and urinary excretion of 17-ketosteroids and estrogen. *Ann. Surg.,* 122:1031–1041.
25. Huggins, C., and Yang, N. C. (1962): Induction and extinction of mammary cancer. *Science,* 137:257–262.
26. Kees, O. S. R. (1964): Clinical improvement following estrogenic therapy in a case of primary adenocarcinoma of the seminal vesicle. *J. Urol.,* 91:665–670
27. Kelley, R. M., and Baker, W. H. (1961): Progestational agents in treatment of carcinoma of endometrium. *N. Engl. J. Med.,* 264:216–222.
28. Kim. U., and Furth, J. (1960): Relation of mammary tumors to mammotropes. II. Hormone responsiveness of 3-methylcholanthrene induced mammary carcinomas. *Proc. Soc. Exp. Biol. Med.,* 103:643–645.
29. Kirkman, H. (1959): Estrogen-induced tumors of the kidney. III. Growth characteristics in the Syrian hamster. *Natl. Cancer Inst. Monogr.,* 1:1–58.
30. Lacassagne, A. (1932): Apparition de cancers de la mamelle chez la souris mâle soumise à des injections de folliculine. *Compt. Rend.,* 195:630–632.
31. Landau, R. L., Ehrlich, E. N., and Huggins, C. (1962): Estradiol benzoate and progesterone in advanced human-breast cancer. *J.A.M.A.,* 182:632–636.
32. Lathrop, A. E. C., and Loeb, L. (1916): Further investigations on the origin of tumors in mice. III. On the part played by internal secretion in the spontaneous development of tumors. *J. Cancer Res.,* 1:1–19.
33. Maisin, J., and Coolen, M.-L. (1936): Au sujet du pouvoir cancèrigéne du méthyl-cholanthrène. *Compt. Rend. Soc. Biol.,* 123:159–160.
34. Maisin, J., Meerseman, F., and Maldague, P. (1956): Cancers de la mamelle chez le rat, oestrogenes et irradiation totale. *Acta Unio Intern. Contra Cancrum,* 12:661–664.

35. Mühlbock, O. (1958): Studies on the hormone dependence of experimental breast tumors in mice. In: *Endocrine Aspects of Breast Cancer,* edited by A. R. Currie, p. 291. Williams & Wilkins, Baltimore.
36. Noble, R. L., and Collip, J. B. (1941): Regression of estrogen-induced mammary tumors in female rats following removal of the stimulus. *Can. Med. Assoc. J.,* 44:1–5.
37. Noble, R. L., and Cutts, J. H. (1959): Mammary tumors of the rat. A review. *Cancer Res.,* 19:1125–1139.
38. Pearson, O. H., Eliel, L. P., Rawson, R. W., Dobriner, K., and Rhoads, C. P. (1949): ACTH- and cortisone-induced regression of lymphoid tumors in man. *Cancer,* 2:943–945
39. Pearson, O. H., Li, M. H., Maclean, J. P., Lipsett, M. B., and West, C. D. (1955): The use of hydrocortisone in cancer. *Ann. N.Y. Acad. Sci.,* 16:393–396.
40. Rees, E. D., and Huggins, C. (1960): Steroid influences on respiration, glycolysis, and levels of pyridine nucleotide-linked dehydrogenases of experimental mammary cancers. *Cancer Res.,* 20:963–971.
41. Rous, P. (1911): A sarcoma of the fowl transmissible by an agent separable from the tumor cells. *J. Exp. Med.,* 13:397–411.
42. Shay, H., Aegerter, E. A., Gruenstein, M., and Komarov, S. A. (1949): Development of adenocarcinoma of the breast in the Wistar rat following the gastric instillation of methylcholanthrene. *J. Natl. Cancer Inst.,* 10:255–266.
43. Shellabarger, C. J., Cronkite, E. P., Bond, V. P., and Lippincott, S. W. (1957): The occurrence of mammary tumors in the rat after sublethal whole-body irradiation. *Radiat. Res.,* 6:501–512.
44. Sydnor, K. L., Butenandt, O., Brillantes, F. P., and Huggins, C. (1962): Race-strain factor related to hydrocarbon-induced mammary cancer in rats. *J. Natl. Cancer Inst.,* 29:805–814.
45. Talwalker, P. K., Meites, J., and Mizuno, H. (1964): Mammary tumor induction by estrogen or anterior pituitary hormones in ovariectomized rats given 7,12-dimethyl-1,2-benzanthracene. *Proc. Soc. Exp. Biol. Med.,* 116:531–534.
46. Warburg, O. (1930): *Metabolism of Tumours.* Constable & Co., London.
47. Wilson, R. H., DeEds, F., and Cox, A. J., Jr. (1941): The toxicity and carcinogenic activity of 2-acetaminofluorene. *Cancer Res.,* 1:595–608.
48. Young, S. (1961): Induction of mammary carcinoma in hypophysectomized rats treated with 3-methylcholanthrene, oestradiol-17β, progesterone and growth hormone. *Nature.* 190:356–357.
49. Young, S., and Cowan, D. M. (1963): Spontaneous regression of induced mammary tumours in rats. *Br. J. Cancer,* 17:85–89.
50. Young, S., Cowan, D. M., and Sutherland, L. E. (1963): The histology of induced mammary tumours in rats. *J. Pathol. Bacteriol.,* 85:331–340.

PITUITARY HORMONES

Endocrine Control in Neoplasia, edited by
R. K. Sharma and W. E. Criss.
Raven Press, New York © 1978.

Abnormal Adrenocorticotropic Hormone Control in Adrenocortical Carcinoma

Rameshwar K. Sharma

Department of Biochemistry and Memphis Regional Cancer Center, University of Tennessee Center for the Health Sciences, Memphis, Tennessee 38163

As is the case with many adrenocortical carcinomas (44,71,76), rat adrenocortical carcinoma 494, which was discovered by Snell and Stewart (101) in 1959, is not stimulated by adrenocorticotropic hormone (ACTH) to synthesize corticosterone. To understand the reason for this we must first understand the basic control mechanism of ACTH in a normal adrenal cell. ACTH is a polypeptide pituitary hormone that regulates the rate of secretion of corticosteroids in the adrenal cortex. Despite rapid advances in our understanding of the control processes in this gland, the critical question of how ACTH triggers the steroidogenic mechanism is still unanswered.

Since the original discovery by Rall and Sutherland and their associates (63) that cyclic adenosine monophosphate (cAMP) mediates the actions of some hormones, the intermediary role of this agent as a second messenger in the regulation of adrenal steroidogenesis has been under continual investigation. According to the second-messenger concept (66,103), a hormone is initially secreted by one type of cell, following which it travels to the target cell. On contact with the target cell, the hormone stimulates the synthesis of a second messenger. According to the classic concept of Sutherland and his associates as modified by the later work of Kuo and Greengard (39), all actions of cAMP are modulated by cAMP-dependent protein kinase. The criteria for acceptance of a second-messenger role for cAMP in adrenal steroidogenesis are the following: (a) ACTH activates adenylate cyclase *in vitro,* (b) ACTH increases cAMP concentration in the adrenal cell, which in turn increases an endogenous cAMP-dependent protein kinase, (c) exogenous cAMP stimulates endogenous protein kinase and steroidogenesis, (d) cyclic nucleotide phosphodiesterase inhibitors potentiate the steroidogenic response of submaximal concentrations of ACTH. We shall weigh the evidence to determine if cAMP meets the preceding criteria.

Adenylate Cyclase

Direct stimulation of adenylate cyclase by ACTH in whole homogenates of rat adrenal glands has been demonstrated; however, it has been found that ACTH concentrations less than 10^{-7} M (approximately 100,000 μU) do not activate adenylate cyclase (77). The concentration of ACTH in the normal rat is less than 5 μU/ml blood (7×10^{-12} M); even after adrenalectomy the ACTH concentration in the rat increases to only 32 μU/ml blood (4×10^{-12} M) (79). It is clear that the concentration of ACTH needed to cause a minimal response of adenylate cyclase is at least 100,000-fold higher than the concentration present in rat blood. Thus these data do not directly demonstrate an association between physiological concentrations of ACTH and activation of adenylate cyclase; rather, they provide evidence that adrenal adenylate cyclase is insensitive to physiological concentrations of the hormone.

cAMP Levels and Steroidogenesis

Haynes (23), using bovine adrenal cortex slices, was the first to demonstrate an increase in cAMP levels in response to ACTH. Subsequent studies in which ACTH was added to incubated rat adrenal quarters or injected into whole animals (18) demonstrated that ACTH-induced steroidogenesis follows the formation of cAMP. The concentration of ACTH used in these *in vitro* studies was 1×10^6 μU/ml, and significant accumulation of cAMP occurred within 1 min of exposure of the adrenal quarters to 1×10^6 μU/ml ACTH (18). Similar results were reported by Beall and Sayers (2) when they used a more sensitive trypsinized cell preparation (74). The concentration of ACTH used by the latter investigators was 10,000 pg (2,000 μU) for the cells isolated from one adrenal gland. These observations apparently support a second-messenger role for cAMP in adrenal steroidogenesis, but the concentrations of ACTH used in these studies were supraphysiological.

On the other hand, other data have been published clearly indicating that submaximal steroidogenic concentrations of ACTH do not increase cAMP levels. Beall and Sayers (2) found that low doses of ACTH, 50 to 250 pg (10–50 μU), stimulated steroidogenesis without causing detectable changes in the concentration of cAMP. They considered the possibility that at low doses of the hormone there might be increases in cAMP at "discrete loci." However, no such discrete loci have yet been reported. Sharma and associates (89) demonstrated that at submaximal steroidogenic concentrations of ACTH (10 μU) there was an increase in endogenous protein kinase activity and steroidogenesis, but there was no corresponding change in the level of cAMP. These data indicated that there was an increase in protein kinase activity but that there was no detectable change in cAMP level.

More recent studies by Perchellet and associates (58) showed that neither submaximal ($<$10 μU) nor supramaximal (100 μU) steroidogenic concentrations of ACTH cause detectable changes in levels of cAMP during the first 30 min, but there is a corresponding rise in endogenous protein kinase activity accompanied by steroidogenesis (Figs. 1 and 2). These results do not support an obligatory role for cAMP in adrenal steroidogenesis at physiological concentrations of the hormone.

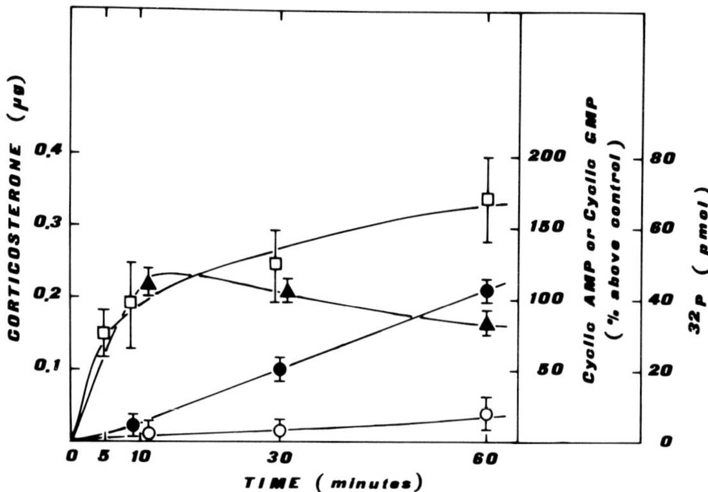

FIG. 1. Time response curve for production of cAMP *(open circles)*, cGMP *(squares)*, corticosterone *(filled circles)*, and phosphorylation *(triangles)* in isolated adrenal cells in response to 5 μU of ACTH. Incubation system: 2×10^6 isolated adrenal cells suspended in 0.8 ml; reagents were dissolved in 0.2 ml of Krebs-Ringer-bicarbonate buffer, pH 7.4, containing 4% albumin and 0.2% glucose, or protein kinase buffer. Total volume of first incubation, 1 ml; second incubation, 0.5 ml. Experiments were conducted in sextuplicates: two of the samples were used for determination of corticosterone, two for measurement of cAMP and cGMP, and two for assay of phosphorylation. 5′-GMP and other noncyclic nucleotides were removed by alumina column. That the separation of cGMP from 5′-GMP was complete was assured by applying to the alumina column a sample containing 10,000 dpm of [^{3}H]cGMP and [^{14}C]5′-GMP and counting an aliquot of the eluate collected, there being no ^{14}C radioactivity in this fraction. The eluate was then adsorbed on a QAE-Sephadex A-25 column in the formate form. A first elution with 7 ml of 0.5 N formic acid yielded cAMP, and a second elution with 7 ml of 4 N formic acid gave cGMP. Recovery of cAMP and cGMP was 60 to 80%. The samples were lyophilized and dissolved in 700 μl water, and the appropriate aliquot was used for measurement of cAMP and cGMP. Results are expressed as mean values (± SD) of six separate determinations from three different experiments. Basal values have been subtracted from experimental results. (Adapted from Perchellet et al., ref. 58.)

Studies from several other laboratories have questioned the existence of an obligatory intermediary role of cAMP in adrenal steroidogenesis. Moyle et al. (51), working with ACTH and its *o*-nitrophenylsulfenyl derivative, demonstrated that although both of these agents elicit the same maximal production of steroids in isolated rat adrenal cells, they have different effects on cAMP synthesis. The ACTH analog was only one-thirtieth to one-hundredth as effective as ACTH in stimulating cAMP accumulation.

Hudson and McMartin (27) investigated the involvement of cAMP in steroidogenesis by using isolated adrenal cell column perfusion. They found that cAMP was released into the perfusate only in response to supramaximal steroidogenic concentrations of ACTH. Steroidogenesis stimulated by cAMP at 0.5, 1.0, and 5 mg/ml showed an inverse relationship between the rate of steroid production

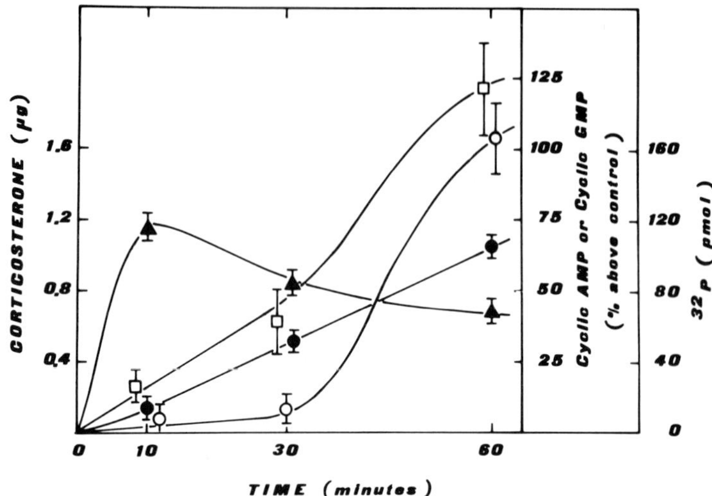

FIG. 2. Time response curve for production of cAMP *(open circles)*, cGMP *(squares)*, corticosterone *(filled circles)*, and phosphorylation *(triangles)* in isolated adrenal cells in response to 100 μU of ACTH. Conditions of the experiment were identical to those in Fig. 1. (Adapted from Perchellet et al., ref. 58.)

and the concentration of cAMP. A correlation between synthesis of cAMP and steroidogenesis existed only over a narrow concentration range of ACTH.

Espiner et al. (9) measured cAMP levels and steroid output in adrenal veins after ACTH stimulation of sheep adrenals *in vivo.* No cAMP output was detected at submaximal steroidogenic concentrations of ACTH, but at extremely high concentrations, the adrenal venous cAMP level rose rapidly before the corresponding rise in cortisol production. At lower supramaximal concentrations of ACTH, the time lags for cortisol production and cAMP production were longer and not distinct. With a second stimulation by ACTH, the output of cAMP was found to be lower, even when ACTH concentration was increased 10-fold.

Exogenous cAMP and Steroidogenesis

The steroidogenic effect of exogenous cAMP or its dibutyryl derivative has been demonstrated in bovine adrenal slices (24), rat adrenal quarters (10,17, 46,106), isolated rat adrenal cells (35,65,75,94), and superfused rat adrenals (80). The kinetics of the steroidogenic responses of quartered rat adrenals (56,57) and isolated adrenal cells (35) to ACTH, cAMP, and dibutyryl cAMP have been examined. A definite lag of 3 to 6 min for both dibutyryl cAMP and ACTH was observed before linear production of steroids commenced.

In a qualitative sense these results tend to support a second-messenger role for cAMP. However, there are two disturbing factors. The first is that exogenous cAMP at less than 100 μM (89) does not stimulate steroidogenesis in isolated adrenal cell preparations, whereas the endogenous rise in cAMP in response to even supramaximal steroidogenic concentrations of ACTH ranges from 100 to 300 nM (2,90). Thus the level of exogenous cAMP required for maximal steroidogenic activity is at least 1,000-fold more than what is endogenously elevated by a maximal steroidogenic concentration of ACTH. The second is that 10 to 100 μM cAMP, which fails to stimulate steroidogenesis, does stimulate protein kinase activity in a typical concentration-related manner (89). These results can be explained only on the basis that cAMP penetrates poorly across the lipid membranes; they further indicate that activation of protein kinase by submaximal steroidogenic concentrations of cAMP is unrelated to the process of steroidogenesis. It should be noted that the degradation of cAMP by phosphodiesterase cannot be the reason for the lack of a cAMP effect since the isolated adrenal cell preparation employed has undetectable phosphodiesterase activity (37).

Phosphodiesterase Inhibitors

Studies with the two phosphodiesterase inhibitors caffeine and theophylline, which are thought to potentiate steroidogenesis by blocking cAMP phosphodiesterase, have been difficult to carry out and have produced varying results. Studies with isolated rat adrenal cells (37) showed that caffeine (10^{-3} to 10^{-2} M) inhibits steroidogenesis induced by either ACTH or dibutyryl cAMP. It was concluded that the inhibition was unrelated to the phosphodiesterase inhibitory activity of caffeine, as no phosphodiesterase activity could be detected in trypsinized adrenal cell preparations, although hydrolysis of the cyclic 3′,5′-phosphates of adenine, guanosine, and inosine was carried out effectively by adrenal tissue homogenates (37). On the other hand, studies with isolated rat adrenal cells prepared by collagenase digestion, which possessed 67% of the phosphodiesterase activity of intact glands, showed that 10^{-3} M theophylline potentiates the steroidogenic effect of submaximal concentrations of ACTH (45). Halkerston et al. (20) concluded that the phosphodiesterase inhibitor theophylline had two antagonistic actions in rat adrenal bisects: (1) a small potentiation of ACTH stimulation of steroidogenesis seen only at certain concentrations of the hormone; (2) a reduction of the stimulatory action of ACTH that was accompanied by partial inhibition of the incorporation of radioactive amino acids into adrenal protein. Studies with 1-methyl-3-isobutyl xanthine, a phosphodiesterase inhibitor 10 times more potent than theophylline, have shown potentiation of ACTH action on increasing rat adrenal cAMP levels and increasing corticosterone production both *in vitro* and *in vivo* (62), but the concentrations of ACTH used in these studies were not physiological.

In conclusion, the studies with phosphodiesterase inhibitors are inconclusive; they do not prove an obligatory second-messenger role for cAMP in adrenal steroidogenesis.

Conclusion

We have surveyed the literature concerning the contention that accumulation of intracellular cAMP is an obligatory intermediate event between ACTH and corticosteroidogenesis by the adrenal gland. In our view, there are three reasons that the evidence in favor of this hypothesis is inadequate: (a) Submaximal steroidogenic ACTH concentrations do not cause a detectable change in the cAMP level, but they do stimulate protein kinase. (b) Neither submaximal nor supramaximal steroidogenic concentrations of ACTH change the levels of cAMP to a detectable degree during the first 30 min, whereas the onset of steroidogenesis is accompanied by the process of phosphorylation. (c) There are technical problems that make it difficult to establish the process of steroidogenesis as stimulated by high and unphysiological concentrations of cAMP. These three arguments against the acceptance of an obligatory second-messenger role for cAMP in adrenal steroidogenesis are strong, but they are not conclusive. Although we are not at this time adherents of the preceding hypothesis, we have no prejudice against its basic appeal, which has attracted many scientists into investigations of the metabolic correlates of adrenal steroidogenesis.

CYCLIC GMP AND ADRENAL STEROIDOGENESIS

In view of the previously mentioned factors indicating that cAMP does not satisfy the criteria for being the sole mediator of ACTH action, Sharma and associates initiated studies on the regulatory role of cyclic GMP (cGMP) in adrenal steroidogenesis. These studies used isolated adrenal cell preparations (35,94) that lacked detectable phosphodiesterase activity (37) and were responsive to as little as 1 μU of ACTH in the synthesis of corticosterone (35). The findings of these studies will now be elaborated. The following discussion will also describe the background conditions that led Sharma and associates to examine the regulatory role of cGMP in adrenal steroidogenesis.

ACTH Stimulation of Adrenocortical Cells and cGMP Levels

Figure 3 shows that in the intact isolated adrenal cell (58,89,90) 2.5 to 10 μU of ACTH do not raise the level of cAMP but do stimulate steroidogenesis. A significant increase in the cAMP level is observed only at concentrations above 10 μU of ACTH. Although 100 μU of ACTH yield the maximum amount of steroidogenesis, the cAMP levels continue to rise as the concentration of the hormone is increased. In contrast, 5 μU of ACTH stimulate peak synthesis of cGMP, with a concomitant rise in corticosterone. More than 5 μU of ACTH causes a dramatic fall in the peak level of cGMP, but corticosterone synthesis continues to rise. These results suggest that ACTH levels of less than 5 μU stimulate steroidogenesis by altering the levels of cGMP but not cAMP. At higher concentrations of ACTH ($>$ 10 μU) there is hormone-concentration-

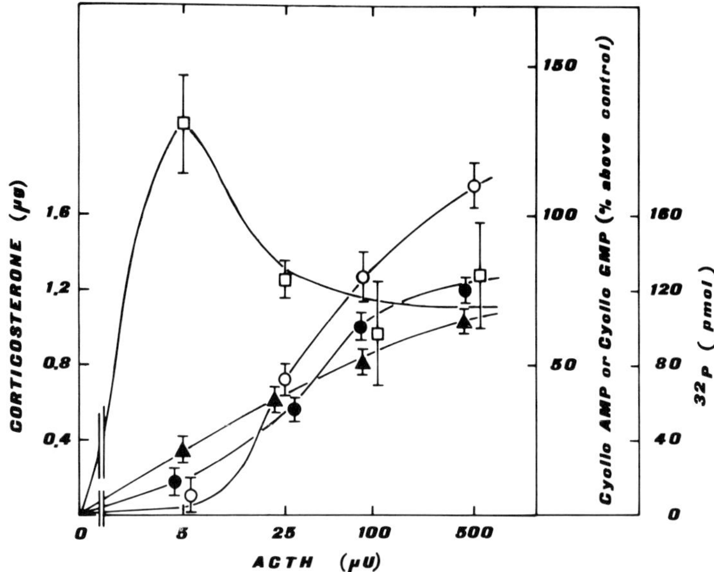

FIG. 3. Concentration response curve for production of cAMP *(open circles),* cGMP *(squares),* corticosterone *(filled circles),* and phosphorylation *(triangles)* in isolated adrenal cells incubated for 60 min in presence of 0 to 500 μU of ACTH. Conditions of the experiment were identical to those in Fig. 1. (Adapted from Perchellet et al., ref. 58.)

dependent synthesis of cAMP, which in turn stimulates corticosterone production. This seems to indicate that stimulation of steroidogenesis by ACTH at low concentrations is mediated by cGMP but not by cAMP. In the absence of ACTH there is basal synthesis of cGMP, and at concentrations of ACTH greater than 10 μU there is a decline of 40 to 50% in the peak synthesis of cGMP.

In reaching a working hypothesis to explain these results, a kinetic model of the regulation of guanylate cyclase by ACTH has been proposed (88). According to this model there are two forms of guanylate cyclase, one of which is hormone-concentration-independent (represented by E); a second form (represented by E') has two sites for ACTH interactions of different affinity. When E' combines with the first molecule of ACTH to form complex C_1', the enzyme becomes active. When a second molecule of ACTH combines with the enzyme to form complex C_3', enzymatic activity is blocked:

$$E + \text{GTP} \rightleftarrows C_1 \rightarrow E + \text{cGMP} + \text{PPi}$$
$$E' + \text{ACTH} \overset{K_1}{\rightleftarrows} C_1'$$
$$C_1' + \text{GTP} \underset{k_2}{\overset{k_1}{\rightleftarrows}} C_2' \overset{k_3}{\rightarrow} C_1' + \text{cGMP} + \text{PPi} \qquad \left[\frac{(k_3 + k_2)}{k_1} = k_{\text{m}}\right]$$
$$C_1' + \text{ACTH} \overset{K_2}{\rightleftarrows} C_3'$$

The rate equation for ACTH-sensitive synthesis of cGMP (those reactants distinguished by superscript primes) would be the following:

$$V = \frac{V_{max} SA}{K_1 K_m + (K_m + S)A + K_m A^2 / K_2} \tag{1}$$

where S and A represent the concentrations of GTP and ACTH, respectively, and K_1 and K_2 are the designated equilibrium constants. In attempting to fit equation (1) to the data of Fig. 3, it was found that this could best be done by assuming that $K_1 > K_2$. This implies that the enzyme combines with the second molecule of ACTH with greater affinity than the first, thus suggesting an allosteric modification of the enzyme structure by the first molecule of bound hormone.

Effect of Exogenous cGMP on Adrenal Steroidogenesis

In order to study the ability of cGMP to stimulate corticosteroidogenesis (89) along with the activation of protein kinase, isolated adrenal cells were incubated with varying concentrations of cGMP. The results (Fig. 4) show that the process of phosphorylation precedes the onset of steroidogenesis, indicating that cGMP-stimulated steroidogenesis proceeds via a cGMP-dependent protein kinase. It should be noted that, to date, a cGMP-dependent protein kinase enzyme has not been isolated from adrenal cortex. There is a preliminary report on the isolation of a crude cGMP-binding protein from the adrenal cortex (16).

Although there is divergence of opinion regarding whether or not cGMP-dependent protein kinase can be dissociated into regulatory and catalytic subunits

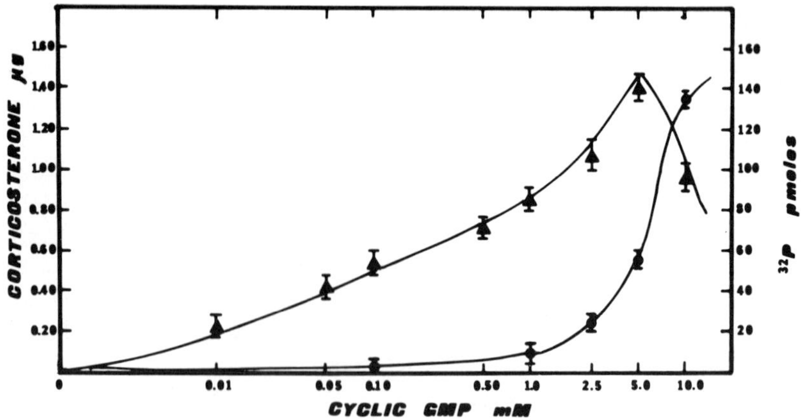

FIG. 4. Corticosterone production *(filled circles)* and phosphorylation *(triangles)* in normal isolated adrenal cells in response to μM and mM cGMP. Incubation system: adrenal cell suspension in 0.8 ml; reagents were dissolved in 0.2 ml Krebs-Ringer-bicarbonate buffer with glucose and albumin or protein kinase buffer. Total volume of first incubation 1 ml; second incubation 0.5 ml. (Adapted from Sharma, et al., ref. 89.)

(40,50,104), the majority of the data indicate that in contrast to cAMP-dependent protein kinase, cGMP-dependent protein kinase is not dissociated into regulatory and catalytic subunits by cGMP (15,43,104).

Relationship of Endogenous Protein Kinase to ACTH-induced cGMP Levels and Corticosterone Synthesis in Isolated Adrenal Cells

In order to determine if induction of corticosteroidogenesis correlates with the state of activation of endogenous levels of cAMP, cGMP, and protein kinase, isolated adrenal cells were incubated with a series of concentrations of ACTH, and the levels of cAMP and cGMP and protein kinase activity were measured (58,89). Figure 3 shows that 2.5 to 10 μU of ACTH do not induce synthesis of cAMP but do stimulate protein kinase activity and steroidogenesis in a typical sigmoid concentration-response manner. It is noteworthy that stimulation of kinase activity occurred well before the onset of steroidogenesis. However, when we examine the activation of steroidogenesis along with the stimulation of cGMP formation and phosphorylation in response to less than 5 μU, good correlation is observed among onsets of cyclic nucleotide synthesis, protein kinase activity, and steroidogenesis.

These results are consistent with the concept that activation of protein kinase is obligatory to ACTH-induced steroidogenesis and that most probably stimulation of endogenous protein kinase by less than 10 μU of ACTH is due to cGMP.

ACTH and cGMP Control Step in Adrenal Steroidogenesis

In adrenal steroidogenesis, the first and rate-limiting step is cleavage of the cholesterol side chain to synthesize pregnenolone and isocaproaldehyde, which is rapidly converted to isocaproic acid (7,32,96,102). The overall rate of cleavage of the cholesterol side chain is dictated by the rate of hydroxylation at C-20 (38,100,105). Studies with bovine adrenal slices (21) have indicated that ACTH, rather than stimulating the transformation of (20S)-20-hydroxycholesterol to cortisol, slightly inhibits this step.

Studies carried out with isolated adrenal cell systems have demonstrated that although cycloheximide inhibits the ACTH-triggered process of steroidogenesis (35,85), presumably from endogenous cholesterol, it does not interfere with the subsequent steroidogenic steps from (20S)-20-hydroxycholesterol (85). Therefore, it is evident that the cycloheximide-sensitive step involved in ACTH-induced steroidogenesis is not cleavage of the cholesterol side chain but rather an event preceding this transformation (85). Various investigators have attempted to further delineate the step that is activated by ACTH (3,29,47,55). These studies have suggested that ACTH control of steroidogenesis is governed by regulation of the size of the mitochondrial precursor pool of cholesterol rather than through a direct effect on the mitochondrial enzyme system that converts

TABLE 1. *Effects of ACTH, cGMP, and cAMP on transformation of exogenous [1,2-$^3H_2$]-cholesterol into corticosterone in presence of NADPH in isolated adrenal cells*[a]

Additions	$^3H/^{14}C$ ratio of corticosterone	Percentage stimulation
Control	14.56	—
+ ACTH	33.80	132
Control	11.61	—
+ cGMP	29.98	158
Control	12.77	—
+ cAMP	34.98	174

[a] $^3H/^{14}C$ ratios of corticosterone were obtained after incubation of [4-^{14}C, 1,2-$^3H_2$] cholesterol + NADPH with isolated adrenal cells. Incubation was carried out in appropriate flasks containing 20 ml isolated adrenal cell preparation as described in "Experimental Procedure" by Sharma and Sawhney (96). Flask 1 (control) contained a mixture of [1,2-$^3H_2$]cholesterol (50 μCi) + [4-^{14}C]cholesterol (5 μCi) ($^3H/^{14}C$ ratio 10.00) + NADPH (1 mM). Flask 2 contained [4-^{14}C]cholesterol (5 μCi) + NADPH (1 mM). Flask 3 contained [1,2-$^3H_2$]cholesterol + NADPH and ACTH (100 μU/ml) or cGMP (10 mM) or cAMP (10 mM). Incubation was for 2.5 hr, and the reaction was stopped by addition of 75 ml of methylene chloride to each flask. Contents of second and third flasks were mixed, and corticosterone was isolated as described in "Experimental Procedure" (96).

Adapted from Sharma and Sawhney (96).

cholesterol to pregnenolone. However, these investigations were indirect because they were carried out with mitochondrial preparations isolated from ACTH- or cAMP-treated animals. Direct studies to demonstrate the ACTH control step in scission of the cholesterol side chain have been hampered because tracer exogenous cholesterol could not be incorporated into the endogenous cholesterol pool of the isolated adrenal cell (52,85).

Neher and Milani provided preliminary evidence that exogenous radioactive cholesterol in the presence of NADPH might equilibrate with the endogenous cholesterol pool and subsequently be converted to corticosterone in an isolated adrenal cell (52). Sharma and Sawhney (96) expanded on those studies and presented evidence that the transformation of exogenous cholesterol to corticosterone in the presence of NADPH is not cycloheximide-sensitive in the isolated adrenal cell. On the other hand, cycloheximide blocks ACTH-induced steroidogenesis from endogenous precursors, presumably cholesterol. ACTH and cGMP activate the transformation of exogenously supplied radioactive cholesterol to corticosterone by more than twofold over that obtained with NADPH alone (Table 1). This effect of ACTH cannot be on cells with damaged membranes, since to date no stimulation of the onset of steroidogenesis by ACTH has been demonstrated in a cell-free system. Similarly, ACTH stimulation in the formation of corticosterone cannot be on the mitochondrial enzymes that may have leaked out due to damaged membranes because ACTH has never been shown to stimulate these enzymes directly. The presence of the intact membrane is a prerequisite for ACTH-induced steroidogenesis. Therefore, this technique has provided the first direct approach for study of the mechanism of steroidogenesis from exogenous cholesterol in intact fasciculata cells.

TABLE 2. *Effects of cycloheximide on ACTH-, cGMP-, and cAMP-stimulated transformation of exogenous [1,2-$^3H_2$]cholesterol into corticosterone in isolated adrenal cells*[a]

Additions	$^3H/^{14}C$ ratio of corticosterone
Control	10.00
+ ACTH	29.24
+ cGMP	32.01
+ cAMP	32.34
+ ACTH + cycloheximide	9.17
+ cGMP + cycloheximide	20.79
+ cAMP + cycloheximide	18.13

[a] $^3H/^{14}C$ ratios of the products were obtained after incubation of [4-^{14}C, 1,2-$^3H_2$] cholesterol + NADPH with isolated adrenal cells. Conditions of the experiment were identical to those of the experiment in Table 1, except that the increased incorporation of [1,2-^3H] cholesterol due to the presence of NADPH was subtracted. This value was calculated from control flask 1, which was then normalized to a $^3H/^{14}C$ ratio of 10.00, corresponding to the initial ratio of cholesterol used in the incubation medium. Flask 1 (control) contained a mixture of [1,2-^3H]cholesterol + [4-^{14}C]cholesterol. Flask 2 contained [4-^{14}C]cholesterol. Flask 3 contained [1,2-$^3H_2$]cholesterol + ACTH or cGMP or cAMP. Flask 4 contained [4-^{14}C]cholesterol. Flask 5 contained [1,2-$^3H_2$]cholesterol + cycloheximide and ACTH or cGMP or cAMP. The contents of the second flask were mixed with those of the third flask, and those of the fourth flask were mixed with those of the fifth flask, and the samples were processed identically.

Adapted from Sharma and Sawhney (96).

It has been shown that cycloheximide inhibits ACTH- and cGMP-activated conversion of exogenously supplied cholesterol to corticosterone (Table 2). These same data further indicate that the stimulation of steroidogenesis obtained with NADPH clearly proceeds via a mechanism that is cycloheximide-independent. In order to determine whether the ACTH-induced cycloheximide-sensitive step is on the premitochondrial or mitochondrial precursor pool of cholesterol, isolated adrenal cells were preincubated with aminoglutethimide, and [^3H]-cholesterol was added along with NADPH and ACTH to transport the cytoplasmic cholesterol pool into mitochondria. After 1 hr of incubation the cells were washed to remove aminoglutethimide. The cells were divided into two groups. One group (control) contained only the cells; the other group contained cells and ACTH or cGMP. The results in Table 3 show that subsequent to the entry of cholesterol into the mitochondria, ACTH and cGMP did not affect cleavage of the cholesterol side chain. These results, taken together with previous findings in which it was shown that the cycloheximide-sensitive step occurs after activation of protein kinase and before synthesis of pregnenolone (84,89), suggest that the ACTH-activated step occurs during entry of cytoplasmic cholesterol into the mitochondria. By inference these data suggest that this very step is under the translational control of the hormone and is mediated by cGMP and cAMP. Although the possibility that a labile protein is involved in such a process is attractive, it remains speculative at this time. To date no such protein has been isolated. The reported (31) sterol carrier protein appears to have a function other than the transport of cholesterol across the mitochondrial membrane. Considering these factors, the mechanism of control of ACTH in

TABLE 3. *Effects of ACTH, cGMP, and cAMP on transformation of mitochondrial [1,2-$^3H_2$]cholesterol into corticosterone in isolated adrenal cells*[a]

Additions	^3H radioactivity of corticosterone
Control	41,030
+ ACTH	39,380
Control	49,200
+ cGMP	47,412
Control	44,312
+ cAMP	44,161

[a] Total ^3H disintegrations per minute of the products were obtained after incubation of mitochondrial [1,2-$^3H_2$]cholesterol with isolated adrenal cells. Isolated adrenal cell preparation (20 ml) obtained from 20 adrenal glands was preincubated with aminoglutethimide (100 μM) for 15 min, and [1,2-$^3H_2$]cholesterol (100 μCi), NADPH (1mM), and ACTH or cGMP or cAMP were added, with the incubation being continued for 1 hr. The cells were centrifuged, washed, and resuspended in 40 ml Krebs-Ringer-bicarbonate buffer containing albumin and glucose. A 20-ml aliquot of cell suspension was added into one flask (control), and the second flask contained a 20-ml aliquot of cell suspension + cycloheximide (10 μM) and ACTH or cGMP (10 mM). Incubation was for 2 hr, and the reaction was stopped by addition of 75 ml of methylene chloride to each flask. Corticosterone was isolated and crystallized as described in "Experimental Procedure" by Sharma and Sawhney (96).

Adapted from Sharma and Sawhney (96).

adrenal steroidogenesis has been proposed as follows:

ACTH binds to the hormone receptor located on the adrenal cell plasma membrane (41). At physiological concentrations the hormone raises the cGMP level, presumably by activating guanylate cyclase enzyme, whereas at supraphysiological concentrations it stimulates the synthesis of cAMP by activating the adenylate cyclase system (18,89,90). The two nucleotides, in turn, activate their respective protein kinase activities (89), which then lead to the translation of a hypothetical preexistent mRNA (8,12). The labile protein thus synthesized controls the entry of the cytoplasmic cholesterol into the mitochondrial precursor pool of cholesterol. This scheme is depicted in Fig. 5.

It is noteworthy that the proposed scheme (Fig. 5) depicting the mechanism of modulation of guanylate cyclase is different in many respects from a concept that is emerging from various other studies conducted on other systems. These investigations have indicated that guanylate cyclase is activated by the following: detergents (11,42,70), sodium azide, presumably via the formation of a catalase–nitric oxide complex (34), unsaturated fatty acids (1); lysolecithin (99), and calcium (107). The isolation of a protein activator required for sodium azide activation has also been reported (49). The mode of activation of guanylate cyclase by these agents appears to proceed by the mechanism depicted below:

stimulus → ↑Ca^{2+} → ↑lipase → ↑arachidonic acid
→ ↑peroxidase (oxygenase, endogenous oxidase, or dismutase to yield superoxide)
→ ↑guanylate cyclase

There are two reasons that this scheme does not appear to be valid in hormonally activated steroidogenesis in the adrenal cell. First, in isolated fasciculata cells less than 10 μU of ACTH increases the cGMP level and endogenous

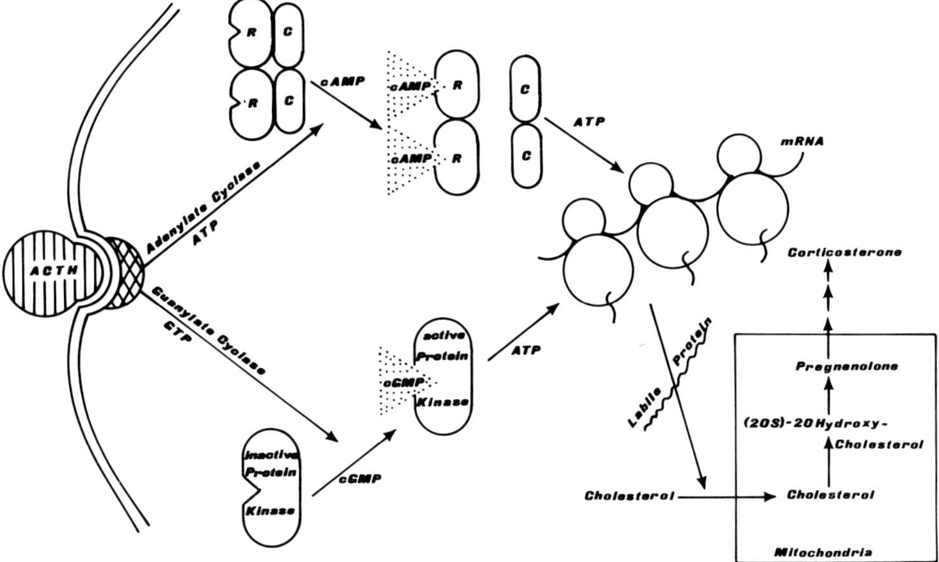

FIG. 5. Postulated model of ACTH-induced steroidogenesis.

protein kinase activity, with concomitant synthesis of corticosterone in a concentration-dependent manner. Exogenous calcium, on the other hand, is unable to do so. Second, no other agent besides ACTH has yet been reported to activate guanylate cyclase and cause a corresponding increase in corticosterone synthesis. This shows that in an adrenal cell guanylate cyclase is specifically activated by a single polypeptide hormone: ACTH.

It is obvious that more work on the preliminary properties of the guanylate cyclase system must be done before a detailed analysis of its hormonal modulation can be undertaken. In the adrenal gland the picture is even more complex, since previous studies (48) have not been successful in detecting a hormonally sensitive adrenal guanylate cyclase. Since studies in the same laboratory have shown no elevation of cGMP by ACTH (109), the importance of performing the initial studies on the intact fasciculata cells, which are devoid of cyclic nucleotide phosphodiesterase activity, cannot be overemphasized. Guanylate cyclase then must be isolated from these cells and not from the intact adrenal gland. Once the hormonally sensitive guanylate cyclase activity is demonstrated in the cell-free system, the functional role of guanylate cyclase in the regulation of steroidogenesis will become clearer. It should be interesting to determine how this enzyme's activity is integrated with other membrane components and cellular events such as ion fluxes, compartmentalization, changes in microfilaments, membrane fluidity, phosphodiesterases, and regulatory processes of protein kinases. If the data accumulated for adenylate cyclase are analogous, it should be pertinent to explore the relationship between the guanylate cyclase enzyme and receptor molecules themselves, a topic of recent hot debate in regard to adenylate cyclase (25,41,60,67). It should be significant to consider the presumption that physiological coupling exists between receptor and guanylate cyclase, but such curiosities cannot be profitable unless we begin systematically to dissect the hormonally active guanylate cyclase system, such as that present in the fasciculata cells.

Subsequent to a report by Sharma et al. (90) indicating a positive correlation between synthesis of cGMP and induction of corticosterone synthesis, various other laboratories independently reported similar findings. Hohn and Chavin (26) showed that porcine ACTH and caiman ACTH elevate cGMP levels and concomitantly decrease cAMP levels in adrenal glands isolated from crocodiles. They emphasized the intermediary role of cGMP in adrenal steroidogenesis. Another laboratory (69) showed a rise in cGMP level in response to ACTH in isolated bovine adrenal cells. They showed a small drop in cGMP level in response to 500 μU of ACTH at 5 min, which reversed to a twofold to threefold increase by 30 min. After a 5-min interval they found an increase in cAMP level. Their cell system did not respond to less than 50 μU of ACTH for stimulation of steroidogenesis. With 50 and 500 μU of ACTH they observed stimulation of corticosterone production from 0.02 to 0.04 μg and from 0.02 to 0.16 μg, respectively. Evidently the cell preparation used by these investigators was far less sensitive than the isolated rat adrenal cell preparation that, in response to 50 μU of ACTH, gave a 65-fold rise in corticosterone levels from 0.02 to 1.37 μg (35). Nussdorfer et al. (54) reported an *in vivo* rise in cGMP level in the rat adrenal cortex in response to ACTH. All of these results *in vitro* and *in vivo* are in sharp contrast to those obtained by Whitley et al. (109), who injected 50 to 200 μU of ACTH in hypophysectomized rats and found decreases in cGMP levels. Of special importance is the evidence presented by Harrington et al. (22); it corroborates the results obtained by Sharma et al. regarding the importance of cGMP in mediation of adrenal steroidogenesis. Harrington et al. (22) studied the effects of low concentations of ACTH on the activation of cAMP and cGMP synthesis, as well as formation of progesterone and 11-deoxycorticosterone. They measured the latter steroids by a cospecific antibody to deoxycorticosterone—a method about five times more sensitive than synthesis of corticosterone as an index of steroidogenesis. Dose–response studies using porcine ACTH showed close correlation between cGMP and progesterone and deoxycorticosterone levels for incubation periods of 10, 20, 40, and 60 min. The authors concluded that their data strongly implicate cGMP as a major component initiating the steroidogenic response to ACTH at doses of ACTH well below those required to detect any change whatever in cAMP.

The preceding discussion on control of steroidogenesis by ACTH was not intended to provide a comprehensive survey of the literature. Much important work has not been mentioned. Only references pertinent to discussion of the contrasting ideas proposed by various laboratories regarding hormonal regulation have been cited. It is interesting to note that several recent reviews (19,73,79) covering the work of many eminent researchers in the field have not seriously considered the possibility of cGMP being the mediator of ACTH in adrenal steroidogenesis.

ABNORMAL ACTH CONTROL IN ADRENOCORTICAL CARCINOMA CELLS

Snell and Stewart were the first workers to detect rat adrenocortical carcinoma, and their discovery refuted an old belief that adrenal cortical tumors rarely occur in the rat (101). These authors suggested that the occurrence of adrenal tumors in rats may be indicative of a general endocrine imbalance, since tumors of the adrenal gland, ovary, mammary gland, and pituitary gland are often found in the same animal. They were able to maintain this adrenocortical carcinoma cell line by transplantation into intact mature male and female Osborne-Mendel rats. Snell and Stewart designated this tumor line adrenocortical carcinoma 494 and demonstrated that it maintained a consistent histologic pattern of cords of uniform polygonal cells.

In 1961 Johnston et al. (28) published an article in which they compared the metabolism of progesterone and 11-deoxycorticosterone in adrenocortical carcinoma 494 with that in the adrenal gland of the normal rat (28). They found sixfold higher levels of radioactive progesterone incorporation into deoxycorticosterone and fourfold lower incorporation into corticosterone in the tumor slices as compared with normal rat adrenal slices. This finding led them to suggest that there is a blockade of the 11β-hydroxylation step of deoxycorticosterone. This article initiated the first systematic approach to examination of abnormal steroid metabolism in adrenocortical carcinoma 494.

At the present time various laboratories are using this carcinoma cell line as a model system in an attempt to locate the specific molecular lesions that may be responsible for the absence of ACTH-induced steroidogenesis. All of these studies are centering on the idea that cAMP and/or cGMP in some manner play an obligatory role in the process of steroidogenesis. The discussion to follow will examine the status of this research. For the sake of simplicity, this discussion will be divided into three parts. The first part will discuss the ultrastructural characteristics of the cells. The second part will examine the ACTH-activated cAMP- and cGMP-regulated reactions; in this part, the synthesis and degradation of the cyclic nucleotides along with their regulatory processes will be discussed. The third part will examine the steroidogenic pathway from (20S)-20-hydroxycholesterol to corticosterone.

Ultrastructural Characteristics

Sharma and Hashimoto examined the ultrastructural characteristics of adrenocortical carcinoma cells (93). The tumor cells were round to oval and uniform in size, measuring about 15 to 20 μm. They were solidly packed together and were connected with interdigitation of numerous short villi projecting from the cell membranes. Desmosome-like junctional devices were occasionally seen, but they were not necessarily present between each pair of cells. No cell was covered with a basal lamina. Lipid granules, if present, were not numerous, usually occurring only 1 or 2 per cell. Their diameters varied from very small (0.5 μm) to very large (4 to 5 μm). About one-half of the tumor cells did not contain lipid granules. Occasionally, membranous bodies that were dense and whorled as described in the fasciculata cells of normal and stimulated rat adrenal cortex (64) appeared to penetrate the granules in a corkscrew fashion. The majority of the lipid granules were not surrounded with smooth-surface endoplasmic reticulum, and they even lacked delimiting membrane.

Smooth-surface endoplasmic reticulum and Golgi apparatus were fairly well developed in most tumor cells, and numerous small vesicles derived from these organelles were seen. Stacks of smooth endoplasmic reticulum-forming bundles were found in the cytoplasm. They were free from mitochondria and lipid granules. Mitochondria were round to oval; on the average of 15 to 20 were seen in a section through the middle of the cell. Large bizarrely shaped mitochondria, as seen in normal rat adrenal cortex (64), were absent. Mitochondrial cristae were thin and tubular, and no vesicular cristae were observed. Mitochondrial matrix (sap) filling the spaces between the cristae was electron-light. Many mitochondria contained dense myelinated bodies. Most mitochondria were surrounded with only a few layers to several layers of smooth-surface endoplasmic reticulum.

Rough-surface endoplasmic reticulum was present in varying amounts, and polysomes were abundant. Glycogen particles were scarce. No lipofuscin pigment granules were observed. The nucleus had a thin rim of heterochromatin, and 1 to 3 nucleoli were present. Neither nuclear nor cytoplasmic structures suggestive of viral inclusions were seen. Later studies with adrenocortical carcinoma cultured cells showed essentially the same characteristics (5). Kimmel and associates repeated these studies and reported similar results (33).

ACTH Control of Steroidogenesis before Cholesterol Side Chain Cleavage

Adenylate Cyclase Activity

Ney and associates were the first workers to undertake studies seeking to determine the reasons for ACTH unresponsiveness of adrenal carcinoma 494 (53). They raised the following questions: Does ACTH normally increase cAMP concentrations in the tumor? Does cAMP, in turn, accelerate steroidogenesis in the carcinoma as it does in the normal adrenal cortex?

They injected 20 U ACTH (5×10^6 pg) in the femoral veins of tumor-bearing rats and found negligible increases in cAMP, as compared with 50-fold increases in cAMP levels in nontumorous adrenals of the same animals. Similar results were found when tumor slices and quartered adrenals were incubated *in vitro* with ACTH at 1 U/ml (5×10^6 pg). In contrast, there were 20-fold increases in cAMP levels in the normal adrenal glands. Although these results suggested a hormonally unresponsive adenylate cyclase system, this was not the case, since the investigators found a threefold rise in adenylate cyclase activity in tumor homogenate (53). The concentration of ACTH used was 0.66 U/ml (3.3×10^6 pg).

Sharma and Hashimoto (93) described a trypsinized cell preparation of adrenocortical carcinoma cells that was prepared in a fashion similar to that of normal isolated adrenal cells (35,74,94). Thus the two cell systems, normal and malignant, could be used advantageously to compare steroidogenic metabolic properties. Like their normal counterparts, the trypsinized malignant cells have no detectable cAMP or cGMP phosphodiesterase activity (88). The metabolism of these cyclic nucleotides can therefore be studied in a direct fashion. The changes in levels of cAMP and cGMP in an intact cell will therefore reflect the adenylate and guanylate cyclase activities.

The studies conducted with isolated adrenocortical carcinoma cells (93) showed that, in contrast to the stimulatory effect of 10 to 50 μU of ACTH (50–250 pg) on synthesis of cAMP and steroidogenesis in the normal cell (59,97), the hormone does not activate synthesis of cAMP. In a normal adrenal cell 50 μU of ACTH gives a near maximal response for synthesis of corticosterone (35). However, a maximal steroidogenic concentration of ACTH, 100 μU, in the malignant cell increases the level of cAMP twofold (59). These results appear to suggest that tumor adenylate cyclase, unlike normal cell cyclase, is relatively unresponsive to ACTH.

Péron and associates prepared tumor cells simply by mincing the tissue and centrifuging the cells at low speed (61). They did not use trypsin for their cell preparation. They could not detect a rise in cAMP level in response to ACTH without the addition of a phosphodiesterase inhibitor (theophylline). In the presence of theophylline they did observe concentration-dependent increases in levels of cAMP caused by ACTH at 100 to 1,400 μU (500–7,000 pg). However, the authors claimed that tumor adenylate cyclase for ACTH is approximately 10 times more sensitive than that of the normal adrenal cell (61). The isolated adrenal cell preparation of Péron et al. did not respond to less than 300 μU of ACTH (1,500 pg) for synthesis of cAMP.

In subsequent studies Schorr et al. made the interesting observation that the centrifuged ($1,000 \times g$) particle preparation of adrenal tumor homogenate responded to various other hormones in addition to ACTH in the formation of cAMP (77,78). The concentration of ACTH used in these experiments was 0.25 U/ml (1.25×10^6 pg). That the specificity of the ACTH receptor is not altogether lost has been shown, since the hormones vasopressin, glucagon, insulin, growth hormone, and parathyroid hormone did not stimulate adenylate cyclase activity. In contrast to these results *in vitro,* studies by Péron et al. (61) using intact tumor cells showed more than a fourfold increase in adenylate cyclase activity in response to glucagon (50 μg/10^6 cells) (61). The concentration of glucagon used by Schorr et al. was 0.35 mg/ml of centrifuged ($1,000 \times g$) particle preparation.

The studies by Sharma and associates with plasma membrane preparations prepared from cultured adrenocortical carcinoma cells not only confirmed the

TABLE 4. *Adenyl cyclase activity of tumor plasma membranes stimulated by epinephrine and ACTH*[a]

Fraction	Addition	Radioactivity (dpm) incorporated into cAMP	Fold stimulation	p^b
Purified (700 × g) particles	—	12,710 ± 530 (4)	1.00	
	10 μM epinephrine	26,400 ± 1,130 (5)	2.08	<0.001
	460 mu ACTH	16,800 ± 610 (4)	1.32	0.001

[a] See "Materials and Methods" as described by Brush et al. (5) for the technique used in preparing cellular particulate fractions.
[b] Probability that there is no significant difference between the listed mean for each purified subcellular fraction and the mean for the same fraction obtained with no additions.
Adapted from Brush et al. (5).

observations of Schorr et al. (77,78) but also showed greater stimulation of membrane adenylate cyclase activity by epinephrine as compared to ACTH (Table 4).

The significance of these findings is not clear at this time since neither the submaximal nor maximal steroidogenic concentrations of ACTH in normal adrenal cells had stimulatory effects on adenylate cyclase activity either in the cell-free system (5) or in the intact tumor cell (59,97). The basal levels of cAMP in the carcinoma tissue and the normal adrenal gland were found to be comparable. This suggests that adrenal tumor 494 has a relatively ACTH-insensitive adenylate cyclase system for synthesis of cAMP.

Guanylate Cyclase Activity

In order to determine if endogenous levels of cGMP formed in response to ACTH correlate with varying concentrations of ACTH, isolated adrenocortical carcinoma cells were incubated with a series of concentrations of ACTH, and the levels of corticosterone and cGMP and protein kinase activity were measured (59). The results (Fig. 6) show that in intact isolated adrenocortical carcinoma cells, ACTH at concentrations up to 50 μU raises the cGMP level without corresponding increases in corticosterone formation and protein kinase activity. In isolated adrenal cells, less than 10 μU of ACTH raises the level of cGMP, with a concomitant increase in protein kinase activity, followed by activation of steroidogenesis (58,89,90). These results indicate that, in contrast to an active adenylate cyclase, the tumor possesses a hormonally dependent guanylate cyclase system. In tumor cells the defective step or steps responsible for lack of stimulation of steroidogenesis by submaximal steroidogenic concentrations of ACTH active in normal cells appear to occur after the events that activate guanylate cyclase. Previously (93) it was shown that exogenous cGMP also lacks steroidogenic activity in the tumor cell *(vide infra)*. These results taken together indicate

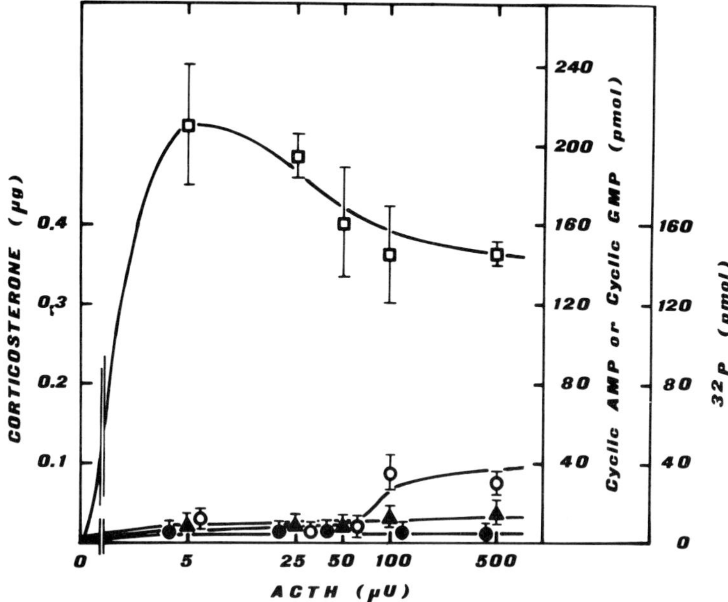

FIG. 6. Corticosterone response curve for production of cAMP *(open circles)*, cGMP *(squares)*, corticosterone *(filled circles)*, and phosphorylation *(triangles)* in isolated adrenocortical carcinoma cells incubated for 10 min in presence of 0 to 500 µU of ACTH. Conditions of the experiment were similar to those in Fig. 1. Basal values have been substracted from experimental results. (Adapted from Perchellet and Sharma, ref. 59.)

the possibility of a defective cGMP-dependent protein kinase, but no such enzyme has yet been isolated from normal adrenal cortex, although there is a preliminary report (16) on the isolation of cGMP-binding protein.

Exogenous Cyclic Nucleotides and Steroidogenesis

Studies with freshly prepared isolated adrenocortical carcinoma cells (93) and with cultured adrenocortical carcinoma cells (5) showed that, in contrast to the situation with normal adrenal cells (35), neither ACTH nor cAMP stimulates corticosterone synthesis (Table 5). These studies confirmed earlier results obtained with adrenal tumor slices (53). The investigators then questioned whether or not the tumors had developed other cyclase systems that might show specificity to other cyclic-nucleotide-activated processes of steroidogenesis (93). However, no response to cGMP, cyclic inosine 3′,5′-monophosphate (cIMP), cyclic uridine 3′,5′-monophosphate (cUMP), or cyclic thymidine 3′,5′-monophosphate (cTMP) was found (91) (Table 5). Since adenylate cyclase activity of the adrenal tumor is stimulated by high concentrations of other hormones such as epinephrine, norepinephrine, and thyroid-stimulating hormones, as well

TABLE 5. *Effects of various cyclic nucleotides on formation of corticosterone in isolated adrenal tumor cells*[a]

Additions	Concentrations	Corticosterone (μg/2 hr)[b]
Pregnenolone		0.328
ACTH	100 μU	0.025
cAMP	10 mM	0.005
Dibutyryl cAMP	1 mM	0.007
cGMP	10 mM	0.003
cIMP	10 mM	0.000
cUMP	10 mM	0.001
cTMP	10 mM	0.001
cCMP	10 mM	0.003
NADPH		0.003
ACTH + NADPH		0.008
cAMP + NADPH		0.003
Dibutyryl cAMP + NADPH		0.020

[a]Incubation system: adrenal cell suspension 0.8 ml; pregnenolone dissolved in 0.20 ml of Krebs-Ringer-bicarbonate buffer. Total volume of incubation, 1 ml.

[b]Average of three observations. Baseline value has been subtracted.

Adapted from Sharma and Hashimoto (93).

as by ACTH, Sharma and Hashimoto, in an attempt to correlate the nonspecificity of the adrenal tumor receptor to corticosteroidogenesis, studied the effects of the hormones epinephrine, glucagon, insulin, and proinsulin on isolated adrenal tumor cells (93). All four hormones were devoid of any stimulatory activity.

These studies indicate that the lack of stimulation of corticosterone formation by ACTH in adrenocortical carcinoma cells cannot be explained merely on the basis of the lesions in membrane cyclases. Indeed, the apparent guanylate cyclase system is intact in the tumor (59), and the adenylate cyclase system is relatively unresponsive (97). These factors, taken together with observations that both exogenous cGMP and cAMP are unable to stimulate steroidogenesis in the adrenocortical carcinoma cell, indicate that there may be lesions in the cyclic-nucleotide-dependent regulatory signals. One of the obvious possibilities is a defective kinase system. Although the relationship between the cGMP-dependent protein kinase system and the abnormal adrenocortical carcinoma steroid metabolism has not been studied in detail, Sharma and associates initiated studies to investigate the possibility of a defective cAMP-binding protein kinase. The possibility that the lack of steroidogenic activity to exogenously supplied cAMP could be due to accelerated cAMP phosphodiesterase activity of the tumor cells can be ruled out, since the trypsinized tumor cells do not possess any such activity (88). Even the tumor tissue has been shown to possess only 20% of the cAMP and cGMP phosphodiesterase activities of normal adrenal cells (83). Furthermore, the steroidogenic pathway from (20S)-20-hydroxycholesterol to corticosterone, although impaired, has been found to be intact in tumor cells.

Endogenous Protein Kinase Activity and Steroidogenesis

In order to correlate the inability of exogenous cyclic nucleotides to stimulate corticosterone synthesis in adenocortical carcinoma cells with endogenous protein kinase activity, isolated adrenocortical carcinoma cells were incubated with varying concentrations of cAMP and cGMP (97). The results depicted in Figs. 7 and 8 show that the concentrations of cAMP and cGMP that stimulate corticosterone synthesis in normal adrenal cells do not activate the onset of steroidogenesis; however, they stimulate protein kinase activity in a typical concentration–response manner in tumor cells. This signifies a lack of association of the process of phosphorylation with steroidogenesis in the tumor cell. cAMP- and cGMP-activated protein kinase is not inhibited by cycloheximide or by actinomycin D (Table 6), which indicates that cyclic-nucleotide-dependent activation of the kinase is not under transcriptional or translational control. Significantly, cGMP (1–10 μM) does not stimulate protein kinase activity, whereas cAMP is quite effective in doing so (Fig. 9). This, again, is in contrast to the situation with the normal adrenal cell, where both cyclic nucleotides in this concentration range stimulate phosphorylation but do not stimulate steroidogenesis (89). This indicates an additional defect in the cGMP-dependent protein kinase of the tumor cells. It is to be emphasized that at these concentrations of the cyclic

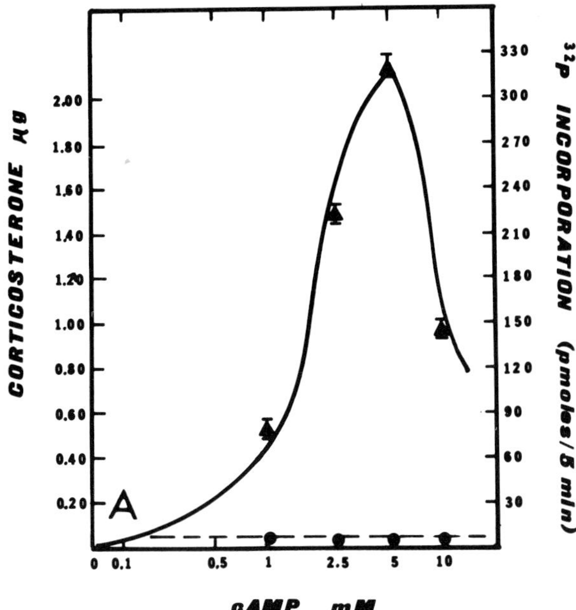

FIG. 7. Corticosterone production *(filled circles)* and phosphorylation *(triangles)* in isolated adrenocortical carcinoma cells in response to cAMP (mM concentrations). Conditions of the experiment were similar to those in Fig. 4. (Adapted from Sharma et al., ref. 97.)

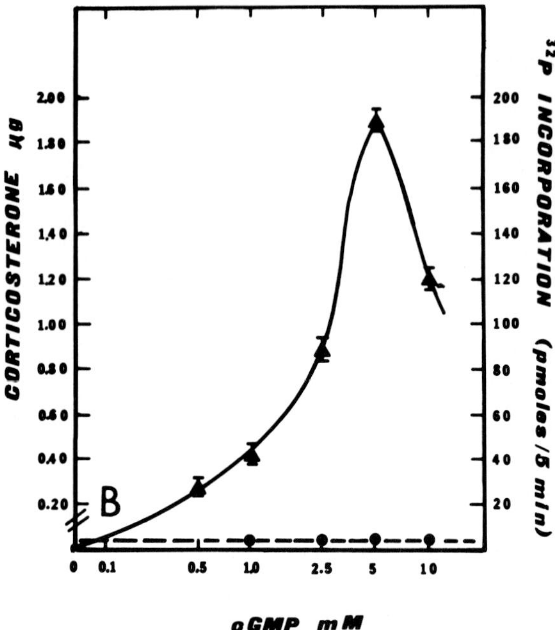

FIG. 8. Corticosterone production *(filled circles)* and phosphorylation *(triangles)* in isolated adrenocortical carcinoma cells in response to cGMP (mM concentrations). The conditions of the experiment were similar to those in Fig. 4. (Adapted from Sharma et al., ref. 97.)

TABLE 6. *Effects of cycloheximide and actinomycin D on cAMP- and cGMP-induced phosphorylation in adrenocortical carcinoma cells*[a]

Cyclic nucleotides (mM)	^{32}P incorporation (pmoles/5 min)					
	cAMP			cGMP		
	Control	+ cycloheximide	+ actinomycin D	Control	+ cycloheximide	+ actinomycin D
0.5				27	23	24
1.0	80	69	72	42	37	50
2.5	222	216	218	88	104	94
5.0	320	339	337	189	182	194
10	145	135	138	121	127	115

[a] Incubation system: adrenal cell suspension 0.8 ml; reagents dissolved in 0.2 ml of Krebs-Ringer-bicarbonate buffer, pH 7.4, containing 4% albumin and 0.2% glucose, or protein kinase buffer. Total volume of first incubation, 1 ml; second incubation, 0.5 ml. Results are averages of six observations. Basal values have been subtracted from experimental results.No stimulation of steroidogenesis was observed in any of the experiments. The average basal value of corticosterone was 0.05 μg per incubation tube and, for phosphorylation, 395 pmoles.

Adapted from Sharma et al. (97).

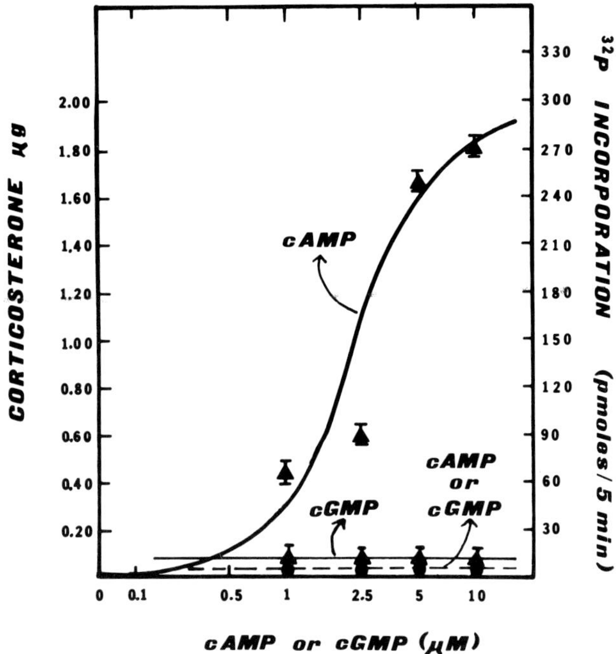

FIG. 9. Corticosterone production *(filled circles)* and phosphorylation *(triangles)* in isolated adrenocortical carcinoma cells in response to cAMP and cGMP (µM concentrations). The conditions of the experiment were similar to those in Fig. 4. (Adapted from Sharma et al., ref. 97.)

nucleotides, the process of phosphorylation does not result in steroidogenesis in a normal adrenal cell.

Modified Protein Kinase

Based on the premise that a cAMP-dependent protein kinase (13) is involved in cAMP-activated steroidogenesis, it was proposed (92) that the defect in the tumor might be due to one of the following factors: (a) cAMP does not bind to the regulatory subunit of the protein kinase, which indicates a defective cAMP-binding receptor; (b) cAMP binds to the regulatory subunit of the protein kinase, but it is unable to dissociate the catalytic subunit; (c) a catalytic subunit of the protein kinase lacks kinase activity and is therefore unable to stimulate ATP-dependent phosphorylation of the appropriate substrate. This, in turn, could result in the lack of hypothetical mRNA translation. One or a combination of these events may be responsible for lack of control of the rate-limiting enzyme in cAMP-activated steroidogenesis.

Sharma et al. have described (98) the partial purification and characterization

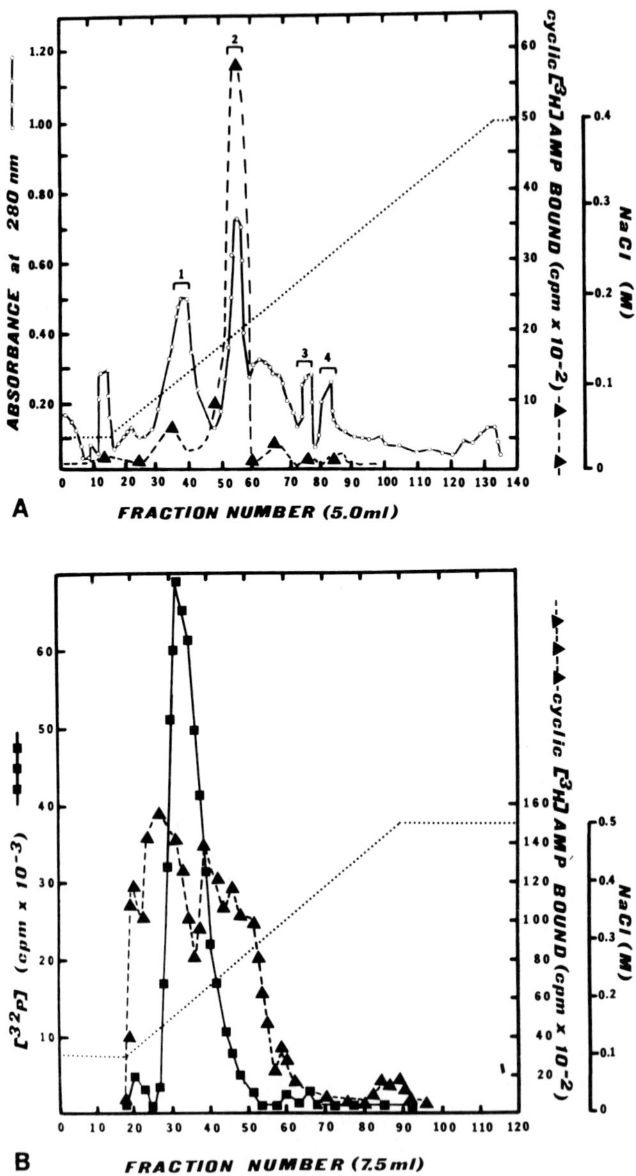

FIG. 10. A: DEAE-52 cellulose chromatography of adrenocortical carcinoma cAMP-binding protein kinases. Column was equilibrated with 100 ml of 20 mM Tris-HCl buffer (pH 7.5) containing 5 mM β-mercaptoethanol and eluted with a gradient of NaCl (0.04–0.4 M). Fractions (5 ml) were collected. Absorbance at 280 nm *(open circles)* and cAMP-binding activity *(triangles)* of the fractions in parallel tubes were determined. **B:** DEAE-52 cellulose chromatography of normal adrenal cAMP-binding protein kinase. Column was equilibrated as in A and eluted with a gradient of NaCl (0.1–0.5 M). Fractions (7.5 ml) were collected. cAMP-binding activity *(triangles)* and cAMP-dependent protein kinase activity *(squares)* of the fractions were determined. (Adapted from Sharma et al., ref. 98.)

TABLE 7. *Effects of various nucleotides on binding of [³H]cAMP to adrenocortical tumor protein kinase*

Sample number	Various nucleotides added	Nucleotide concentration (fold excess)	[³H]cAMP bound[a] (%)
1	None		100 ± 0[b]
2	cAMP	500	29 ± 1
3	cGMP	500	97 ± 2
4	cIMP	500	69 ± 2
5	cUMP	500	100 ± 0
6	cCMP[c]	500	100 ± 0
7	ADP	500	100 ± 0
8	ATP	500	100 ± 0

[a]The value of 100% represents 0.08 pmole of bound [³H]cAMP.
[b]Mean ± SD.
[c]cCMP: cyclic cytidine 3′,5′-monophosphate.
Adapted from Sharma et al. (98).

of defective cAMP-binding protein kinase from adrenocortical carcinoma and compared it with that obtained from normal adrenal gland.

Figure 10A shows that peak 2 eluted from the DEAE-52 cellulose column contained cAMP-binding activity. This binding was specific. The data in Table 7 clearly demonstrate that of all the cyclic nucleotides tested, only cIMP competed to a small extent with the receptor of cAMP.

Table 8 shows that cAMP does not stimulate protein kinase activity of the

TABLE 8. *Effect of cAMP concentration on histone phosphorylation by adrenocortical carcinoma protein kinase enzyme*[a]

Concentration of cAMP (μM)	³²P incorporation (% of control)[b]
0.005	107 ± 3[c]
0.010	108 ± 3
1	108 ± 4
5	108 ± 5
10	106 ± 3
5,000	108 ± 4
10,000	108 ± 5

[a]Incubation system: protein kinase buffer comprised of 50 mM sodium β-glycerate (pH 6.0), 10 mM magnesium acetate, 20 mM NaF, 0.3 mM EGTA, 250 μg histone, 100 μM [γ-³²P]ATP (1 μCi), 20 μg tumor protein kinase enzyme, and various concentrations of cAMP. Total volume of incubation mixture was 0.5 ml, and samples were processed as described in "Materials and Methods" (98). Results are averages of six observations.
[b]The control value (120 pmoles/5 min/20 μg) was obtained by running the assay in the absence of cAMP.
[c]Mean ± SD.
Adapted from Sharma et al. (98).

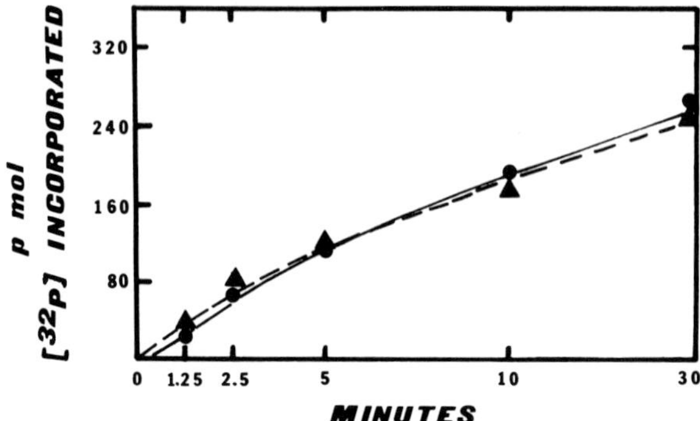

FIG. 11. Time course of endogenous phosphorylation of adrenocortical carcinoma protein kinase enzyme in the presence *(filled circles)* and absence *(triangles)* of 5 μM cAMP. Conditions of the experiment were similar to those in Table 8, except that no histone was added to the reaction mixture. The reaction blank at 0 time (< 10 pmoles) was substracted from each determination. (Adapted from Sharma et al., ref. 98.)

tumor enzyme in the phosphorylation of the histones. These results are in contrast to those for the cAMP-dependent protein kinase enzyme found in the normal adrenal gland, which binds cAMP and catalyzes phosphorylation of histones (14). This indicates that the catalytic subunit of the protein kinase enzyme either is absent or, if intact, is unable to be dissociated from the regulatory subunit by cAMP. A careful analysis of the cAMP-dependent kinase activity of the fractionated protein peaks was made, but no such activity was detected in any fraction. However, in normal adrenal extract, cAMP-dependent protein kinase activity was observed (Fig. 10B).

That the enzyme has endogenous kinase activity is shown by the results in Fig. 11. In this experiment the tumor enzyme was incubated with [γ-^{32}P]ATP for different time intervals ranging from 1.25 to 30 min. However, the addition of cAMP did not affect the rate of phosphorylation. This confirms the results discussed earlier showing that cAMP is unable to activate the protein kinase. The process of endogenous phosphorylation was previously observed in intracellular membranes of liver (95) and with the protein kinase enzyme isolated from bovine heart (68).

This crude protein kinase enzyme was purified to homogeneity (81,82) by hydrophobic chromatography, affinity chromatography, and gel filtration. The enzyme was found to have a molecular weight of 85,000 d. SDS polyacrylamide gel chromatography of photoaffinity labeled cAMP linked with the enzyme revealed a molecular weight of 42,000 d, indicating that it consists of two identical subunits. Stoichiometry of cAMP binding with the enzyme showed that it binds two cAMP molecules. This suggests that each subunit binds one molecule of cAMP. In contrast to the cAMP-dependent protein kinase enzyme found in the normal adrenal gland, this enzyme did not catalyze phosphorylation of exogenous histone. However, the enzyme showed the property of autophosphorylation, which again was in contrast to the situation with the normal enzyme.

In view of these findings and earlier observations (91,92), showing that the biosynthetic steps from (20S)-20-hydroxycholesterol to corticosterone are at least partly intact in the tumor, it is evident that the original hypothesis of Sharma et al. (92), which related lack of stimulation of steroidogenesis by exogenous cAMP to the defective protein kinase enzyme, may be further narrowed down.

In the current hypothesis it is proposed that the biochemical lesion in the tumor responsible for the lack of exogenously added cAMP-activated steroidogenesis is in the defective protein kinase enzyme. The indirect evidence in favor of a defective cGMP-dependent protein kinase system in the adrenocortical carcinoma cell has also been presented recently (59,97). However, at this time the relationship between carcinogenesis and these defects in cyclic-nucleotide-mediated regulatory processes in endocrine neoplasia is not clear. But if the tumor indeed possesses a defective cGMP-dependent protein kinase system in addition to the defective cAMP-dependent protein kinase system, then the abnormal regulation due to the lesions in protein kinases might be a generality accompanied by malignancy in adrenocortical carcinoma. The result of this change in cyclic nucleotide metabolism might be useful to the survival of the malignant cell, but the consequences to the normal cell would be catastrophic.

The proposed model depicting the lesion in the cAMP-dependent protein kinase system that can account for the lack of cAMP-activated steroidogenesis is shown in Fig. 12.

Abnormal ACTH Control of Steroidogenesis after Rate-limiting Step

Altered Control System

Experiments (84) with double-labeled (^{3}H and ^{14}C) radioactive precursors of pregnenolone, progesterone, and deoxycorticosterone show that, in contrast to the situation with the normal adrenal cell, ACTH strongly inhibits the incorporation of pregnenolone and progesterone into deoxycorticosterone and corticosterone in the malignant cell (Tables 9 and 10). Furthermore, when the experiments are repeated using cAMP instead of ACTH, cAMP (in contrast to ACTH) has little effect on transformation of pregnenolone to deoxycorticosterone, but it does inhibit incorporation of deoxycorticosterone into corticosterone (Table 11). These results not only demonstrate important differences between ACTH and cAMP control in adrenal tumor cells but also provide further evidence that cAMP may not be the sole mediator of ACTH action.

Other effects of ACTH, cAMP, and cGMP on membrane mechanisms will be discussed presently. These effects, which undoubtedly modify intracellular steroid concentrations and thereby enzyme reaction rates, may eventually help to explain some of these results.

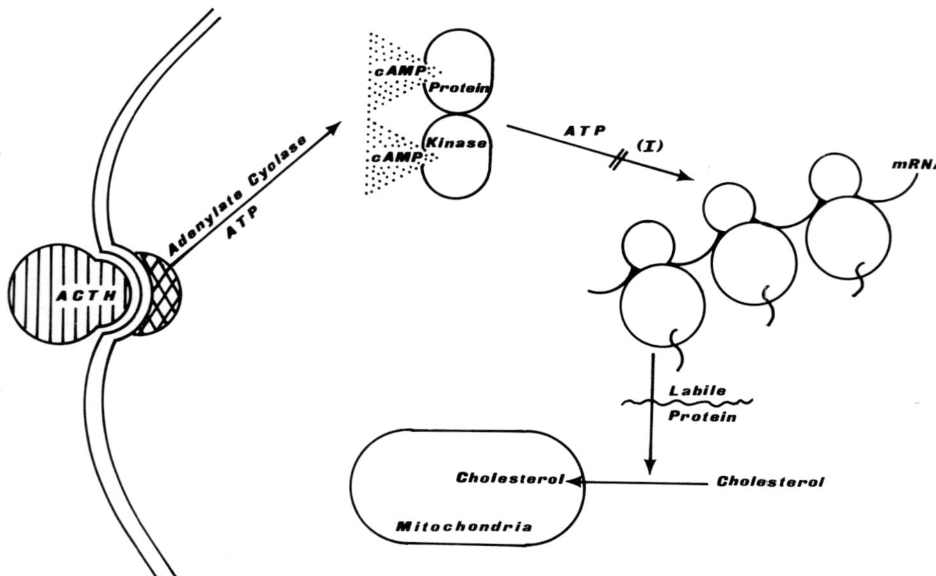

FIG. 12. Postulated defective step (I) responsible for loss of cAMP control in adrenocortical carcinoma cells.

TABLE 9. *Effects of adrenocorticotropin on incorporation of [^3H]pregnenolone into deoxycorticosterone and corticosterone in adrenocortical carcinoma cells*[a]

Compound	Crystallization	$^3H/^{14}C$ ratio of compound in Flask 1	Flasks 2 + 3
Deoxycorticosterone acetate	Crude product	15.60	6.20
	1st	16.80	6.39
Corticosterone	1st	18.88	5.94
	2nd	17.93	5.72
	3rd	17.72	5.74

[a] $^3H/^{14}C$ ratios of products (and their derivatives) were obtained after incubation of [4-^{14}C, 7α-^3H]pregnenolone in adrenocortical carcinoma cells. Incubation was carried out in three flasks containing 20 ml isolated adrenocortical carcinoma cell preparation as described in "Materials and Methods" by Sharma (84). Flask 1 contained a mixture of [7α-^3H]pregnenolone (20 μCi) + [4-^{14}C]pregnenolone (1 μCi) ($^3H/^{14}C$ ratio 20.00). Flask 2 contained [7α-^3H]-pregnenolone (20 μCi) + adrenocorticotropin (200 μU/ml). Flask 3 contained [4-^{14}C]pregnenolone (1 μCi). Incubation was for 2.5 hr, and the reaction was stopped by addition of 25 ml methylene chloride to each flask. Contents of second and third flasks were mixed, and deoxycorticosterone and corticosterone were isolated as described in "Materials and Methods" (84).

Adapted from Sharma (84).

TABLE 10. *Effects of adrenocorticotropin on incorporation of [^3H]progesterone into deoxycorticosterone and corticosterone in adrenocortical carcinoma cells*[a]

Compound	Crystallization	$^3H/^{14}C$ ratio of compound in Flask 1	Flasks 2 + 3
Deoxycorticosterone acetate	Crude product	20.45	12.34
	1st	17.05	10.05
	2nd	18.18	10.55
Corticosterone	1st	18.47	7.87
	2nd	19.78	8.25
	3rd	20.12	8.27

[a] $^3H/^{14}C$ ratios of products (and their derivatives) were obtained after incubation of [4-^{14}C, 7α-^3H]progesterone in adrenocortical carcinoma cells. Conditions of the experiment were similar to those in the experiment in Table 9.

Adapted from Sharma (84).

11β-Hydroxylase Activity

Studies with adrenocortical carcinoma cells using radioactive precursors such as (20S)-20-hydroxycholesterol have indicated that these cells synthesize at least fourfold more deoxycorticosterone than corticosterone (5,91,92). In the normal isolated adrenal cell these steroids are formed in the same concentrations (85,92). Whether or not this is a general property of all types of adrenal tumor cells has yet to be determined.

TABLE 11. *Effects of cAMP on incorporation of [^3H]pregnenolone into deoxycorticosterone and corticosterone in adrenocortical carcinoma cells*[a]

Compound	Crystallization	$^3H/^{14}C$ ratio of compound in	
		Flask 1	Flasks 2 + 3
Deoxycorticosterone acetate	Crude product	17.79	15.67
	1st	17.41	15.91
	2nd	17.49	16.11
Corticosterone	1st	19.36	14.86
	2nd	19.78	14.61
	3rd	19.17	14.55

[a] $^3H/^{14}C$ ratios of products (and their derivatives) were obtained after incubation of [4-^{14}C, 7α-^3H]pregnenolone in adrenocortical carcinoma cells. Conditions of the experiment were similar to those in the experiment in Table 9. Flask 1 contained [4-^{14}C, 7α-^3H]pregnenolone. Flask 2 contained [7α-^3H]pregnenolone and cAMP. Flask 3 contained [4-^{14}C]pregnenolone. Adapted from Sharma (84).

Evidence has been provided (85) that corticosterone biosynthesis in the normal isolated adrenal cell involves two slow biosynthetic steps. The first step, controlled by ACTH, is conversion of cholesterol to (20S)-20-hydroxycholesterol; the second step, not controlled by ACTH, is transformation of deoxycorticosterone to corticosterone. However, in the adrenal tumor cell the latter step appears to be considerably slower than in the normal cell (5,91,92).

Different Modes of Membrane Effects by ACTH, cAMP, and cGMP

ACTH stimulates (87) incorporation of exogenous deoxycorticosterone into corticosterone in isolated adrenal and adrenocortical carcinoma cells (Table 12). Indirect evidence has been provided (87) that this requires interposition of the plasma membrane, since preloading the cells eliminates hormonal stimulation (Table 13). Therefore, this effect probably is dependent on deoxycorticosterone transport across the plasma membrane of normal and malignant adrenal cells.

cAMP, dibutyryl cAMP, cGMP, and cIMP duplicate the stimulatory effect of ACTH in normal cells (72,87) (Tables 14–16); as with the latter agent, stimulation of deoxycorticosterone incorporation into corticosterone by these cyclic nucleotides is most probably at the plasma membrane, since preloading the cells eliminates the cyclic nucleotide stimulation (72,87) (Tables 17 and 18). These results indicate that ACTH, cAMP, cGMP, and cIMP, the agents that stimulate steroidogenesis (35) in an isolated adrenal cell, also stimulate the transport phenomenon of deoxycorticosterone across the plasma membrane. In the tumor, however, ACTH stimulates the membrane effect (87), but the cyclic nucleotides are incapable of doing so (72). Previously it was shown (93) that ACTH, cAMP, cGMP, and cIMP were not able to stimulate corticosterone

TABLE 12. *Effects of ACTH on incorporation of [^3H]deoxycorticosterone into corticosterone in normal isolated adrenal and adrenocortical carcinoma cells*[a]

Isolated cells from	Crystallization	$^3H/^{14}C$ ratio of corticosterone from: Flask 1	Flasks 2 + 3
Normal adrenal	1st	20.00	24.12
	2nd	20.06	25.70
	3rd	20.59	26.49
Adrenocortical carcinoma	1st	19.97	27.96
	2nd	17.76	26.71
	3rd	16.40	25.40

[a] $^3H/^{14}C$ ratios of corticosterone were obtained after incubation of [4-^{14}C, 1,2-$^3H_2$]deoxycorticosterone with isolated adrenal and adrenocortical carcinoma cells. Incubation was carried out in three flasks containing 20 ml isolated adrenal or adrenocortical carcinoma cell preparation. Flask 1 contained a mixture of [1,2-$^3H_2$]deoxycorticosterone (4.0 μCi) + [4-^{14}C]-deoxycorticosterone (0.20 μCi) ($^3H/^{14}C$ ratio 20.00). Flask 2 contained [1,2-$^3H_2$]deoxycorticosterone (4.0 μCi) + ACTH (200 μU/ml). Flask 3 contained [4-^{14}C]deoxycorticosterone (0.20 μCi). Incubation was for 2.5 hr, and the reaction was stopped by adding 75 ml methylene chloride to each flask. Contents of second and third flasks were mixed, and corticosterone was isolated as described in "Materials and Methods" by Sharma (87).

Adapted from Sharma (87).

TABLE 13. *Effects of ACTH on incorporation of [^3H]deoxycorticosterone into corticosterone in preloaded normal isolated adrenal and adrenocortical carcinoma cells*[a]

Isolated cells from	Compound	Crystallization	^3H dpm of compound from: Control	+ ACTH
Normal adrenal	Deoxycorticosterone acetate	Crude	1,239,000	1,245,000
		1st	1,230,000	1,240,000
	Corticosterone	1st	206,500	243,000
		2nd	202,000	222,000
		3rd	200,400	219,000
Adrenocortical carcinoma	Deoxycorticosterone acetate	1st	1,962,000	1,905,000
	Corticosterone	1st	69,500	66,100
		2nd	68,400	60,300

[a] Total ^3H dpm of products (and their derivatives) were obtained after incubation of [1,2-$^3H_2$] deoxycorticosterone with isolated adrenal and adrenocortical carcinoma cells. Isolated adrenal cell preparation (20 ml) obtained from adrenals of 32 rats or the same amount of cell suspension obtained from 1.5 g adrenal tumor was preincubated with 5 mg of nonradioactive deoxycorticosterone + [1,2-$^3H_2$]deoxycorticosterone (8.0 μCi) for 30 min. The cells were washed and resuspended in 40 ml of Krebs-Ringer-bicarbonate buffer containing albumin and glucose. A 20-ml aliquot of cell suspension was added to one flask, and the second flask contained a 20-ml aliquot of cell suspension + ACTH (200 μU/ml). Incubation was for 2.5 hr, and the reaction was stopped by adding 75 ml methylene chloride to each flask. Deoxycorticosterone and corticosterone were isolated as described in "Materials and Methods" by Sharma (87).

Adapted from Sharma (87).

TABLE 14. *Effects of dibutyryl cAMP on incorporation of [^3H]deoxycorticosterone into corticosterone in normal isolated adrenal and adrenocortical carcinoma cells*[a]

Isolated cells from	Crystallization	$^3H/^{14}C$ ratio of corticosterone in	
		Flask 1	Flasks 2 + 3
Normal adrenal	1st	20.04	25.47
	2nd	20.06	27.11
	3rd	20.35	28.49
Adrenocortical carcinoma	1st	20.00	21.47
	2nd	19.91	22.72
	3rd	19.86	22.57

[a] $^3H/^{14}C$ ratios of products were obtained after incubation of [4-^{14}C, 1,2-$^3H_2$]deoxycorticosterone with isolated adrenal and adrenocortical carcinoma cells. Conditions of the experiment were similar to those in the experiment in Table 12, except that dibutyryl cAMP was used in place of ACTH.

Adapted from Sharma (87).

synthesis in tumor cells. Taken together with the findings that the tumor does not contain any detectable amount of normal cAMP-binding protein kinase enzyme, but instead possesses an altered protein kinase that binds cAMP and undergoes autophosphorylation, but is unable to activate the cAMP-dependent phosphorylation process, these results suggest that the inability of the cyclic

TABLE 15. *Effects of cGMP on incorporation of [^3H]deoxycorticosterone into corticosterone in normal isolated adrenal and adrenocortical carcinoma cells*[a]

Isolated cells from	Crystallization	$^3H/^{14}C$ ratio of corticosterone from		Percentage stimulation
		Flask 1	Flasks 2 + 3	
Normal adrenal	1st	25.18	43.05	
	2nd	25.63	42.33	
	3rd	25.97	43.70	68
Adrenocortical carcinoma	1st	25.03	26.13	
	2nd	25.88	27.17	
	3rd	26.70	27.76	0

[a] $^3H/^{14}C$ ratios of corticosterone were obtained after incubation of [1,2-$^3H_2$, 4-^{14}C]deoxycorticosterone with isolated adrenal and adrenocortical carcinoma cells. Incubation was carried out in three flasks containing 20 ml isolated adrenal or adrenocortical carcinoma cell preparation, as described in "Materials and Methods" (72). Flask 1 contained a mixture of [1,2-$^3H_2$]deoxycorticosterone (25 μCi) + (4-^{14}C]deoxycorticosterone (1 μCi) ($^3H/^{14}C$ ratio 25.00). Flask 2 contained [1,2-$^3H_2$]deoxycorticosterone (25 μCi) + cGMP (10 mM). Flask 3 contained [4-^{14}C]deoxycorticosterone (1 μCi). Incubation was for 2.5 hr, and the reaction was stopped by addition of 75 ml methylene chloride to each flask. Contents of second and third flasks were mixed, and corticosterone was isolated as described in "Materials and Methods" by Sawhney and Sharma (72).

Adapted from Sawhney and Sharma (72).

TABLE 16. *Effects of cIMP on incorporation of [^{3}H]deoxycorticosterone into corticosterone in normal isolated adrenal and adrenocortical carcinoma cells*[a]

Isolated cells from	Crystal-lization	$^{3}H/^{14}C$ ratio of corticosterone in: Flask 1	Flasks 2 + 3	Percentage stimulation
Normal adrenal	1st	25.18	88.13	
	2nd	25.63	89.28	
	3rd	25.97	90.89	250
Adrenocortical carcinoma	1st	25.03	25.44	
	2nd	25.88	25.12	
	3rd	26.70	25.63	0

[a] $^{3}H/^{14}C$ ratios of products were obtained after incubation of [1,2-$^{3}H_2$, 4-^{14}C]deoxycorticosterone with isolated adrenal and adrenocortical carcinoma cells. Conditions of the experiment were similar to those of the experiment in Table 15.
Adapted from Sawhney and Sharma (72).

nucleotides to influence the membrane transport process in the malignant cell is due to lack of a cyclic-nucleotide-dependent phosphorylation phenomenon.

Therefore these studies indicate that the two types of membrane transport processes are different in malignant and normal cells, and they also indicate that the ACTH-activated transport system is quite distinct from the cyclic-nucleotide-stimulated system in a normal cell. In the tumor, where there is a defective protein kinase system, ACTH does stimulate the membrane-dependent transport system, but the cyclic nucleotides do not. This indicates that in contrast to the cyclic nucleotide system, the ACTH-stimulated membrane phenomenon does not involve the obligatory protein kinase system. These factors have been depicted in Fig. 13.

TABLE 17. *Effects of dibutyryl cAMP on incorporation of [^{3}H]deoxycorticosterone into corticosterone in preloaded normal isolated adrenal cells*[a]

Compound	Crystallization	^{3}H dpm of compound from: Control	+ Dibutyryl cAMP
Deoxycorticosterone acetate	Crude	1,177,000	1,182,000
	1st	1,169,000	1,178,000
Corticosterone	1st	187,800	178,800
	2nd	183,500	177,600
	3rd	182,300	184,000

[a] Total ^{3}H dpm of products (and their derivatives) were obtained after incubation of [1,2-$^{3}H_2$] deoxycorticosterone with isolated adrenal cells. Conditions of the experiment were similar to those of the experiment in Table 13.
Adapted from Sharma (87).

TABLE 18. *Effects of cGMP and cIMP on incorporation of [^{3}H]deoxycorticosterone into corticosterone in preloaded normal isolated adrenal cells*[a]

Compound	Crystallization	^{3}H dpm of compound from: Control	+ cGMP	+ cIMP
Deoxycorticosterone acetate	1st	182,192	168,968	178,330
Corticosterone	1st	21,820	18,640	20,100
	2nd	20,130	17,090	19,250
	3rd	18,040	16,600	18,210

[a]Total ^{3}H dpm of products (and their derivatives) were obtained after incubation of [1,2-$^{3}H_2$] deoxycorticosterone with isolated adrenal cells. Isolated adrenal cell preparation (20 ml) obtained from adrenals of 32 rats was preincubated with 50 μCi of [1,2-$^{3}H_2$]deoxycorticosterone for 30 min. The cells were washed and resuspended in 60 ml of Krebs-Ringer-bicarbonate buffer containing albumin and glucose. Flask 1, used as a control, contained a 20-ml aliquot of cell suspension. Flask 2 contained a 20-ml aliquot of cell suspension + cGMP (10 mM). To Flask 3, in addition to cell suspension (20 ml), cIMP (10 mM) was added. Incubation was for 2.5 hr, and the reaction was stopped by addition of 75 ml methylene chloride to each flask. Deoxycorticosterone and corticosterone were isolated and purified by thin-layer chromatography and were crystallized to constant specific activity as described in "Materials and Methods" by Sawhney and Sharma (72).

Adapted from Sawhney and Sharma (72).

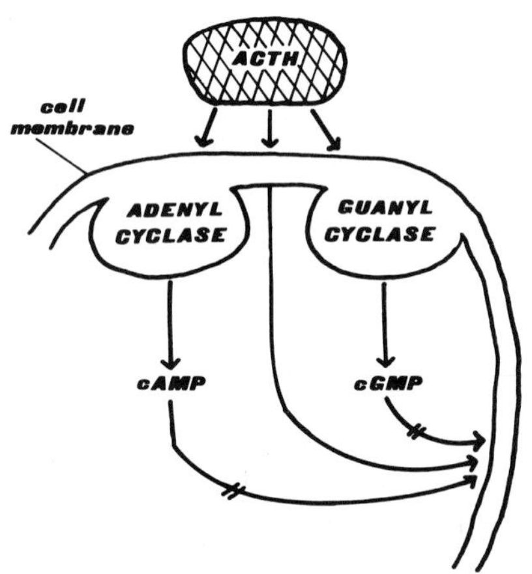

FIG. 13. Triggering of other membrane effects, possibly transport, by ACTH, cAMP, and cGMP. Postulated plasma membrane defects in adrenocortical carcinoma cells *(arrows with cross-bars).*

CONCLUSION

The preceding discussion indicates that the adrenal tumor control system differs from that in the normal adrenal cell. Various biochemical lesions in the tumor cell have been located. These abnormalities in the control mechanism exist both before and after the steps of cholesterol side chain cleavage. One such predominant lesion in the cAMP-binding protein kinase enzyme has been localized. No detectable amount of normal cAMP-binding protein kinase enzyme was found in the tumor. Instead, a novel autophosphorylating cAMP binding protein kinase was found in the adrenocortical carcinoma. This enzyme has been purified to homogeneity. It has a molecular weight of 85,000 d and consists of two identical subunits. Stoichiometry of cAMP binding with the enzyme shows that it binds two cAMP molecules, which indicates that each subunit binds one molecule of cAMP. This enzyme undergoes autophosphorylation, but it is unable to activate the cAMP-dependent phosphorylation process. This suggests that the lack of cAMP-dependent phosphorylation by this enzyme may explain the nonstimulatory effect of cAMP in regulation of steroidogenesis in adrenocortical carcinoma 494 cells.

Other defects in the control system after the cholesterol side chain cleavage step have been shown. One such abnormal control step probably resides in the plasma membrane. The latter lesion in the tumor may be due to the membrane cyclic-nucleotide-dependent phosphorylation system. Future studies designed to elucidate the cause–effect relationship of these regulatory steps in adrenocortical carcinoma will contribute to our basic understanding of the influence of hormones in neoplasia.

ACKNOWLEDGMENTS

Appreciation is expressed to Dr. J. S. Brush for his assistance in evaluating the kinetic data pertaining to the interrelationship of ACTH and cGMP in steroidogenesis, to Dr. A. Roberts and Dr. W. Y. Cheung for critical comments, and to Dr. G. Shanker, Dr. J.-P. Perchellet, Dr. R. S. Sawhney, and Ms. Helga Ahrens, research fellows, whose dedicated research made possible the completion of this chapter. The excellent typing assistance of Ms. Frances Lassiter is also greatly appreciated.

Portions of the experimental work described in this chapter were supported by grants from the National Cancer Institute (CA-16091) and the Damon Runyon Memorial Fund for Cancer Research (DRG-1237).

I would like to dedicate this research to my parents, who worked so hard to prepare me for this work.

REFERENCES

1. Asakawa, T., Scheinbaum, I., and Ho, R. (1976): Stimulation of guanylate cyclase activity by several fatty acids. *Biochem. Biophys. Res. Commun.*, 73:141–148.

2. Beall, R. J., and Sayers, G. (1972): Isolated adrenal cells: Steroidogenesis and cyclic AMP accumulation in response to ACTH. *Arch. Biochem. Biophys.*, 148:70–76.
3. Bell, J. J., and Harding, B. W. (1974): The acute action of adrenocorticotropic hormone on adrenal steroidogenesis. *Biochim. Biophys. Acta,* 348:285–298.
4. Bennet, V., O'Keefe, E., and Cuatrecasas, P. (1976): Mechanism of action of cholera toxin and the mobile receptor theory of hormone receptor–adenylate cyclase interactions. *Proc. Natl. Acad. Sci. U.S.A.,* 72:33–37.
5. Brush, J. S., Sutliff, L. S., and Sharma, R. K. (1974): Metabolic regulation and adenyl cyclase activity of adrenocortical carcinoma cultured cells. *Cancer Res.,* 34:1495–1502.
6. Constantopoulos, G., Satoh, P. S., and Tchen, T. T. (1961): Cleavage of cholesterol side chain by adrenal cortex III. Identification of 20α-22ξ-dihydroxycholesterol as an intermediate. *Biochem. Biophys. Res. Commun.,* 8:50–55.
7. Constantopoulos, G., and Tchen, T. T. (1961): Cleavage of cholesterol side chain by adrenal cortex: Cofactor requirement and product of cleavage. *J. Biol. Chem.,* 236:65–67.
8. Davis, W. W., and Garren, L. D. (1968): On the mechanism of action of adrenocorticotropic hormone. The inhibitory site of cycloheximide in the pathway of steroid biosynthesis. *J. Biol. Chem.,* 243:5153–5157.
9. Espiner, E. A., Livesey, J. J., Ross, J., and Donald, R. A. (1974): Dynamics of cyclic adenosine 3′,5′-monophosphate release during adrenocortical stimulation *in vivo. Endocrinology,* 95:838–846.
10. Farese, R. V., Linarelli, L. G., Glinsmann, W. H., Ditzion, B. R., Paul, M. I., and Pauk, G. L. (1969): Persistence of the steroidogenic effect of adenosine-3′,5′-monophosphate *in vitro:* Evidence for a third factor during the steroidogenic effect of ACTH. *Endocrinology,* 85:867–874.
11. Fujimoto, M., and Okabayasin, T. (1975): Proposed mechanisms of stimulation and inhibition of guanylate cyclase with reference to the actions of chlorpromazine, phospholipases and Triton X-100. *Biochem. Biophys. Res. Commun.,* 67:1332–1336.
12. Garren, L. D., Gill, G. N., Masui, H., and Walton, G. M. (1971): On the mechanism of action of ACTH. *Recent Prog. Horm. Res.,* 27:433–478.
13. Gill, G. N., and Garren, L. D. (1969): On the mechanism of action of adrenocorticotropic hormone. The binding of cyclic 3′,5′-adenosine monophosphate to an adrenal cortical protein. *Proc. Natl. Acad. Sci. U.S.A.,* 63:512–519.
14. Gill, G. N., and Garren, L. D. (1970): A cyclic 3′,5′-adenosine monophosphate dependent protein kinase from the adrenal cortex. Comparison with a cyclic AMP binding protein. *Biochem. Biophys. Res. Commun.,* 39:335–343.
15. Gill, G. N., Holdy, K. E., Walton, G. M., and Kanstein, C. B. (1976): Purification and characterization of 3′:5′-cyclic GMP-dependent protein kinase. *Proc. Natl. Acad. Sci. U.S.A.,* 73:3918–3922.
16. Gill, G. N., and Kanstein, C. B. (1975): Guanosine 3′,5′-monophosphate receptor protein: Separation from adenosine 3′,5′-monophosphate receptor protein. *Biochem. Biophys. Res. Commun.,* 63:1113–1122.
17. Glinsmann, W. H., Hern, E. P., Linarelli, L. G., and Farese, R. V. (1969): Similarities between effects of adenosine 3′,5′-monophosphate and guanosine 3′,5′-monophosphate on liver and adrenal metabolism. *Endocrinology,* 85:711–719.
18. Grahme-Smith, D. G., Butcher, R. W., Ney, R. L., and Sutherland, E. W. (1967): Adenosine 3′,5′-monophosphate as the intracellular mediator of the action of adrenocorticotropic hormone on the adrenal cortex. *J. Biol. Chem.,* 242:5535–5541.
19. Halkerston, I. D. K. (1975): Cyclic AMP and adrenocortical function. In: *Advances in Cyclic Nucleotide Research, Vol. 14,* edited by P. Greengard and G. A. Robison, pp. 99–136. Raven Press, New York.
20. Halkerston, I. D. K., Feinstein, M., and Hechter, O. (1966): An anomalous effect of theophylline on ACTH and adenosine 3′,5′-monophosphate stimulation. *Proc. Soc. Exp. Biol. Med.,* 122:896–900.
21. Hall, P. F., and Young, D. G. (1968): Site of action of tropic hormones upon the biosynthetic pathways to steroid hormones. *Endocrinology,* 82:559–568.
22. Harrington, C. A., Femimore, D. C., and Farmer, W. (1977): Coupled dose related responses of guanosine 3′,5′-cyclic monophosphate and progesterone plus desoxycorticosterone in isolated rat adrenocortical cells. In: *59th Annual Meeting, Endocrine Society, Chicago.* (abstract 170).

23. Haynes, R. C., Jr. (1958): The activation of adrenal phosphorylase by the adrenocorticotropic hormone. *J. Biol. Chem.*, 233:1220–1222.
24. Haynes, R. C., Koritz, S. B., and Péron, F. G. (1959): Influence of adenosine 3′,5′-monophosphate on corticoid production by rat adrenal glands. *J. Biol. Chem.*, 234:1421–1423.
25. Helmrich, E. J. M., Zenner, H. P., Pfeuffer, T., and Cori, C. F. (1976): Signal transfer from hormone receptor to adenylate cyclase. *Curr. Top. Cell. Regul.*, 10:41–87.
26. Hohn, K. V., and Chavin, W. (1975): ACTH control of adrenocortical c-GMP. *Gen. Comp. Endocrinol.*, 26:374–381.
27. Hudson, A. M., and McMartin, C. (1975): An investigation of the involvement of adenosine 3′:5′-cyclic monophosphate in steroidogenesis by using isolated adrenal cell column perfusion. *Biochem. J.*, 148:539–544.
28. Johnson, D. F., Snell, K. C., François, D., and Heftmann, E. (1961): *In vitro* metabolism of progesterone-4-^{14}C in an adrenocortical carcinoma of the rat. *Acta Endocrinol.*, 37:329–335.
29. Kahnt, F. W., Milani, A., Steffen, H., and Neher, R. (1974): The rate-limiting step of adrenal steroidogenesis and adenosine 3′:5′-monophosphate. *Eur. J. Biochem.*, 44:243–250.
30. Kahnt, F. W., and Neher, R. (1966): Über die Adrenale Steroid-biosynthese in Vitro. III. Selektive Hemmung der Nebennierenrindenfunktion. *Helv. Chim. Acta*, 49:725–732.
31. Kan, K. W., and Ungar, F. (1973): Characterization of an adrenal activator for cholesterol side chain cleavage. *J. Biol. Chem.*, 248:2868–2875.
32. Karaboyas, G. C., and Koritz, S. B. (1965): Identity of the site of action of 3′,5′-adenosine monophosphate and adrenocorticotropic hormone in corticosteroidogenesis in rat adrenal and beef adrenal cortex slices. *Biochemistry*, 4:462–468.
33. Kimmel, G. L., Péron, F. G., Haskar, A., Bedigan, E., Robidaux, W. F., Jr., and Lin, M. T. (1974): Ultrastructure, steroidogenic potential, and energy metabolism of the Snell adrenocortical carcinoma 494. *J. Cell Biol.*, 62:152–163.
34. Kimura, H., Mittal, C. K., and Murad, F. (1975): Activation of guanylate cyclase from rat liver and other tissues by sodium azide. *J. Biol. Chem.*, 250:8016–8022.
35. Kitabchi, A. E., and Sharma, R. K. (1971): Corticosteroidogenesis in isolated adrenal cells of rats. I. Effect of corticotropins and 3′,5′-cyclic nucleotides on corticosterone production. *Endocrinology*, 88:1109–1116.
36. Kitabchi, A. E., Sharma, R. K., and West, W. H. (1971): A sensitive bioassay method for ACTH using isolated rat adrenal cells. *Horm. Metab. Res.*, 3:133–134.
37. Kitabchi, A. E., Wilson, D. B., and Sharma, R. K. (1971): Steroidogenesis in isolated adrenal cells of rat. II. Effect of caffeine on ACTH and cyclic nucleotide-induced steroidogenesis and its relation to cyclic nucleotide phosphodiesterase (PDE). *Biochem. Biophys. Res. Commun.*, 44:898–904.
38. Koritz, S. B. (1962): The effect of calcium ions and freezing on the *in vitro* synthesis of pregnenolone by rat adrenal preparations. *Biochim. Biophys. Acta*, 56:63–75.
39. Kuo, J. F., and Greengard, P. (1969): Cyclic nucleotide-dependent protein kinase. IV. Widespread occurrence of adenosine 3′,5′-monophosphate dependent protein kinase in various tissues and phyla of the animal kingdom. *Proc. Natl. Acad. Sci. U.S.A.*, 64:1349–1355.
40. Kuo, J. F., Kuo, W., Shoji, M., Davis, C. W., Seery, V. L., and Donnely, T. E., Jr. (1976): Purification and general properties of guanosine 3′:5′-monophosphate-dependent protein kinase from guinea pig fetal lung. *J. Biol. Chem.*, 251:1759–1766.
41. Lefkowitz, R. J., Roth, J., Pricer, W., and Pastan, I. (1970): ACTH receptors in the adrenal: Specific binding of ACTH-^{125}I and its relation to adenyl cyclase. *Proc. Natl. Acad. Sci. U.S.A.*, 65:745–752.
42. Limbird, L. E., and Lefkowitz, R. J. (1975): Myocardial guanylate cyclase: Properties of the enzyme and effects of cholinergic agonists in vitro. *Biochim. Biophys. Acta*, 377:186–196.
43. Lincoln, T. M., Dills, W. L., Jr., and Corbin, J. D. (1977): Purification and subunit composition of guanosine 3′:5′-monophosphate-dependent protein kinase from bovine lung. *J. Biol. Chem.*, 252:4269–4275.
44. Lipsett, M. B., Hertz, R., and Ross, G. T. (1963): Clinical and pathophysiological aspects of adrenocortical carcinoma. *Am. J. Med.*, 35:374–383.
45. Mackie, C., and Schulster, D. (1973): Phosphodiesterase activity and the potentiation by theophylline of adrenocorticotropin stimulated steroidogenesis and adenosine 3′,5′-monophosphate levels in isolated rat adrenal cells. *Biochem. Biophys. Res. Commun.*, 53:545–551.
46. Mahaffee, D., and Ney, R. L. (1970): Effects of nucleotides possessing a 3′,5′-cyclic monophosphate on adrenal steroidogenesis. *Metabolism*, 19:1104–1108.

47. Mahaffee, D., Reitz, R. C., and Ney, R. L. (1974): The mechanism of action of adrenocorticotropic hormone. The role of mitochondrial cholesterol accumulation in the regulation of steroidogenesis. *J. Biol. Chem.,* 249:227–233.
48. McMilan, B. H., Ney, R. L., and Schorr, I. (1971): Adenyl cyclase activity in normal adrenals and a corticosterone producing adrenal cancer of the rat. *Endocrinology,* 89:281–283.
49. Mittal, C. K., Kimura, H., and Murad, F. (1977): Purification and properties of a protein required for sodium azide activation of guanylate cyclase. *J. Biol. Chem.,* 252:4384–4390.
50. Miyomoto, E., Kuo, J. F., and Greengard, P. (1969): Adenosine 3′,5′-monophosphate-dependent protein kinase from brain. *Science,* 165:63–65.
51. Moyle, W. R., Kong, Y. C., and Ramchandran, J. (1973): Steroidogenesis and cyclic adenosine 3′,5′-monophosphate accumulation in rat adrenal cells. Divergent effects of adrenocorticotropin and its *o*-nitrophenyl sulfenyl derviative. *J. Biol. Chem.,* 248:2409–2417.
52. Neher, R., and Milani, A. (1974): Steroidogenesis in adrenal cells. *J. Steroid Biochem.,* 5:811–816.
53. Ney, R. L., Hochella, N. J., Grahme-Smith, D. G., Dexter, R. N., and Butcher, R. W. (1969): Abnormal regulation of adenosine 3′,5′-monophosphate and corticosterone formation in an adrenocortical carcinoma. *J. Clin. Invest.,* 46:1733–1739.
54. Nussdorfer, G. G., Neri, G., and Mazzochi, G. (1977): Effects of ACTH on the intracellular levels of cyclic AMP and cyclic GMP in the rat adrenal cortex. In: *3rd International Conference on Cyclic Nucleotides, New Orleans.* (abstract THA-226).
55. Paul, D. P., Gallant, S., Orme-Johnson, N. R., Orme-Johnson, W. H., and Brownie, A. C. (1976): Temperature dependence of cholesterol binding to cytochrome P-450_{SCC} of the rat adrenal. Effect of adrenocorticotrophic hormone and cycloheximide. *J. Biol. Chem.,* 251:7120–7126.
56. Pearlmutter, A. F., Rapino, E., and Saffran, M. (1971): ACTH and cyclic adenine nucleotides do not provoke identical adrenocortical responses. *Endocrinology,* 89:963–968.
57. Pearlmutter, A. F., Rapino, E., and Saffran, M. (1973): Comparison of steroidogenic effects of cAMP and dbc AMP in the rat adrenal gland. *Endocrinology,* 92:679–686.
58. Perchellet, J.-P., Shanker, G., and Sharma, R. K. (1978): Regulatory role of guanosine 3′,5′-monophosphate in adrenocorticotropin hormone-induced adrenal steroidogenesis. *Science,* 199:311–312.
59. Perchellet, J.-P., and Sharma, R. K. (1977): Metabolic regulation of steroidogenesis in isolated adrenocortical carcinoma cells. ACTH regulation of guanosine cyclic 3′:5′-monophosphate. *Biochem. Bophys. Res. Commun.,* 78:676–683.
60. Perkins, J. P. (1973): Adenyl cyclase. In: *Advances in Cyclic Nucleotide Research, Vol. 3,* edited by P. Greengard and G. A. Robison, pp. 1–64. Raven Press, New York.
61. Péron, F. G., Maudsley, D. V., and Haskar, A. (1975): Cyclic AMP response of isolated Snell adrenocortical carcinoma 494 cells to trophic hormones and other substances. *Endocrine Res. Commun.,* 2:403–417.
62. Peytreman, A., Nicholson, W. E., Liddle, G. W., Hardman, J. G., and Sutherland, E. W. (1973): Effects of methylxanthines on adenosine 3′,5′-monophosphate and corticosterone in the rat adrenal. *Endocrinology,* 92:525–530.
63. Rall, T. W., Sutherland, E. W., and Berthet, J. (1957): The relationship of epinephrine and glucagon to liver phosphorylase. IV. Effect of epinephrine and glucagon on the reactivation of phosphorylase in liver homogenates. *J. Biol. Chem.,* 224:463–475.
64. Rhodin, J. A. G. (1971): The ultrastructure of the adrenal cortex of rat under normal and experimental conditions. *J. Ultrastruct. Res.,* 344:23–71.
65. Rivkin, I., and Chasin, M. (1971): Nucleotide specificity of the steroidogenic response of rat adrenal cell suspensions prepared by collagenase digestion. *Endocrinology,* 88:664–670.
66. Robison, G. A., Butcher, R. W., and Suterland, E. W. (editors) (1971): *Cyclic AMP.* Raven Press, New York.
67. Rodbell, M. (1972): Cell surface receptor sites. In: *Current Topics in Biochemistry,* edited by C. B. Anfinsen, R. F. Goldberger, and A. N. Schechter, pp. 187–218. Academic Press, New York.
68. Rosen, O. M., Erlichman, J., and Rubin, C. S. (1974): Molecular characterization of cyclic AMP-dependent protein kinases derived from bovine heart and human erythrocytes. In: *Metabolic Interconversion of Enzymes, Vol. 13,* edited by E. H. Fischer, E. G. Krebs, H. Neurath, and E. R. Stadtman, pp. 143–154. Springer-Verlag, New York.

69. Rubin, R. P., Laychock, S. G., and End, D. W. (1977): On the role of cyclic AMP and cyclic GMP in steroid production by bovine cortical cells. *Biochim. Biophys. Acta,* 496:329–338.
70. Rudland, P. S., Gospodarowicz, D., and Seifert, W. (1974): Activation of guanyl cyclase and intracellular cyclic GMP by fibroblast growth factor. *Nature,* 250:741–742, 773–774.
71. Saez, J. M., Dazord, M. A., and Gallet, D. (1975): ACTH and prostaglandins receptors in human adrenocortical tumors. *J. Clin. Invest.,* 56:536–547.
72. Sawhney, R. S., and Sharma, R. K. (1976): Different plasma membrane effects of adrenocorticotropic hormone and cyclic nucleotides in normal and malignant adrenal cells. *F.E.B.S. Lett.,* 70:163–166.
73. Sayers, G., Beall, R. J., and Seelig, S. (1974): Modes of action of ACTH. In: *Biochemistry of Hormones, Vol. 8,* edited by H. V. Rickenberg, pp. 26–60. University Park Press, Baltimore.
74. Sayers, G., Swallow, R. L., and Giordano, N. D. (1971): An improved technique for the preparation of isolated rat adrenal cells: A sensitive, accurate, and specific method for the assay of ACTH. *Endocrinology,* 88:1063–1068.
75. Scarpa, A., and Inesi, G. (1972): Ionophore mediated equilibration of calcium ion gradients in fragmented sarcoplasmic reticulum. *F.E.B.S. Lett.,* 22:273–276.
76. Schimmer, B. P. (1972): Adenylate cyclase activity in adrenocorticotropic hormone-sensitive and mutant adrenocortical tumor cell lines. *J. Biol. Chem.,* 247:3134–3138.
77. Schorr, I., and Ney, R. L. (1971): Abnormal hormone responses of an adrenocortical cancer adenyl cyclase. *J. Clin. Invest.,* 50:1295–1300.
78. Schorr, I., Rathnam, P., Saxena, B. B., and Ney, R. L. (1971): Multiple specific hormone receptors in the adenylate cyclase of an adrenocortical carcinoma. *J. Biol. Chem.,* 246:5806–5811.
79. Schulster, D. (1974): Adrenocorticotrophic hormone and the control of adrenal corticosteroidogenesis. In: *Steroid Biochemistry and Pharmacology,* edited by M. H. Briggs and G. A. Christie, pp. 233–295. Academic Press, New York.
80. Schulster, D., Tait, S. A. S., Tait, J. F., and Mortek, J. (1970): Production of steroids by *in vitro* superfusion of endocrine tissue. III. Corticosterone output from rat adrenals stimulated by adrenocorticotropin or cyclic 3′,5′-adenosine monophosphate and the inhibitory effect of cycloheximide. *Endocrinology,* 80:487–502.
81. Shanker, G., and Sharma, R. K.: unpublished data.
82. Shanker, G. (1977): Novel protein kinases in adrenocortical carcinoma. Ph.D. dissertation, University of Tennessee Center for the Health Sciences, Memphis, Tennessee.
83. Sharma, R. K. (1972): Studies on adrenocortical carcinoma of rat. Cyclic nucleotide phosphodiesterase activities. *Cancer Res.,* 32:1734–1736.
84. Sharma, R. K. (1973): Metabolic regulation of steroidogenesis in adrenocortical carcinoma of rat. Effect of adrenocorticotropin and adenosine cyclic 3′,5′-monophosphate on corticosteroidogenesis. *Eur. J. Biochem.,* 32:506–512.
85. Sharma, R. K. (1973): Regulation of steroidogenesis by adrenocorticotropic hormone in isolated adrenal cells of rat. *J. Biol. Chem.,* 248:5473–5476.
86. Sharma, R. K. (1974): Metabolic regulation of steroidogenesis in isolated adrenal cells of rat. Effect of actinomycin D on cyclic GMP-induced steroidogenesis. *Biochem. Biophys. Res. Commun.,* 59:992–1003.
87. Sharma, R. K. (1974): ACTH control of steroidogenesis in adrenocortical carcinoma cells of rat. Effect of adrenocorticotropic hormone and adenosine cyclic 3′:5′-monophosphate on the plasma membrane. *F.E.B.S. Lett.,* 38:197–201.
88. Sharma, R. K. (1976): Regulation of steroidogenesis in adrenocortical carcinoma. In: *Control Mechanisms in Cancer,* edited by W. E. Criss, T. Ono, and J. R. Sabine, pp. 109–124, Raven Press, New York.
89. Sharma, R. K., Ahmed, N. K., and Shanker, G. (1976): Metabolic regulation of steroidogenesis in isolated adrenal cells of rat. Relationship of adrenocorticotropin-, adenosine 3′:5′-monophosphate-, and guanosine 3′:5′-monophosphate-stimulated steroidogenesis with the activation of protein kinase. *Eur. J. Biochem.,* 70:427–433.
90. Sharma, R. K., Ahmed, N. K., Sutliff, L. S., and Brush, J. S. (1974): Metabolic regulation of steroidogenesis in isolated adrenal cells of the rat. ACTH regulation of cGMP and cAMP levels and steroidogenesis. *F.E.B.S. Lett.,* 45:107–110.
91. Sharma, R. K., and Brush, J. S. (1973): Metabolic regulation of steroidogenesis in isolated ad-

renal and adrenocortical carcinoma cells of rat. The incorporation of (20S)-20-[7-^{3}H]hydroxycholesterol into deoxycorticosterone and corticosterone. *Arch. Biochem. Biophys.,* 156:560–562.
92. Sharma, R. K., and Brush, J. S. (1974): Metabolic regulation of steroidogenesis in adrenocortical carcinoma cells of rat. Effect of adrenocorticotropin and adenosine cyclic 3′:5′-monophosphate on the incorporation of (20S)-20-hydroxy[7α-^{3}H]cholesterol into deoxycorticosterone and corticosterone. *Biochem. Biophys. Res. Commun.,* 56:256–263.
93. Sharma, R. K., and Hashimoto, K. (1972): Ultrastructural studies and metabolic regulation of isolated adrenocortical carcinoma cells of rat. *Cancer Res.,* 32:666–674.
94. Sharma, R. K., Hashimoto, K., and Kitabchi, A. E. (1972): Steroidogenesis in isolated adrenal cells of rat. III. Morphological and biochemical correlation of cholesterol and cholesterol ester content in ACTH and N^6-2′-*O*-dibutyryl-adenosine-3′,5′-monophosphate activated adrenal cells. *Endocrinology,* 91:994–1003.
95. Sharma, R. K., McLaughlin, C. A., and Pitot, H. C. (1976): Protein phosphorylation of the smooth and rough endoplasmic reticulum in normal and neoplastic liver of the rat. *Eur. J. Biochem.,* 65:577–586.
96. Sharma, R. K., and Sawhney, R. S. (1978): Metabolic regulation of steroidogenesis in isolated adrenal cell. Investigation of the adrenocorticotropic hormone-, guanosine 3′:5′-monophosphate- and adenosine 3′,5′-monophosphate-control step. *Biochemistry,* 17:316–321.
97. Sharma, R. K., Shanker, G., and Ahmed, N. K. (1977): Metabolic regulation and relationship of endogenous protein kinase activity and steroidogenesis in isolated adrenocortical carcinoma cells of the rat. *Cancer Res.,* 37:472–475.
98. Sharma, R. K., Shanker, G., Ahrens, H., and Ahmed, N. K. (1977): Partial purification and characterization of the defective cyclic adenosine 3′:5′-monophosphate binding protein kinase from adrenocortical carcinoma. *Cancer Res.,* 37:3297–3300.
99. Shier, W. T., Baldwin, J. H., Hamilton, N., Hamilton, N., Hamilton, R. T., and Thanasi, N. (1976): Regulation of guanylate and adenylate cyclase activities by lysolecithin. *Proc. Natl. Acad. Sci. U.S.A.,* 73:1586–1590.
100. Shimizu, K., Hayano, M., Gut, M., and Dorfman, R. I. (1961): The transformation of 20α-hydroxycholesterol to isocoproic acid and C_{21} steroids. *J. Biol. Chem.,* 236:695–699.
101. Snell, K. C., and Stewart, H. L. (1959): Variations in histological pattern and functional effects of a transplantable adrenal cortical carcinoma in intact, hypophysectomized and newborn rats. *J. Natl. Cancer Inst.,* 22:1119–1132.
102. Stone, D., and Hechter, O. (1954): Studies on ACTH action in perfused bovine adrenals: The site of action of ACTH in corticosteroidogenesis. *Arch. Biochem. Biophys.,* 51:457–469.
103. Sutherland, E. W., and Rall, T. W. (1960): The relation of adenosine-3′,5′-phosphate and phosphorylase to the actions of catecholamines and other hormones. *Pharmacol. Rev.,* 12:265–299.
104. Takai, Y., Nakaya, S., Inoue, M., Kishimoto, A., Nishiyama, K., Hirohai, Y., and Nishizuka, Y. (1976): Comparison of mode of activation of guanosine 3′:5′-monophosphate-dependent and adenosine 3′:5′ -monophosphate-dependent protein kinases from silkworm. *J. Biol. Chem.,* 251:1481–1487.
105. Tchen, T. T. (1968): Conversion of cholesterol to pregnenolone in the adrenal cortex: Enzymology and regulation. In: *Functions of the Adrenal Cortex, Vol. 1,* edited by K. W. McKerns, pp. 3–26. Appleton-Century-Crofts, New York.
106. Tsang, C. P. W., and Péron, F. G. (1971): Effects of adenosine-3′,5′-monophosphate on steroidogenesis and glycolysis in the rat adrenal gland incubated *in vitro. Steroids,* 17:453–469.
107. Wallach, D., and Pastan, I. (1976): Stimulation of membranous guanylate cyclase by concentrations of calcium that are in the physiological range. *Biochem. Biophys. Res. Commun.,* 72:859–865.
108. Walton, G. M., and Gill, G. N. (1973): Adenosine 3′,5′-monophosphate and protein kinase dependent phosphorylation of ribosomal protein. *Biochemistry,* 12:2604–2611.
109. Whitley, T. H., Stowe, N. W., Ong, S., Ney, R. L., and Steiner, A. L. (1975): Control and localization of rat adrenal cyclic guanosine-3′,5′-monophosphate. Comparison with adrenal cyclic adenosine-3′,5′-monophosphate. *J. Clin. Invest.,* 56:146–154.

Endocrine Control in Neoplasia, edited by
R. K. Sharma and W. E. Criss.
Raven Press, New York © 1978.

Human Adrenocortical Tumors: Alterations in Membrane-Bound Hormone Receptors and cAMP Protein Kinases

José M. Saez, Guy P. Tell, and Alice Dazord

Unité de Recherches sur le Contrôle Hormonal des Activités Cellulaires, INSERM U 162, Hôpital Debrousse, 29 Rue Soeur Bouvier, 69322 Lyon Cedex 1, France

In normal adrenals ACTH is essential for maintenance of adrenal cortex structure and function (57). In most steroid-secreting adrenocortical tumors in man these primordial effects of ACTH seem to be lacking, since steroidogenesis and tumor growth appear to proceed without regulatory control (25). The biochemical abnormalities responsible for this tumoral ACTH insensitivity are largely unknown.

The ACTH and prostaglandin E_1 (PGE_1) receptors (5,7,39,40), as well as the cAMP-dependent protein kinase (10,39) of normal human adrenal cortex, have been under investigation in our laboratory for several years, and recently we have studied a number of human adrenocortical tumors using the same method. In this chapter we shall describe some aspects of the biochemical abnormalities observed in 20 human adrenocortical tumors.

STEROIDOGENIC REFRACTORINESS TO ACTH IN HUMAN ADRENOCORTICAL TUMORS

In most patients with adrenocortical tumors, steroid output is not modified either by ACTH stimulation or by dexamethasone suppression (25). The results of an ACTH stimulation test in 20 human adrenocortical tumors are summarized in Table 1. Interpretation of these tests in patients with adrenocortical tumors is difficult for two reasons: (a) the output of steroids may vary from one day to another in the same patient by as much as 100% (38); (b) in some patients with adrenocortical tumors the contralateral adrenal can respond normally to ACTH. Theoretically these two difficulties can be overcome by studying the responsiveness of isolated adrenocortical cells prepared by the same method as that used for rat adrenals (21,43).

Steroidogenesis of normal human adrenal cells is maximally stimulated by 10^{-9} M ACTH, 6×10^{-8} PGE_1, and 1 mM dibutyryl cAMP (DbcAMP) (Fig.

TABLE 1. In vivo *responsiveness to ACTH of human adrenocortical tumors (20 cases)*

Responsiveness	Number
Normal response	3
Borderline response	4
No response	9
Not studied	4

1). The responses of isolated cells from 14 human adrenocortical tumors to these stimuli are summarized in Table 2. The tumors fell into five categories: (a) tumors that responded to the three stimuli, (b) tumors in which steroidogenesis was stimulated by both PGE_1 and DbcAMP but not by ACTH, (c) one tumor that responded to ACTH and DbcAMP but not to PGE_1, (d) one tumor that responded only to DbcAMP, (e) two tumors in which steroidogenesis was not modified by any of the three stimuli tested. It must be pointed out that *in vivo* and *in vitro* the last two tumors secreted large amounts of steroids, including cortisol.

According to the postulated mechanism of action of ACTH, as illustrated in Fig. 2, the abnormality in tumors of categories b, c, and d might be localized at the membrane receptor level, whereas in group e the abnormality might be localized beyond cAMP formation.

In order to investigate further the alterations of membrane receptors, hormonal responsiveness of adenylate cyclase and the ACTH and PGE_1 binding receptors of tumoral crude plasma membranes were studied.

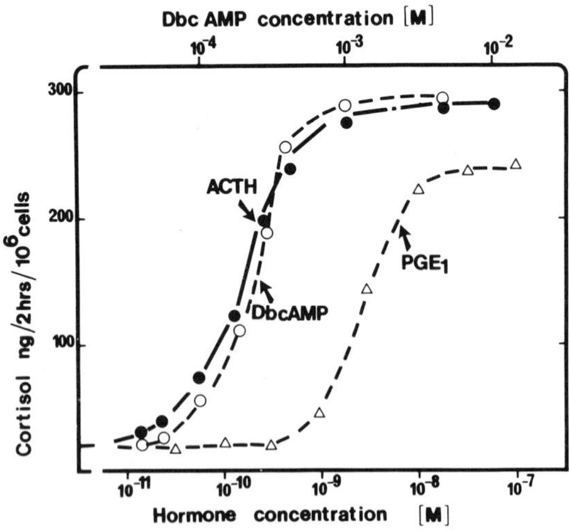

FIG. 1. Steroidogenesis of normal human adrenal cells in presence of increasing concentrations of ACTH, PGE_1, and DbcAMP.

TABLE 2. In vitro *steroidogenic responsiveness of isolated cells from human adrenals to various stimuli*[a]

Stimulus	Normal adrenal	Tumors A ($n=2$)	B ($n=8$)	C ($n=1$)	D ($n=1$)	E ($n=2$)
ACTH 10^{-8} M	+	+	−	+	−	−
PGE_1 6×10^{-6} M	+	+	+	−	−	−
DbcAMP 1 mM	+	+	+	+	+	−

[a] Isolated adrenal cells from normal adrenals and tumors were prepared by a modification (21) of the method described by Sayers et al. (43), and steroid production by the isolated adrenal cells was measured in the presence or in the absence of hormones after incubation for 2 hr at 37°C. Cortisol and 3β-hydroxyandrost-5-en-17-one (DHA) concentrations were measured by a sensitive radioimmunoassay.

ADENYLATE CYCLASE RESPONSIVENESS OF CRUDE ADRENAL PLASMA MEMBRANES

Crude plasma membranes from normal and tumoral adrenals were prepared, and adenylate cyclase activity was determined by methods described previously (5,7,59). Adenylate cyclase from normal human adrenal is stimulated by ACTH, PGE, and NaF (Fig. 3). ACTH and PGE_1 at maximal concentrations have additive effects in the normal adrenal (7) as well as in tumors that are normally sensitive to both hormones (38). Among the 20 tumors in which responsiveness was studied, four groups were isolated (Fig. 3):

Group I. Group I included 10 tumors in which adenylate cyclase activity was stimulated by ACTH, PGE_1, and NaF. Steroidogenesis of isolated adrenal

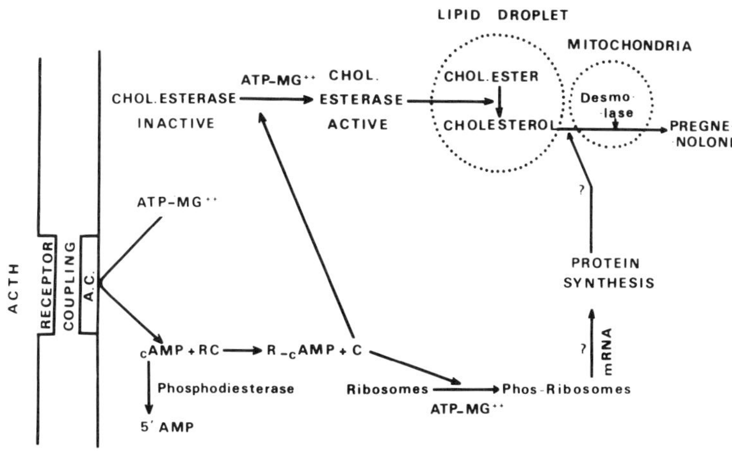

FIG. 2. Schematic representation of mechanism of ACTH action on steroidogenesis.

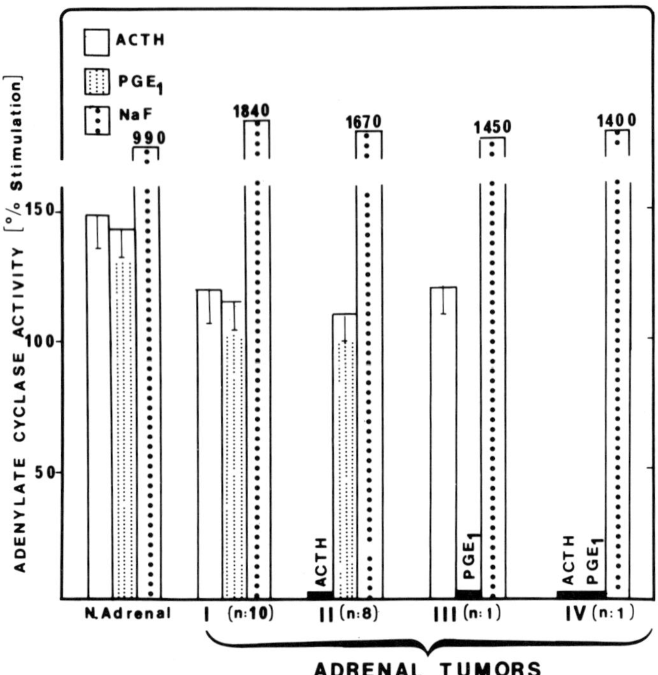

FIG. 3. Percentage stimulation of adenylate cyclase activity of crude membranes (20,000 × *g* pellet) of normal and tumoral human adrenals by several stimuli.

cells could be studied in only four cases in this group. Two tumors (Table 2, group A) responded to the three stimuli; the other two (Table 2, group E) did not. This indicates that the first two tumors normally respond to hormones, whereas the last two may present a block beyond cAMP formation. In the other six tumors of group I, we could not study steroidogenesis in isolated cells, but we did obtain indirect evidence that they were sensitive to ACTH, since (a) the *in vivo* responses to ACTH stimulation were normal (3 cases) or borderline (3 cases) and (b) the binding characteristics of ACTH *(vide infra)* to the plasma membranes prepared from these tumors were normal.

Group II. Group II included tumors in which adenylate cyclase activity was stimulated by both PGE_1 and NaF but not by ACTH. This was to be expected, since steroidogenesis in these tumors was stimulated by PGE_1 and DbcAMP but not by ACTH (Table 2, group B).

Group III. Group III contained one tumor whose adenylate cyclase activity responded to ACTH and NaF but not to PGE_1. PGE_1 steroidogenesis refractoriness was also observed in this tumor (Table 2, group C), which confirmed the alteration of the sole PGE receptor.

Group IV. Group IV contained one tumor in which only NaF was able to stimulate adenylate cyclase activity. This correlates with the fact that no steroidogenic response was observed in the presence of ACTH or PGE_1 (Table 2, group D).

BINDING OF ^{125}I-$ACTH_{1-24}$ AND ^{125}I-$ACTH_{11-24}$ TO NORMAL AND TUMORAL ADRENAL CRUDE MEMBRANES

The results presented thus far for ACTH-insensitive tumors of groups II and IV suggest that the biochemical abnormality is localized either at the ACTH binding site or at the putative coupling system between the hormone binding site and the adenylate cyclase catalytic subunit. Both hypotheses have been postulated to explain the ACTH refractoriness in a mutant of mouse adrenocortical cell line (44,45). Specific ACTH binding sites have been demonstrated in membranes prepared from normal adrenal (18,23,38,39,62) in several species, including man. Studies of the ACTH structure–function relationship using several ACTH analogs (5,17,18,35,39,40,50) have shown that the peptide sequence necessary for the binding is located in the COOH-terminal fragment of ACTH ($ACTH_{11-24}$) (18,39) and that the NH_2-terminal sequence is essential for the steroidogenic action (5,17,18,35,50). However, because the binding affinity of the COOH-terminal sequence $ACTH_{11-24}$ or $ACTH_{11-20}$ amide to the normal adrenal receptor is much lower than that of $ACTH_{1-24}$ and $ACTH_{1-20}$ amide (18,40) and because $ACTH_{1-10}$ at high concentrations can displace bound ^{125}I-$ACTH_{1-24}$ but not bound ^{125}I-$ACTH_{11-24}$ (39,40), it has been suggested that the NH_2-terminal sequence ($ACTH_{1-10}$) contributes to the binding also by increasing the binding affinity of the ACTH molecule (39,40).

ACTH binding studies with membrane preparations from human adrenocortical tumors have shown that all tumors specifically bind both ^{125}I-$ACTH_{1-24}$ and ^{125}I-$ACTH_{11-24}$. However, the apparent binding affinity of $ACTH_{1-24}$ for ACTH-insensitive tumors (groups II and IV) is about 10 times lower than that measured for the normal adrenal or for tumors in which adenylate cyclase activity is stimulated by ACTH (Fig. 4 and Table 3). On the other hand, the binding affinities of ^{125}I-$ACTH_{11-24}$ are similar in normal and ACTH-sensitive and -resistant tumors (Fig. 5). In addition, in the three ACTH-insensitive tumors of group II, we have found that $ACTH_{1-10}$ is not able to displace bound $ACTH_{1-24}$. These results strongly suggest that the biochemical abnormality in this group of tumors is due to loss or modification of the receptor site that binds the NH_2-terminal sequence of ACTH.

BINDING OF [^{3}H]PGE_1 TO CRUDE NORMAL AND TUMORAL ADRENAL MEMBRANES

The presence of a specific functional receptor for PGE_1 in normal human adrenals has been proven by the existence of specific binding sites and the ability of PGE_1 to stimulate adenylate cyclase (7) and increase production of cortisol in isolated adrenal cells (Fig. 1). The binding affinity of [^{3}H]PGE_1 to

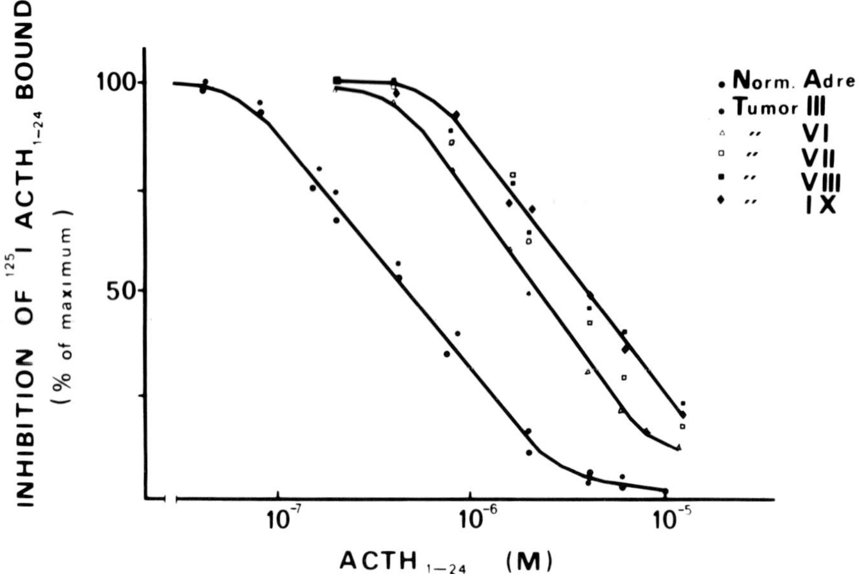

FIG. 4. Displacement of bound ^{125}I-ACTH$_{1\text{-}24}$ by ACTH$_{1\text{-}24}$ on plasma membranes obtained from normal human adrenals, a tumor of group I (ACTH-sensitive tumor III), and four tumors of group II (ACTH-insensitive tumors VI, VII, VIII, and IX). (From Saez et al., ref. 38, with permission.)

tumors of groups I, II, and V ($K_D = 1$ to 4×10^{-8} M) was similar to that observed with normal adrenals (7). On the other hand, no specific binding was found in PGE$_1$-resistant tumors (groups III and IV). These results suggest that the PGE$_1$ refractoriness may be due to loss of the PGE$_1$ binding site.

All the results presented thus far concerning ACTH and PGE receptors in normal and tumoral human adrenals can be explained by the model presented in Fig. 6. In this model it is proposed that the ACTH and PGE$_1$ receptors are independent. It is also postulated that the ACTH receptor is composed of two binding sites, one of which binds the 11–24 sequence of the hormone and the other the 1–10 sequence. The 11–24 sequence is responsible for high-affinity binding of ACTH, and it will facilitate binding of the 1–10 sequence to the second site. Only when this second site is occupied will adenylate cyclase be

TABLE 3. *Apparent dissociation constants of ACTH$_{1\text{-}24}$ and ACTH$_{11\text{-}24}$ of membranes obtained from human normal and tumoral adrenals*

	ACTH$_{1\text{-}24}$ (μM)	ACTH$_{11\text{-}24}$ (μM)
Normal adrenal	0.32 ± 0.18	4.3 ± 1.6
Tumor: group I	0.43 ± 0.19	4.7 ± 1.8
groups II–IV	4.1 ± 1.2	5.1 ± 2.3

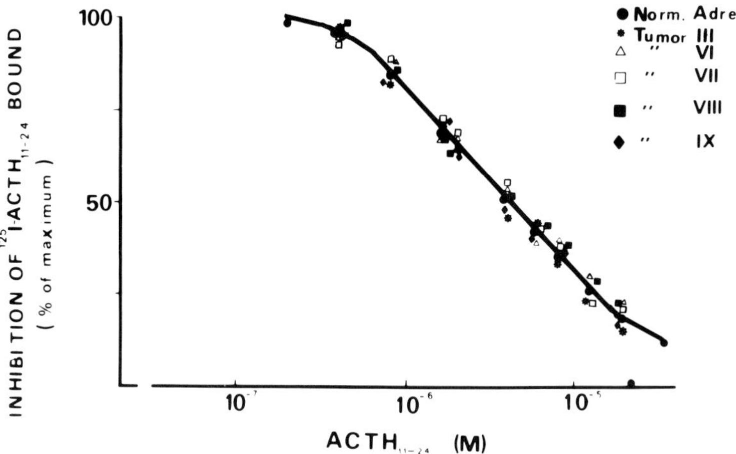

FIG. 5. Displacement of bound ^{125}I-ACTH$_{11\text{-}24}$ by ACTH$_{11\text{-}24}$ on plasma membranes. (From Saez et al., ref. 38, with permission.)

stimulated. The model also explains why ACTH and PGE$_1$ have additive stimulatory effects on adenylate cyclase of normal adrenal and why adenylate cyclase and steroidogenesis in ACTH-insensitive tumors (group II) are still stimulated by PGE$_1$ and the PGE$_1$-insensitive tumor (group III) is stimulated by ACTH.

EFFECT OF GTP AND ITS ANALOGS ON NORMAL AND TUMORAL ADRENAL ADENYLATE CYCLASE

The modifications of membrane receptors that have been described cannot rule out an associated alteration of the coupling system that conveys information from the hormone binding site to the adenylate cyclase. Recently it has been postulated that the guanyl nucleotide GTP and its derivatives play an important

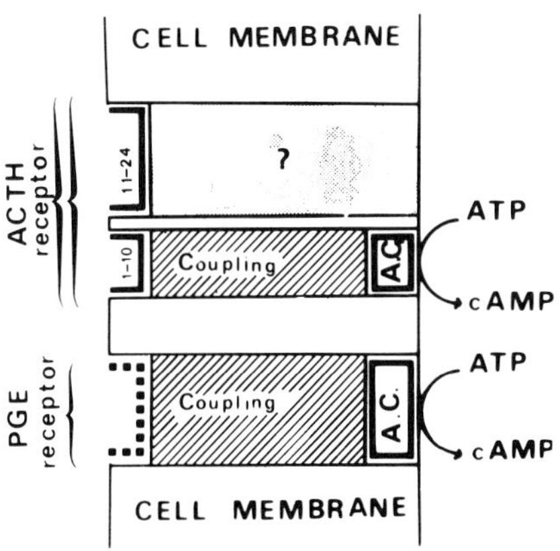

FIG. 6. Postulated model for interaction of ACTH and PGE with their adrenal receptors. (From Saez et al., ref. 38, with permission.)

TABLE 4. *Adenylate cyclase responses to GTP and Gpp(NH_2)p in presence and absence of ACTH or PGE_1 in normal and tumoral human adrenals*

Additions	Normal adrenal	Tumors ACTH-resistant group II ($n=3$)	Tumors PGE_1-resistant group III ($n=1$)
None	15 ± 2[a]	16 ± 3	16 ± 2
ACTH 10^{-6} M	32 ± 4	15 ± 3	31 ± 3
PGE_1 10^{-5} M	26 ± 3	35 ± 5	15 ± 2
GTP 10^{-5} M	24 ± 4	29 ± 4	26 ± 2
Gpp(NH_2)p 10^{-5} M	53 ± 6	52 ± 5	48 ± 4
ACTH + Gpp (NH_2)p	97 ± 10	55 ± 4	75 ± 6
PGE_1 + Gpp (NH_2)p	65 ± 8	90 ± 10	49 ± 5

[a] Mean ± SD of triplicate replications.

role in transmission of the hormonal message and in the functional state of membrane hormone receptors (24,37). GTP and its derivative Gpp (NH_2)p are potent stimulants of normal human adrenal adenylate cyclase, and they enhance adrenal responses to ACTH and to PGE_1 (14,59). In ACTH-resistant tumors GTP and its derivatives enhance basal and PGE_1-stimulated adenylate cyclase, but they do not reveal any ACTH responsiveness (Table 4). On the other hand, in PGE_1-resistant tumors, guanyl nucleotides are effective in increasing basal and ACTH adenylate cyclase activities, but no further stimulation is observed in the presence of PGE_1. These results show that guanyl nucleotides cannot reverse the absence of responsiveness to ACTH or to PGE_1. In addition, since basal adenylate cyclase activity and the response to NaF and guanyl nucleotides were no less in tumors than in normal adrenals, it is tempting to speculate that in these tumors the GTP site may be more closely associated with the enzyme catalytic subunit than with the hormone binding sites.

cAMP-DEPENDENT PROTEIN KINASE OF NORMAL AND TUMORAL HUMAN ADRENALS

The first event after cAMP formation is binding of this nucleotide to the regulatory unit of protein kinase. This interaction leads to dissociation of the cAMP regulatory subunit complex from the fully activated kinase (2,12). Half-maximal stimulation of protein kinase from normal human adrenal is obtained with about 5×10^{-9} M cAMP, and the maximal rate of phosphorylation is obtained with 5×10^{-7} M cAMP (10). As in most tissues (3), the cytosol protein kinase of human adrenals is resolved into two cAMP-dependent protein kinases (Fig. 8, upper panel, peaks I and II) and one cAMP-independent protein kinase, the latter being eluted at low ionic strength.

The cAMP stimulation of cytosol protein kinase activities in four human adrenocortical tumors is shown in Fig. 7. Tumor III was sensitive to ACTH. Indeed, the steroidogenic response of isolated cells from this tumor to ACTH was significantly higher than that of normal adrenal. Tumors IX and X were

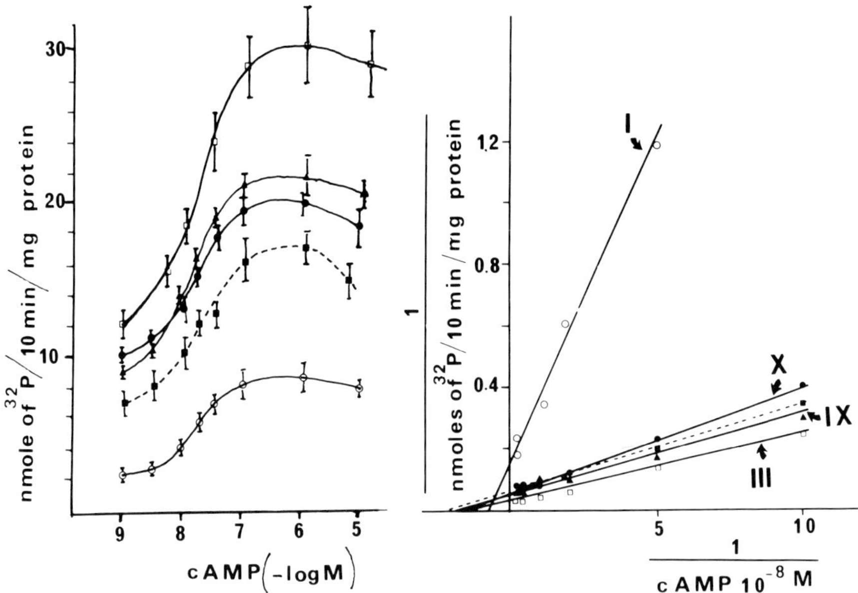

FIG. 7. Left: Protein kinase activities measured in presence of increasing amounts of cAMP: *Filled squares,* normal adrenal; *open circles,* tumor I (cAMP-resistant); *open squares,* tumor III (ACTH-sensitive); *triangles,* tumor IX, and *filled circles,* tumor X (both ACTH-insensitive). **Right:** Lineweaver-Burk representation of same data. (From Riou et al., ref. 36, with permission.)

ACTH-insensitive due to a modification of the ACTH receptor. Tumor I represents one of the two cases in which the adenylate cyclase responded to both ACTH and PGE_1, whereas steroidogenesis was not influenced by any of the stimuli (Table 2, group E).

The most significant findings of this study (Fig. 7) were that the K_m for cAMP and the maximal velocity of tumor I protein kinase were statistically different from the values observed in normal adrenal. On the other hand, the basal activity and the maximal velocity of protein kinase of tumor III were higher than in normal adrenal.

The elution pattern of cytosol protein kinase from tumor I following DEAE cellulose chromatography was very different from that of normal human adrenals (Fig. 8). The cAMP-independent kinase activity was eluted at the same molarity as that of normal adrenal. There was also a peak of kinase activity eluted at about the same molarity as peak I of normal adrenal, but the activity was almost cAMP-independent. In addition, no cAMP binding or kinase activities were found in the area corresponding to peak II of the normal adrenals, which indicates loss of this isoenzyme in tumor I.

Abnormal protein kinase activities have been described in lymphoma cells (1,4), in some hepatoma cell lines (15), and in rat adrenocortical tumor 494 (56). Ion-exchange chromatography has demonstrated abnormal elution patterns

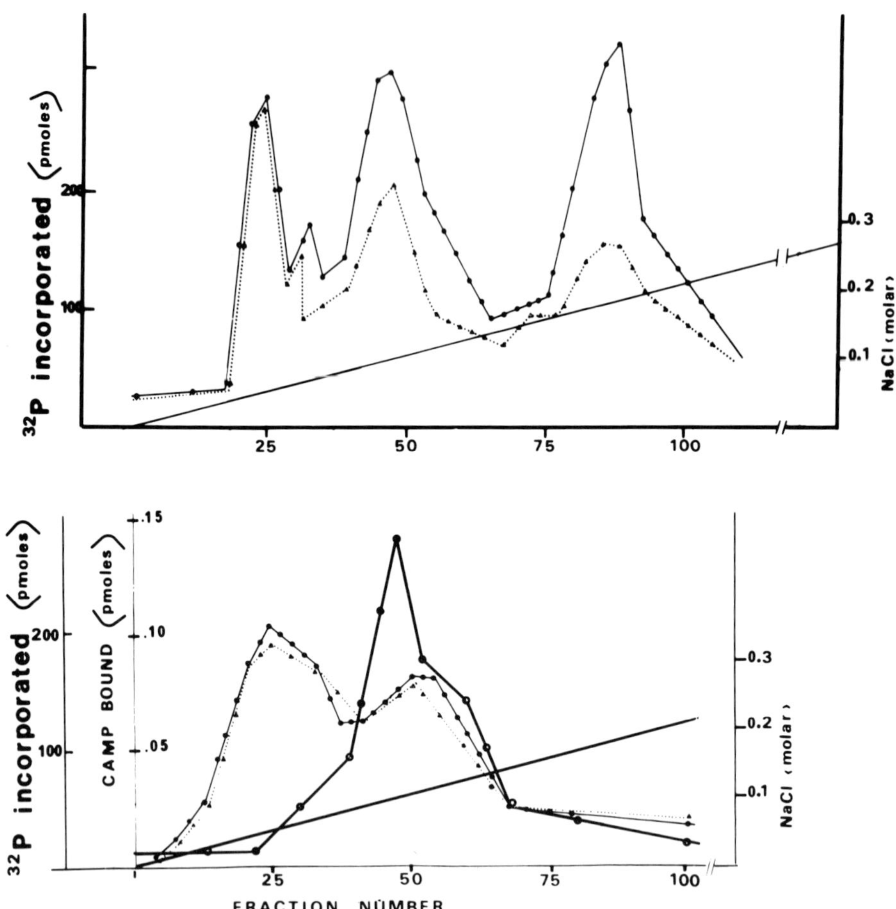

FIG. 8. DEAE cellulose chromatography of protein kinase from normal human adrenal **(top)** and tumor I **(bottom).** Symbols indicate protein kinase activities in presence *(filled circles)* and absence *(triangles)* of cAMP. (From Riou et al., ref. 36, with permission.)

in the three cases. It has been postulated that the abnormal protein kinase could in the first two cases be responsible for failure of cAMP to induce specific enzyme, to stop growth (1,4,15), and to increase steroidogenesis in the adrenocortical tumor (56).

EFFECTS OF ACTH ON ADRENAL CELL DNA SYNTHESIS

In vivo ACTH stimulates DNA synthesis (12,41), but the mechanism by which the hormone exerts this effect is still not well understood. On the other hand, *in vitro* ACTH inhibits DNA synthesis of normal and tumoral adrenal cells (13,19,28). To explain these contradictory results it has been postulated

TABLE 5. *Effects of ACTH analogs, insulin, and DbcAMP on human fetal adrenocortical cells*[a]

	[^{3}H]thymidine incorporation (cpm/μg protein)	Cortisol production (μg/day)
Control (0.5% FCS)	12 ± 5	0.52 ± 0.10
FCS 10%	550 ± 40	0.55 ± 0.12
FCS 10% + $ACTH_{1\text{-}24}$ 10^{-8} M	60 ± 8	9.40 ± 0.45
FCS 10% + $ACTH_{11\text{-}24}$ 10^{-7} M	490 ± 40	0.58 ± 0.15
FCS 10% + NPS-$ACTH_{1\text{-}24}$ 10^{-6} M	58 ± 10	8.92 ± 0.55
FCS 10% + $ACTH_{1\text{-}10}$ 10^{-4} M	160 ± 19	3.42 ± 0.31
FCS 10% + DbcAMP 10^{-3} M	45 ± 8	9.82 ± 0.50
FCS 10% + insulin 10^{-7} M	690 ± 30	0.49 ± 0.09

[a] Adrenal cells from human fetus (3 months) were isolated (21) and cultured in F-10 medium containing 10% fetal calf serum (FCS) at 37°C in humidified atmosphere (5% CO_2, 95% air). Three days after the third passage, cell growth was arrested by incubation in F-12 medium containing 0.5% FCS; growth was reinitiated by changing to fresh F-12 containing 10% FCS. After 20 hr cells were pulsed with [^{3}H]thymidine (6 μCi/dish) for 6 hr. At the end of the incubation time the medium was removed; the cells were washed and then collected. The cell suspension was combined with an equal volume of 10% trichloroacetic acid, and the acid-insoluble material was collected on glass fiber filters. Values are means ± SD of three dishes.

that the inhibitory effects of ACTH *in vitro* could be due to accumulation of both glucocorticoids and cAMP (41) in the medium. The *in vivo* situation may be different, as the release of both cAMP and glucocorticoids into the bloodstream would prevent their accumulation and therefore their potential inhibitory effect on cell growth.

The effects of several ACTH analogs and DbcAMP on DNA synthesis and cortisol produced by synchronized human fetal adrenocortical cells are shown in Table 5. Only those compounds that increased steroidogenesis were able to block the stimulatory effects of fetal calf serum on DNA synthesis. Likewise, in one ACTH- and PGE_1-sensitive tumor (one tumor of group A, Table 2),

TABLE 6. *Effects of ACTH analogs DbcAMP and PGE_1 on adrenocortical cells from human tumors*[a]

	Tumor I		Tumor II	
	[^{3}H]thymidine incorporation (cpm/μg protein)	Cortisol (μg/day)	[^{3}H]thymidine incorporation (cpm/μg protein)	Cortisol (μg/day)
Control (10% FCS)	680 ± 70	3.1 ± 0.4	430 ± 40	1.9 ± 0.12
$ACTH_{1\text{-}24}$ 10^{-8} M	101 ± 15	28.6 ± 1.1	450 ± 60	2.1 ± 0.15
$ACTH_{11\text{-}24}$ 10^{-7} M	620 ± 82	3.9 ± 0.8	410 ± 30	2.2 ± 0.14
$ACTH_{1\text{-}10}$ 10^{-4} M	230 ± 26	14.3 ± 0.9	504 ± 70	1.8 ± 0.10
DbcAMP 10^{-3} M	68 ± 12	34.6 ± 2.2	65 ± 11	19.2 ± 0.84
PGE_1 10^{-7} M	180 ± 40	18.4 ± 1.2	170 ± 22	12.2 ± 0.92

[a] Adrenal cells from tumors were cultured as indicated in the footnote to Table 5. After the third passage the cells were studied using the protocol described in Table 5.

$ACTH_{1-24}$, $ACTH_{1-10}$, PGE_1, and DbcAMP were able to increase cortisol production and inhibit DNA synthesis, but $ACTH_{11-24}$ did not modify either of these two parameters (Table 6, tumor I). On the other hand, in one ACTH-resistant PGE_1-sensitive tumor (one tumor of group B, Table 2), ACTH analogs had no effect on either cortisol secretion or DNA synthesis, whereas both DbcAMP and PGE_1 modified these two parameters (Table 6, tumor II).

These results suggest that initial and complete interaction of ACTH with its receptor, which commits cells to increase cAMP and steroid production, is necessary to express *in vitro* ACTH inhibitory effect on adrenal DNA synthesis.

CONCLUSION AND PROSPECTS

The essential feature of tumor cells that distinguishes them from their normal counterparts is their ability to grow without recognized control and invade normal tissue (34). Moreover, tumor cells also often present abnormalities of regulation of their specific function. These changes are accompanied by frequent modification of cell components, including surface receptors (34). However, in most cases these abnormalities have not been well correlated with a particular modification of a specific cell function. Tumors from endocrine glands could be a great model to establish such correlations when tumor cells present specific alterations of hormone membrane receptors.

Modifications of adenylate cyclase responsiveness to several hormonal stimuli have been described in pituitary adenomas (29,47), parathyroid adenomas, pheochromocytomas (47), thyroid carcinomas (8,11), and adrenocortical tumors (16,31,38). The abnormalities observed were of two types: in some tumors the adenylate cyclase was stimulated by several hormones, indicating the presence of ectopic receptors (16,29,31,47); in others there was lack of response to their specific hormones (8,11,16). However, since no binding tests were performed in these studies, precise localization of the abnormalities was not possible. In one independent study a lower binding affinity of thyroid-stimulating hormone (TSH) for thyroid carcinoma than for normal tissue has been reported (20).

With respect to thyroid tumors, it is interesting to note that in one experimental thyroid tumor it has been demonstrated that TSH refractoriness is associated with almost complete loss of TSH binding sites (26,27). Recently it has been postulated that the binding site loss was due to a decrease in ganglioside content of plasma membranes, specifically loss of GM_1 ganglioside (30).

Abnormalities in steroidogenic pathways of human adrenocortical tumors have been widely reported (9). However, few studies have been reported that dealt with biochemical alteration in hormonal regulation of steroidogenesis in these tumors (16,31,38). Hinshaw and Ney (16) studied four adrenocortical tumors. In two of them, adenylate cyclase was insensitive to ACTH; in the other two, ACTH as well as TSH induced a significant increase in enzymatic activity. Ectopic receptors in one adrenocortical feminizing tumor were described by Millington et al. (31). Adenylate cyclase and *in vitro* steroidogenesis of this tumor were stimulated by ACTH, luteinizing hormone (LH), follicle-stimulating hormone (FSH), prolactin, and human placental lactogen. In five ACTH-sensitive tumors (group I) and six ACTH-resistant tumors (group II) we studied adenylate cyclase responsiveness to norepinephrine, glucagon, and TSH; in none of them could we observe any effect.

Some insights into the biochemical alterations responsible for the lack of action of ACTH have been obtained from studies performed in experimental adrenocortical tumors. Schimmer described two ACTH-resistant mutant adrenal cell lines (Y-6 and OS-3) derived from the mouse ACTH-sensitive Y-1 cell line (44,45). In the ACTH-resistant cells, ACTH was not able to stimulate either adenylate cyclase or steroidogenesis. However, adenylate cyclase was increased by NaF, and steroidogenesis was stimulated by cAMP. Therefore it appears that this tumor has the same defect as those of our group II. However, since no ACTH binding studies have been performed with these mouse tumor cell lines, precise localization of the abnormality has not been achieved. It is interesting to note that in one ACTH-resistant mutant (Y-6) restoration of ACTH responsiveness was obtained after *Mycoplasma* infection and animal passage (46), but the molecular mechanisms of this recovery are not understood.

Another experimental adrenocortical tumor with interesting properties is rat adrenocorticocarcinoma 494, first described by Snell and Stewart (58). In contrast to the adenylate cyclase response of the normal rat adrenal, which is stimulated only by ACTH, the tumor cyclase is also stimulated by TSH, LH, FSH, and catecholamines (16,33). These results suggest that the tumor has specific binding sites for several hormones, but only those for catecholamines have been confirmed by binding studies (61). More intriguing was that in spite of the fact that ACTH increased cAMP production, no increase in corticosterone production was induced by the hormone (33,54). Moreover, cAMP and its derivatives were not able to increase steroidogenesis (33,54). Since the phosphodiesterase activity was even lower than in normal adrenal (51), and since the tumor was able to convert pregnenolone into corticosterone (52–54), it was suggested that the main biochemical abnormality responsible for the lack of action of ACTH was localized beyond cAMP formation (54). Recently, Sharma et al. (56) have shown that this is the case, since the tumor 494 has no cAMP-dependent protein kinase. In DEAE cellulose chromatography there was only one peak of cAMP binding activity without kinase activity. Therefore the anomaly seems to be different from what we have found in a human adrenocortical tumor.

Recently the role of cAMP as the obligatory intracellular mediator of ACTH action on adrenal has been under close scrutiny (32,55). However, the results obtained in both human and experimental tumors strongly suggest that cAMP may well be the obligatory mediator for most (but not for all) actions of ACTH in adrenal cortex (6).

Our studies clearly indicate that in human adrenocortical tumors, loss of sensitivity to hormones can be related to a variety of biochemical abnormalities. Despite apparent heterogeneity, the results allow a better understanding of the mechanism by which ACTH controls steroidogenesis in normal adrenals. For the future the most promising areas of this research appear to be isolation of specific macromolecules containing the receptor from normal and tumoral membranes and establishment of cell lines from hormone-sensitive and -resistant tumors. Both topics could shed light on the role of membrane-bound hormones in control of cell growth.

SUMMARY

The biochemical abnormalities responsible for the failure of ACTH and PGE_1 to increase steroidogenesis in some human adrenocortical tumors have been investigated. According to the adenylate cyclase responses to ACTH, PGE_1, and NaF and to the *in vitro* steroidogenesis response to the same hormones and DbcAMP, the tumors fall into five categories: (I) 8 tumors in which adenylate cyclase and steroidogenesis were stimulated by both ACTH and PGE_1, as is the case in normal adrenals; (II) 10 tumors that responded to PGE_1, DbcAMP, and NaF, but in which ACTH had no effect (although these tumors bound ACTH specifically, binding affinity was about 10 times lower than that of normal human adrenals; binding studies with several ACTH fragments suggested the possibility of modification or loss of the receptor site that binds the NH-terminal sequence of ACTH; the putative GTP membrane active site was normal); (III) one tumor that was PGE_1-resistant due to loss of PGE_1 binding sites; (IV) one tumor in which anomalies of both receptors, ACTH and PGE_1, were found; (V) two tumors in which the abnormality was located beyond cAMP formation; in one of them the cAMP-dependent protein kinase was abnormal.

ACKNOWLEDGMENTS

This research was supported by grants from Institut National de la Santé et della Recherche Médicale (ATP 24–75–47 and 76–5–473) and the Ligue Nationale Française contre le Cancer.

REFERENCES

1. Bourne, H. R., Tomkins, G. M., and Dion, J. (1973): Regulation of phosphodiesterase synthesis. Requirement for cyclic adenosine monophosphate-dependent protein kinase. *Science,* 181:452–454.
2. Brostrom, M. A., Reimann, E. M., Walsh, D. A., and Krebs, E. G. (1970): A cyclic 3′,5′-AMP-stimulated protein kinase from cardiac muscle. In: *Advances in Enzyme Regulation, Vol. 8,* edited by G. Weber, pp. 191–203. Pergamon Press, Oxford.
3. Corbin, J. D., Kelly, S. L., and Park, C. R. (1975): The distribution and dissociation of cyclic adenosine 3′,5′-monophosphate dependent protein kinases in adipose cardiac and other tissues. *J. Biol. Chem.,* 250:218–225.
4. Daniel, V., Littwack, G., and Tomkins, G. A. (1973): Induction of cytolysis of cultured lymphoma cells by adenosine 3′5′-cyclic monophosphate and the isolated or resistant variant. *Proc. Natl. Acad. Sci. U.S.A.,* 70:76–80.

5. Dazord, A., Gallet, D., and Saez, J. M. (1975): Adenyl cyclase activity in rat, ovine, and human adrenal preparations. *Horm. Metab. Res.,* 7:184–189.
6. Dazord, A., Gallet, D., and Saez, J. M. (1977): Protein degradation in adrenal cells in culture is inhibited by ACTH and cyclic AMP. *F.E.B.S. Lett.,* 83:307–310.
7. Dazord, A., Morera, A. M., Bertrand, J., and Saez, J. M. (1974): Prostaglandin receptors in human and ovine adrenal glands: Binding and stimulation of adenyl cyclase in subcellular preparations. *Endocrinology* 95:352–359.
8. DeRubertis, F., Yamashita, K., Dekker, A., Larsen, P. R., and Field, J. B. (1972): Effects of thyroid stimulating hormone on adenyl cyclase activity and intermediary metabolism of cold thyroid nodules and normal human thyroid tissues. *J. Clin. Invest.,* 51:1109–1117.
9. Dorfman, R. I., and Ungar, F. (1965): *Metabolism of Steroid Hormones,* pp. 22–110. Academic Press, New York.
10. Evain, D., Riou, J. P., and Saez, J. M. (1977): Adenosine 3′,5′-monophosphate-dependent protein kinase from normal human adrenal. *Mol. Cell. Endocrinol.,* 6:191–201.
11. Field, J. B., Larsen, P. R., Yamashita, K., Mashiter, K., and Dekker, R. (1973): Demonstration of iodide transport defect but normal iodide organification in nonfunctioning nodules of human thyroid glands. *J. Clin. Invest.,* 52:2404–2410.
12. Garren, L. D., Gill, G. N., Masui, H., and Walton, G. M. (1971): On the mechanism of action of ACTH. *Recent Prog. Horm. Res.,* 27:433–478.
13. Gill, G. N., and Weidman, E. R. (1977): Hormonal regulation of initiation of DNA synthesis and of differentiated function in Y-1 adrenal cortical cells. *J. Cell. Physiol.,* 92:65–76.
14. Glossman, H., and Gips, H. (1975): Bovine adrenal cortex adenylate cyclase properties of the particulate enzyme and effects of guanyl nucleotide. *Naunyn Schmiedebergs Arch. Pharmacol.,* 289:77–97.
15. Granner, D. K., Sellers, L., Lee, A., Butters, C., and Kutina, L. (1975): A comparison of the uptake metabolism and action of cyclic adenosine nucleotides in cultured hepatoma cells. *Arch. Biochem. Biophys.,* 169:601–615.
16. Hinshaw, H. T., and Ney, R. L. (1974): Abnormal hormonal control in the neoplastic adrenal cortex. In: *Hormones and Cancer,* edited by K. W. McKerns, pp. 309–332. Academic Press, New York.
17. Hofmann, K., Montibeller, I. A., and Finn, F. M. (1974): ACTH antagonists. *Proc. Natl. Acad. Sci. U.S.A.,* 71:80–83.
18. Hofmann, K., Wingender, W., and Finn, F. M. (1970): Correlation of adrenocorticotropic activity of ACTH analogs with degree of binding to an adrenal cortical particulate preparation. *Proc. Natl. Acad. Sci. U.S.A.,* 67:829–836.
19. Hornsby, P. J., and Gill, G. N. (1977): Hormonal control of adrenocortical cell proliferation. Desensitization to ACTH and interaction between ACTH and fibroblast growth factor in bovine adrenocortical cell cultures. *J. Clin. Invest.,* 60:342–352.
20. Ichikawa, Y., Saito, E., Abe, Y., Homma, M., Muraki, T., and Ito, K. (1976): Presence of TSH receptors in thyroid neoplasms. *J. Clin. Endocrinol. Metab.,* 42:395–398.
21. Kitabchi, A. E., and Sharma, R. K. (1974): Corticosteroidogenesis in isolated adrenal cells of rats. I. Effect of corticotropins and 3′,5′-cyclic nucleotides on corticosterone production. *Endocrinology,* 88:1109–1116.
22. Lefkowitz, R. J. (1975): Guanosine triphosphate binding sites in solubilized myocardium. Relation to adenylate cyclase activity. *J. Biol. Chem.,* 250:1006–1011.
23. Lefkowtiz, R. J., Roth, J., Pricer, W., and Pastan, I. (1970): ACTH receptors in the adrenal: Specific binding of ACTH-^{125}I and its relation to adenyl cyclase. *Proc. Natl. Acad. Sci. U.S.A.,* 65:745–752.
24. Leray, F., Chambaut, A. M., and Hanoune, J. (1972): Role of GTP in epinephrine and glucagon activation of adenyl cyclase on liver plasma membranes. *Biochem. Biophys. Res. Commun.,* 48:1385–1391.
25. Lipsett, M. B., Hertz, R., and Roos, G. T. (1963): Clinical and pathophysiologic aspects of adrenocortical carcinoma. *Am. J. Med.,* 35:374–383.
26. Macchia, V., Meldolesi, M. F., and Chiariello, M. (1972): Adenyl cyclase in a transplantable thyroid tumor: Loss of ability to respond to TSH. *Endocrinology,* 90:1483–1491.
27. Mandato, E., Meldolesi, M. F., and Macchia, V. (1975): Diminished binding of thyroid-stimulating hormone in a transplantable rat thyroid tumor as a possible cause of hormone unresponsiveness. *Cancer Res.,* 35:3089–3093.

28. Masui, H., and Garren, L. D. (1971): Inhibition of replication in functional mouse adrenal tumor cells by adrenocorticotropic hormone mediated by adenosine 3′:5′-cyclic monophosphate. *Proc. Natl. Acad. Sci. U.S.A.,* 68:3206–3210.
29. Matsukura, S., Kakita, T., Hirata, Y., Yoshimi, H., Fukase, M., Iwasaki, Y., Kato, Y., and Imura, H. (1977): Adenylate cyclase of GH and ACTH producing tumors of human: Activation by nonspecific hormones and other bioactive substances. *J. Clin. Endocrinol. Metab.,* 44:392–397.
30. Meldolesi, M. F., Fishman, P. H., Aloj, S. M., Kohn, L. D., and Brady, R. D. (1976): Relationship of gangliosides to the structure and function of thyrotropin receptors: Their absence on plasma membranes of a thyroid tumor defective in thyrotropin receptor activity. *Proc. Natl. Acad. Sci. U.S.A.,* 73:4060–4064.
31. Millington, D. S., Golder, M. P., Conley, T., London, D., Roberts, U., Butt, W. R., and Griffiths, K. (1976): In vitro synthesis of steroids by a feminizing adrenocortical carcinoma: Effect of prolactin and other protein hormones. *Acta Endocrinol. (Kbh),* 82:561–571.
32. Moyle, W. R., MacDonald, G. J., and Garfink, J. E. (1976): Role of histone kinases as mediators of corticotropin-induced steroidogenesis. *Biochem. J.,* 160:1–9.
33. Ney, R. L., Hochella, N. J., Grahme-Smith, D. G., Dexter, R. N., and Butcher, R. W. (1969): Abnormal regulation of adenosine 3′,5′-monophosphate and corticosterone formulation in an adrenocortical carcinoma. *J. Clin. Invest.,* 48:1733–1739.
34. Nicolson, G. L., and Poste, G. (1976): The cancer cell: Dynamic aspects and modifications in cell surface organization. *N. Engl. J. Med.,* 295:197–203, 253–258.
35. Ramachandran, J., and Li, C. H. (1967): Structure-activity relationships of the adrenocorticotropins and melanotropins: The synthetic approach. *Adv. Enzymol.,* 29:391–477.
36. Riou, J. P., Evain, D., Perrin, F., and Saez, J. M. (1977): Adenosine 3′,5′-cyclic monophosphate-dependent protein kinase in human adenocortical tumors. *J. Clin. Endocrinol. Metab.,* 44:413–419.
37. Rodbell, M., Lin, M. C., Salomon, Y., Londos, C., Harwood, J. P., Martin, B. R., Rendell, M., and Berman, M. (1974): The role of adenine and guanine nucleotides in the activity and response of adenylate cyclase systems to hormones: Evidence for multi-site transition states. *Acta Endocrinol. (Kbh),* 77[Suppl. 191]:11–37.
38. Saez, J. M., Dazord, A., and Gallet, D. (1975): ACTH and prostaglandin receptors in human adrenocortical tumors. *J. Clin. Invest.,* 56:536–547.
39. Saez, J. M., Dazord, A., Morera, A. M., and Bataille, P. (1975): Interactions of adrenocorticotropic hormone with its adrenal receptors. *J. Biol. Chem.,* 250:1683–1689.
40. Saez, J. M., Morera, A. M., Dazord, A., and Bataille, P. (1974): Interactions of ACTH with its adrenal receptors: Specific binding of $ACTH_{1-24}$, its *O*-nitrophenyl sulfenyl derivative and $ACTH_{11-24}$. *J. Steroid Biochem.,* 5:925–933.
41. Saez, J. M., Morera, A. M., and Gallet, D. (1977): In vivo opposite effects of ACTH and glucocorticoids on adrenal DNA synthesis. *Endocrinology,* 100:1268–1275.
42. Sand, G., Sortay, A., Pochet, R., and Dumont, J. E. (1976): Adenylate cyclase and protein phosphokinase activities in human thyroid. Comparison of normal glands, hyperfunctional nodules and carcinomas. *Eur. J. Cancer,* 12:447–453.
43. Sayers, G., Swallow, R. L., and Giordano, N. O. (1971): An improved technique for the preparation of isolated rat adrenal cells: A sensitive, accurate and specific method for the assay of ACTH. *Endocrinology,* 88:1063–1068.
44. Schimmer, B. P. (1969): Phenotypically variant adrenal tumor cell cultures with biochemical lesions in the ACTH-stimulated steroidogenic pathway. *J. Cell. Physiol.,* 74:115–122.
45. Schimmer, B. P. (1972): Adenylate cyclase activity in adrenocorticotropic hormone-sensitive and mutant adrenocortical tumor cell lines. *J. Biol. Chem.,* 247:3134–3138.
46. Schimmer, B. P. (1976): Adenylate cyclase activity and steroidogenesis in phenotypic revertants of an ACTH-insensitive adrenal tumor cell line. *Nature,* 259:482–483.
47. Schorr, I., Hinshaw, H. I., Cooper, M. A., Mahaffee, D., and Ney, R. L. (1972): Adenyl cyclase hormone responses of certain human endocrine tumors. *J. Clin. Endocrinol. Metab.,* 34:447–451.
48. Schorr, I. S., and Ney, R. L. (1971): Abnormal hormone responses of an adrenocortical cancer adenyl cyclase. *J. Clin. Invest.,* 50:1295–1300.
49. Schorr, I. S., Rathnam, P., Saxena, B. B., and Ney, R. L. (1971): Multiple specific hormone receptors in the adenylate cyclase of an adrenocortical carcinoma. *J. Biol. Chem.,* 246:5806–5811.

50. Seelig, S., and Sayers, G. (1973): Isolated adrenal cortex cells: ACTH agonists, partial agonists, antagonists; cyclic AMP and corticosterone production *Arch. Biochem. Biophys.,* 154:230–239.
51. Sharma, R. K. (1972): Studies on adrenocortical carcinoma of rat cyclic nucleotide phosphodiesterase activities. *Cancer Res.,* 32:1734–1736.
52. Sharma, R. K. (1973): Regulation of steroidogenesis by adrenocorticotropic hormone in isolated adrenal cells of rat. *J. Biol. Chem.,* 248:5473–5478.
53. Sharma, R. K. (1973): Metabolic regulation of steroidogenesis in adrenocortical carcinoma cells of rat: Effect of adrenocorticotropin and adenosine cyclic 3′:5′-monophosphate on corticosteroidogenesis. *Eur. J. Biochem.,* 32:506–512.
54. Sharma, R. K. (1976): Regulation of steroidogenesis in adrenocortical carcinoma. In: *Control Mechanisms in Cancer,* edited by W. E. Criss, T. Ono, and J. R. Sabine, pp. 109–124. Raven Press, New York.
55. Sharma, R. K., Ahmed, N. K., and Shanker, G. (1976): Metabolic regulation of steroidogenesis in isolated adrenal cells of rat. Relationship of adrenocorticotropin-, adenosine 3′:5′-monophosphate- and guanosine 3′:5′-monophosphate-stimulated steroidogenesis with the activation of protein kinase. *Eur. J. Biochem.,* 70:427–433.
56. Sharma, R. K., Shanker, G., Ahrens, H., and Ahmed, N. K. (1977): Partial purification and characterization of the defective cyclic adenosine 3′:5′-monophosphate binding protein kinase from adrenocortical carcinoma. *Cancer Res.,* 37:3297–3300.
57. Smith, P. E. (1930): Hypophysectomy and a replacement therapy in the rat. *Am. J. Anat.,* 45:205–209.
58. Snell, K. C., and Stewart, H. L. (1959): Variations in histologic pattern and functional effects of a transplantable adrenal cortical carcinoma in intact, hypophysectomized, and newborn rats. *J. Natl. Cancer Inst.,* 22:1119–1155.
59. Tell, G. P., Cathiard, A. M., and Saez, J. M. (1977): The GTP sensitive adenylate cyclase of ACTH and prostaglandin-resistant human adrenocortical tumour. *Cancer Res.,* 38:955–959.
60. Tell, G. P., Morera, A. M., and Saez, J. M. (1976): Mechanism of ACTH action. In: *Congenital Adrenal Hyperplasia,* edited by P. A. Lee, L. P. Plotnick, A. A. Kowarski, and C. J. Migeon, pp. 33–76. University Park Press, Baltimore.
61. Williams, L. T., Gore, T. B., and Lefkowitz, R. J. (1977): Ectopic β-adrenergic receptor binding sites. Possible molecular basis of aberrant catecholamine responsiveness of an adrenocortical tumor adenylate cyclase. *J. Clin. Invest.,* 59:319–324.
62. Wolfsen, A. R., McIntyre, U. B., and Odell, W. D. (1972): Adrenocorticotropin measurement by competitive binding receptor assay. *J. Clin. Endocrinol. Metab.,* 34:684–689.

Endocrine Control in Neoplasia, edited by
R. K. Sharma and W. E. Criss.
Raven Press, New York © 1978.

Prolactin and Mammary Cancerigenesis

*Clifford W. Welsch and **Joseph Meites

**Department of Anatomy and **Department of Physiology, Michigan State University, East Lansing, Michigan 48824*

In recent years, there has been an unparalleled surge in the investigation of prolactin as a potentially critical hormone in human breast cancerigenesis. The impetus for this investigation derives, at least in part, from the results of a number of studies demonstrating rather convincingly that prolactin is an important factor in murine mammary cancerigenesis (131). In addition, other developments have further increased the volume of information pertaining to the potential role of this pituitary peptide in cancer of the human breast: the recent development of radioimmunoassays to measure serum prolactin in humans (33,36); a method to quantitate prolactin membrane receptors in human and animal tissues (34,35,50,100); drugs that can effectively reduce secretion of prolactin in humans and animals (64,65,133).

The primary purpose of this chapter is to summarize a number of pertinent studies pertaining to the role of prolactin in rodent mammary cancerigenesis, emphasizing the results of studies carried out in our laboratories. In addition, a comparatively short review of studies pertaining to the role of prolactin in human breast cancerigenesis is also provided. Neuroendocrine mechanisms controlling the secretion of prolactin have been discussed in a number of recent reviews (20,75), and therefore they will not be considered here.

ENHANCEMENT BY PROLACTIN OF SPONTANEOUS MAMMARY CANCERIGENESIS IN MICE

As early as 1916 it was reported by Lathrop and Loeb (59) that the hormonal changes of pregnancy were conducive to the development of mammary cancers in mice. Subsequently Loeb and Kirtz (62) in 1939 and Mühlbock and Boot (80) in 1959 demonstrated that multiple pituitary isografts to mice sharply increased the incidence of mammary cancers in that species. In 1950 Desclin (26) reported that pituitary isografts persistently secreted prolactin, an observation that was subsequently confirmed and extended by Everett (30). These studies made clear the potential for involvement of prolactin in the development of mammary cancers in mice. Although it is well known that pituitary isografts secrete large amounts of prolactin, some growth hormone is also secreted by these grafts (73). Since the quantity of growth hormone secreted is considerably less than that secreted by the *in situ* pituitary, it is probable that the amount of growth hormone released from these grafts is unimportant in cancerigenesis in the mouse mammary gland. This is particularly true when only a single pituitary is grafted, a procedure that markedly increases mammary cancerigenesis (61).

Additional support for the theory that prolactin is the key pituitary hormone involved in mouse mammary cancerigenesis came from several sources: Boot et al. (7) showed that daily administration of ovine prolactin to mice increased the incidence of mammary cancers; Lacassagne and Duplan (57) showed that administration of the tranquilizer reserpine to mice resulted in a higher incidence of mammary cancers; Liebelt (60), and Bruni and Montemurro (12) showed that induced hypothalamic lesions increased the incidence of mammary cancers. Reserpine treatment and hypothalamic lesions (median eminence) sharply increased pituitary prolactin secretion (63,133).

From the foregoing evidence it would appear that if prolactin secretion is chronically raised above normal levels in certain strains of mice, invariably there will be an increase in the incidence of mammary cancers. Is the inverse true? Will a secretory level of prolactin that is below normal inhibit the development of mammary cancers in mice? The answer to this question was recently provided by our laboratory (120); it was found that chronic treatment of young nulliparous C3H/HeJ mice with the prolactin-suppressing drug 2-bromo-α-ergocryptine (CB-154) (84,129) virtually prevented the development of mammary cancers (Fig. 1). More than one-fourth of the controls (24 of 90) developed mammary cancers, but only 1 of 90 ergot-treated mice developed mammary cancer. In a subsequent study using another prolactin-suppressing drug (the ergoline derivative 6-methyl-8β-ergoline acetonitrile), mammary cancerigenesis was again sharply reduced (121). Therefore it appears that not only is prolactin

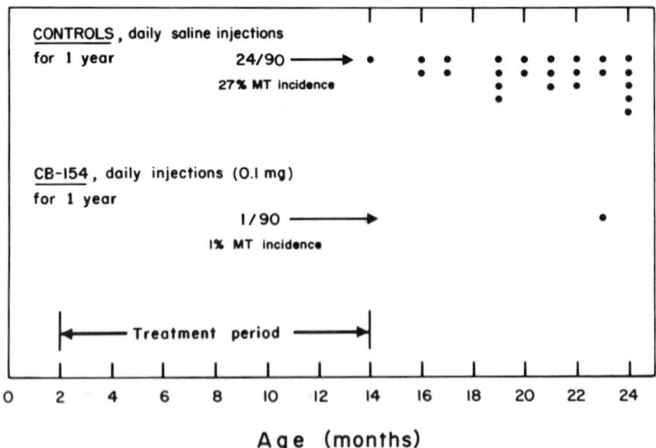

FIG. 1. Effects of CB-154 treatments on incidence of spontaneous mammary cancers in nulliparous C3H/HeJ female mice. Controls versus CB-154, $p < 0.001$. (From Welsch and Gribler, ref. 120, with permission.)

an important hormonal stimulant of mammary cancerigenesis but also it may be an essential hormone for neoplastic transformation of the mouse mammary gland.

Hyperplastic alveolar nodules (HAN) of the mammary gland have been described by a number of investigators and have been established as the precursors of many of the mammary cancers that occur in certain strains of mice, e.g., C3H, BALB/c (25,71). The hormonal responsiveness of these precancerous lesions has been shown in studies demonstrating that hypophysectomy or ovariectomy-adrenalectomy of mammary-cancer-susceptible mice suppresses their development and growth (5). Recently we reported that prolactin appears to be the principal *pituitary* hormone involved in the development, maintenance, and transformation of HAN (114,117,120). For example, chronic treatment of nulliparous and multiparous C3H mice with CB-154 produced a reduction in the incidence of HAN (nulliparous mice), a reduction in the number of HAN (multiparous mice), and a subsequent sharp reduction in mammary cancer incidence (nulliparous and multiparous mice) (120). These results emphasize the striking sensitivity to prolactin that exists during the early developmental stages of spontaneous mouse mammary cancer.

Although the developmental stages of mouse mammary cancer appear to be markedly influenced by secretory levels of prolactin, advanced spontaneous mammary cancers in most strains of mice appear to be prolactin-independent. Treatment of C3H/HeJ female mice bearing advanced spontaneous mammary cancers with the prolactin suppressor CB-154 did not significantly influence the growth of these cancers (120). Furthermore growth of these cancers was not significantly influenced by chronic administration of prolactin (82) or by pituitary isografts (89). Therefore it appears that spontaneous C3H mouse mammary neoplasms gradually but fairly consistently evolve from a stage of prolactin responsiveness to a stage of prolactin independence.

Although the previously mentioned studies have demonstrated a relationship between prolactin secretion and mammary cancerigenesis in mice, measurements of pituitary and/or blood levels of this hormone in mice as a predictive test for mammary cancer susceptibility have not yielded a significant correlation. For example, few consistent patterns were observed in pituitary and blood levels of prolactin among virgin, pregnant, and lactating high- and low-mammary-cancer strains of mice (90,103,104). Furthermore, no differences in serum placental lactogen levels during pregnancy were noted between high-mammary-cancer C3H/He mice and low-mammary-cancer C57BL/6 mice, although mammary growth was much more conspicuous in the former strain than in the latter (137). These results do not negate the possible importance of prolactin in mammary cancerigenesis, but they do suggest that a moderate rate of prolactin secretion may be sufficient to permit cancer development. These observations also imply that the sensitivity of the mammary gland to prolactin is an additional important factor in mammary cancerigenesis, a concept supported by a number of studies reported by Nagasawa and colleagues (90).

One of the most intriguing problems pertaining to hormonal control of mouse mammary cancerigenesis is the nature of the interaction of prolactin and steroid hormones in this neoplastic process. Administration of estrogens to certain strains of mice sharply increases mammary cancer incidence (13,113). This treatment increases prolactin secretion, whereas ovariectomy reduces the secretion of this hormone (74), an observation that led to the well-known concept proposed originally by Furth (37) and colleagues (52) that estrogens are mammary oncogenic primarily because of their stimulatory effect on prolactin secretion. Treatment of hypophysectomized mice with estrogens in an effort to determine whether or not these steroids are capable of inducing spontaneous mammary cancers in animals free of pituitary hormones was not effective because hypophysectomized rodents are generally intolerant of prolonged steroid treatment. However, prolactin secretion can be suppressed in rodents chronically treated with estrogens by concurrent treatment with a number of ergot alkaloids (11,64), despite the stimulatory effect of these steroids on the secretion of this hormone. Recently we reported (10,115) that chronic treatment of female C3H mice with estrogens or with the oral contraceptive Enovid (norethynodrel with mestranol) increased the incidences of mammary hyperplasias and mammary cancers; however, on concurrent prolactin suppression with the ergot drug CB-154, the incidences of hyperplasias and mammary cancers were sharply reduced to levels comparable to those in non-steroid-treated control animals (Figs. 2 and 3). Furthermore, ovariectomy and chronic CB-154-induced prolactin suppression appear to be equally effective in suppressing the spontaneous development of mammary cancers in these mice (124). Thus in these particular studies it appeared that estrogens were mammary cancerigenic primarily because of their stimulatory

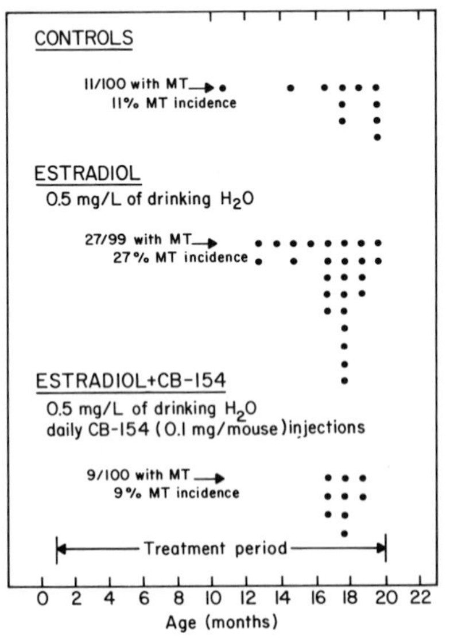

FIG. 2. Effects of 17β-estradiol and 17β-estradiol/CB-154 treatments on incidence of spontaneous mammary cancers in C3H/HeJ female mice. 17β-Estradiol was added to drinking water. 17β-Estradiol versus 17β-estradiol/CB-154 or controls, $p < 0.001$. (From Welsch et al., ref. 115, with permission.)

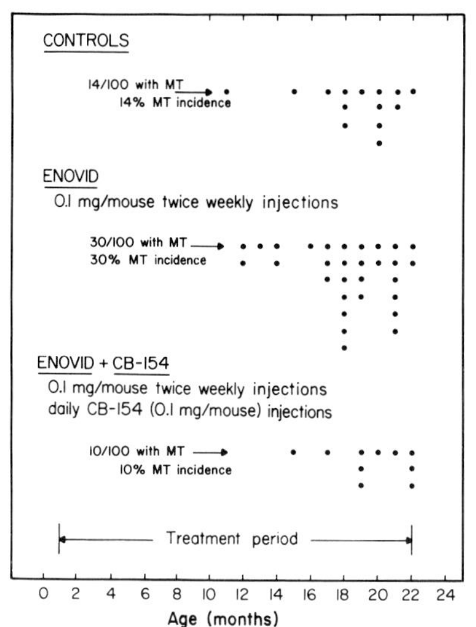

FIG. 3. Effects of Enovid and Enovid/CB-154 treatments on incidence of spontaneous mammary cancers in C3H/HeJ female mice. Envoid was injected subcutaneously twice weekly. Envoid versus Envoid/CB-154 or controls, $p < 0.001$. (From Welsch et al., ref. 115, with permission.)

effect on prolactin secretion. We do not intend to imply that the mammary oncogenic activities of estrogens are mediated solely via the pituitary gland; instead, we wish to emphasize that the indirect activity of the steroid is also a significant factor in estrogen-induced murine mammary cancerigenesis. Although in all probability the induction of murine mammary cancers by estrogen requires a functional pituitary gland, steroid-induced growth of established mammary cancers may not always require pituitary hormones. A recent report indicated that a transplantable mouse (GR/A) mammary cancer regressed following hypophysectomy, but its growth was reactivated by acute administration of estrogen and progesterone (105). As far as we know, this is the only report showing that ovarian steroids can stimulate growth of existing mammary cancers in rodents lacking a functional pituitary gland.

Administration of pituitary hormones to ovariectomized or ovariectomized-adrenalectomized mice also has been attempted in order to determine if these hormones are capable of inducing mammary cancerigenesis in steroid-deficient animals. Prolactin-secreting pituitary isografts have been reported to increase mammary cancer incidence in ovariectomized mice (6) and in intact and orchidectomized male mice (40), which suggests that there may be a primary role for prolactin and a secondary role for ovarian steroids in this process. However, there is no doubt that the adrenal glands contribute significant quantities of steroid hormones to this process. In a more recent study, Yanai and Nagasawa (138) transplanted multiple pituitaries into ovariectomized-adrenalectomized *8-month-old* C3H mice and observed within 8 months a 51% mammary cancer incidence. No mammary cancers were observed in the nongrafted ovariectomized-adrenalectomized control mice. Although the matter of the presence or absence of accessory adrenal tissue in the adrenalectomized animals is unresolved, the results of these studies suggest that very high levels of endogenous secretion of prolactin are capable of enhancing mammary cancerigenesis in sex-hormone-lacking (or, at least, sex-hormone-deficient) female mice. Successful induction by prolactin of spontaneous mammary cancers in rodents ovariectomized-adrenalectomized or orchidectomized-adrenalectomized at a *very young age* has not, to our knowledge, been reported. Therefore it remains to be determined whether or not prolactin can initiate early induction of spontaneous mouse mammary cancers in animals free of steroid (sex) hormones.

RELATION OF PROLACTIN TO CARCINOGEN-INDUCED MAMMARY CANCERIGENESIS IN RATS

Carcinogen-induced mammary cancers in rats have been studied extensively in recent years, and their dependence on prolactin has been clearly established. In general, most treatments that cause hyperprolactinemia in female rats bearing mammary cancers induced by either 7,12-dimethylbenzanthracene (DMBA) or 3-methylcholanthrene (MCA) cause striking increases in the growth of these neoplasms. For example, physiological conditions and treatments that markedly enhance carcinogen-induced mammary cancer growth in female rats and also cause hyperprolactinemia include the following: adrenalectomy (19), pregnancy (24,69), pseudopregnancy (24), pituitary homografts (118), pituitary tumors (52), hypothalamic lesions (119), and hypothalamic implants of steroids (83). A number of drugs that induce hypoprolactinemia cause marked diminution in growth of these cancers (16,84,108,122).

The effects of a number of CNS-influencing drugs on development and growth of carcinogen-induced rat mammary cancers have been investigated in our laboratory. L-DOPA (precursor of catecholamines), iproniazid (monoamine oxidase inhibitor), and ergot drugs (dopamine agonists) inhibited growth of DMBA-induced mammary cancers, whereas drugs such as reserpine, chlorpromazine, haloperidol, and methyldopa (all inhibitors of catecholamine activity) promoted growth of these tumors (9,54,84,94,95). When any of these drugs was given prior to administration of DMBA or for a period after administration of DMBA, it inhibited development of mammary cancers.

Recently we (44) studied several additional CNS-active drugs that had not previously been investigated for their effects on growth of DMBA-induced mammary cancers. Rats bearing these cancers were injected daily for 3 weeks with piribedil (a dopamine agonist), clonidine (a norepinephrine agonist), pimozide (a dopamine receptor blocker), or α-methyl-*p*-tyrosine (an inhibitor of dopamine and norepinephrine synthesis). The results are shown in Fig. 4. It can be seen that pimozide (PIM) and α-methyl-*p*-tyrosine (αMPT) stimulated mammary cancer growth above that observed in the saline-injected controls (SAL), whereas piribedil (PIR), clonidine (CLO), and a combination of PIR and CLO induced regression of mammary cancers. Stimulation or inhibition of mammary cancer

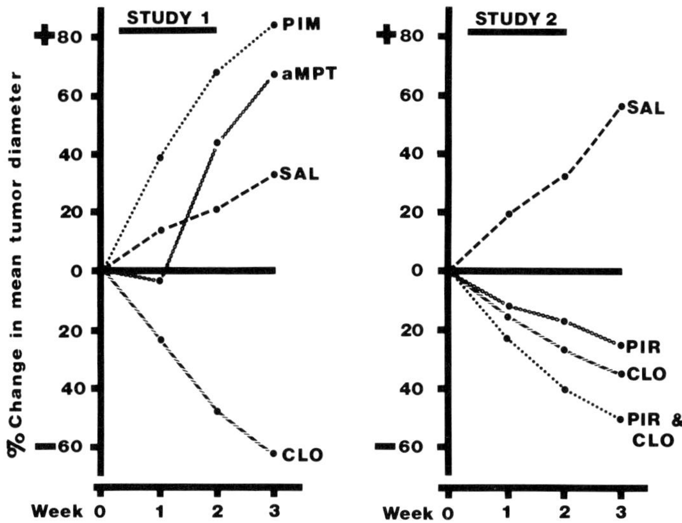

FIG. 4. Changes in mean carcinogen-induced mammary cancer diameter during drug treatment of female rats expressed as percentage change from initial tumor diameter. SAL = 0.85% saline, PIM = pimozide, αMPT = α-methyl-p-tyrosine, CLO = clonidine, PIR = piribedil. (From Hodson et al., ref. 44, with permission.)

growth was related to corresponding increases or decreases in blood serum levels of prolactin (Table 1). These results indicate that chronic stimulation of dopamine or norepinephrine receptors in the hypothalamus results in decreased mammary cancer growth, whereas chronic inhibition of these receptors results in enhancement of mammary cancer growth. Sulpiride, a neuroleptic drug, also was found to raise serum prolactin levels and increase the growth of DMBA-induced mammary cancers in rats (92).

The influence of dietary fat on pituitary prolactin secretion and chemical carcinogenesis in the rat mammary gland has recently received increased attention. In 1970 Carroll and Khor (15) showed that a high intake of dietary fat is stimulatory to carcinogen-induced rat mammary cancerigenesis. More recently, Chan et al. (18) reported that a high-fat diet enhanced chemical-induced carcinogenesis in the rat mammary gland, but in addition it increased pituitary prolactin secretion. They reported higher serum prolactin levels during the afternoon of proestrus in non-cancer-bearing rats fed high-fat diets than in rats fed low-fat diets. In experiments not yet reported we recently confirmed these observations in Sprague-Dawley female rats with existing DMBA-induced mammary cancers. Rats fed a diet consisting of 20% lard or corn oil showed greater growth of mammary cancers than rats fed a diet with 4% fat, and they had significantly higher serum prolactin values than the rats fed the low-fat diet. The mechanism(s) by which a high-fat diet increases pituitary prolactin release remain to be investigated.

TABLE 1. *Changes in serum prolactin levels and body weights during drug treatment*

Treatment	Number of rats	Initial body weight (g)	Final body weight (g)	Serum prolactin (ng/ml)
Study 1				
αMPT[a]	8	292 ± 7[b]	294 ± 12[b]	167.1[b] ± 20.1[c]
PIM	8	276 ± 7	281 ± 5	179.2[b] ± 24.1
CLO	8	281 ± 7	286 ± 8	19.2[b] ± 2.52
SAL	8	270 ± 11	279 ± 8	30.3 ± 2.04
Study 2				
PIR	8	294 ± 8	303 ± 9	16.7[b] ± 2.3
CLO	8	282 ± 9	281 ± 8	18.3[b] ± 1.4
PIR & CLO	8	272 ± 10	281 ± 9	14.6[b] ± 4.1
SAL	8	272 ± 9	290 ± 8	28.7 ± 3.1

[a] αMPT = α-methyl-*p*-tyrosine, SAL = 0.85% saline, PIM = pimozide, CLO = clonidine, PIR = piribedil.

[b] Mean ± SEM.

[c] Significantly different from saline controls ($p < 0.01$).

From Hodson et al. (44), with permission.

The effects of caloric restriction on growth of tumors in general and mammary cancers in particular have been widely investigated. In general, it has been reported that caloric restriction inhibits development and growth of mammary cancers (134). In experiments yet to be reported we attempted to determine if any of the reduced growth of mammary cancers produced by caloric restriction could be accounted for by decreased secretion of estrogen and prolactin. Sprague-Dawley rats with existing DMBA-induced mammary cancers were fed half the complete diet consumed daily by control rats. A second group of control rats were given only half the complete diet. The half-ration experiment rats were injected subcutaneously daily for 5 weeks with 0.2 μg estradiol benzoate, 120 μg haloperidol (to increase serum prolactin), or a combination of the two agents. The full-ration and half-ration control rats were injected daily with corn oil only.

The effects on body weight in these rats are shown in Table 2. It can be seen that at the end of 5 weeks the rats given half rations showed considerable losses in body weight (58–77 g each) as compared to the full-ration rats (8 g each). Table 3 shows that whereas the full-ration rats demonstrated an average gain of 2.1 tumors per rat, the half-ration control rats showed a loss of 2.0 cancers per rat. The half-ration rats injected with estrogen showed a loss of only 0.4 cancers per rat, whereas the rats given haloperidol showed a gain of 1.2 cancers per rat. The rats given the combination of estrogen and haloperidol showed a gain of only 0.4 cancers per rat. Similar results were obtained when average mammary cancer diameter was measured. Thus estrogen and haloperidol were able to overcome the effects of underfeeding for 5 weeks, although the combination of the two substances was no more effective than either alone.

TABLE 2. *Changes in body weight as a result of half rations for mammary-cancer-bearing rats*

Group and number of rats	Treatment	Change of body weight at 2 weeks (g)	Change of body weight at 5 weeks (g)
1 (7)	Full-ration controls	−5 ± 4	−8 ± 10
2 (8)	Half-ration controls	−39 ± 3	−58 ± 7
3 (7)	Half rations + EB[a]	−40 ± 6	−77 ± 8
4 (7)	Half rations + HAL[a]	−36 ± 2	−60 ± 9
5 (5)	Half rations + EB + HAL	−36 ± 4	−69 ± 12

[a] EB = estradiol benzoate, HAL = haloperidol.
(From Bradley and Meites, *unpublished*.)

This shows that at least part of the reason mammary cancers in rats regress during underfeeding is that secretion of estrogen and prolactin is decreased. It has been well demonstrated that reduced food intake results in reduction in secretion of anterior pituitary hormones and in cessation of estrous cycles. We recently reported (14) that underfed rats showed reduced blood levels of prolactin, luteinizing hormone (LH), follicle-stimulating hormone (FSH), thyroid-stimulating hormone (TSH), and growth hormone (GH) as compared to full-ration rats. In addition to the effects on mammary cancers produced by deficiencies in secretion of pituitary and ovarian hormones induced by underfeeding, it is also possible that the limited availability of nutrients may directly influence the growth of mammary cancers.

In another study (Bradley and Meites, *unpublished*) the effects of restricted protein intake and injections of hormone on mammary cancer growth were

TABLE 3. *Effects of underfeeding with or without injections of estradiol benzoate and haloperidol on mammary cancer number*

	Number of tumors per rat per week						
Treatment	0	1	2	3	4	5	Change
Controls, full rations	5.00	5.28	6.14	6.57	6.71	7.14	+2.14
Controls, half relations	4.50	4.50	4.12	3.62	3.00	2.50	−2.00[a]
Half rations + EB[b]	4.00	4.28	3.85	4.00	3.71	3.57	−0.43
Half rations + HAL[b]	4.42	4.42	4.28	4.42	5.00	5.58	+1.16
Half rations + EB + HAL	5.20	5.20	5.00	5.60	5.60	5.60	+0.40

[a] Significantly different change in tumor number from full-ration controls by 5th week of treatment.
[b] EB = estradiol benzoate, HAL = haloperidol.
(From Bradley and Meites, *unpublished*.)

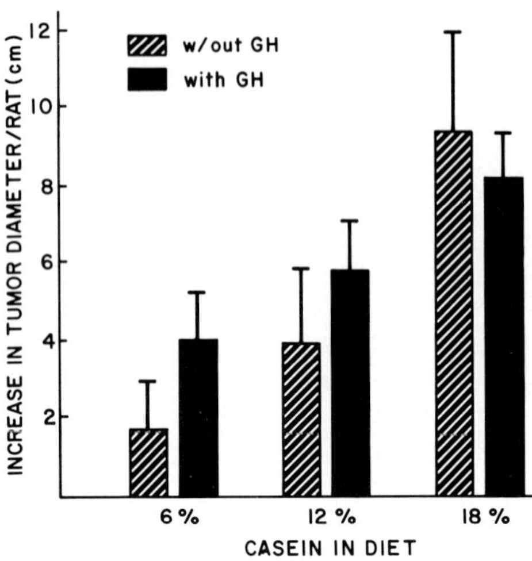

FIG. 5. Effects of restricted dietary protein (casein) and injections of GH on carcinogen-induced mammary cancer growth in female rats. (From Bradley and Meites, *unpublished*.)

studied. Groups of rats carrying DMBA-induced mammary cancers (8 rats per group) were fed semisynthetic diets for 3 weeks containing 6, 12, or 18% casein, but otherwise the diets were isocaloric. Half the rat groups were injected daily subcutaneously with 1 mg NIH-S-10 ovine GH dissolved in physiological saline. The rats were regulated so that each received 13 g of food per day in all treatment groups. The results are shown in Fig. 5. It can be seen that the rats fed the 6% casein diet showed significantly smaller gains in average mammary cancer diameter per rat than the rats fed the 12 and 18% casein diets. Daily injections of GH completely overcame the deficiency in cancer growth induced by the 6% casein diet. Similar effects were observed in mean cancer number. GH had no stimulatory effect on mammary cancer growth in the rats fed 12 and 18% casein, which shows that GH does not directly stimulate mammary cancer growth in rats. These results suggest that the decrease in mammary cancer growth induced by a deficiency of protein can be overcome by injection of GH, presumably because of its ability to conserve protein in the body, even in a starving animal. This is probably the explanation of its mechanism of action, rather than direct stimulation of mammary cancer growth. There is no convincing evidence that GH can increase mammary cancer growth in normally fed rats (48).

Interaction between ovarian hormones and prolactin in the *induction* of carcinogen-induced rat mammary cancers has been the subject of a number of studies. Although under most conditions this interaction is no doubt crucial, this very complicated relationship remains to be elucidated. Ovariectomy of rats 30 days prior to carcinogen treatment prevented the occurrence of mammary cancers (118). Concurrent enhancement of prolactin secretion in these animals did not increase the incidence of these cancers (118). However, if ovariectomy was performed slightly before carcinogen treatment, concurrent treatment with prolactin and GH increased mammary cancer incidence considerably above that seen in the ovariectomized controls (109). Suppression of prolactin secretion prior to carcinogen treatment also sharply reduced mammary cancer incidence in female rats (21), whereas enhanced secretion of this hormone increased mammary cancer incidence in carcinogen-treated male rats (125). Therefore it appears that ovarian hormones and prolactin (or, at least, their residual effects) are critical, perhaps essential, in chemical transformation of the epithelium of the rat mammary gland; but it appears that pituitary hormones alone can promote the growth of these transformed cells even in the absence of ovarian function, resulting in substantial mammary cancer growth. Alternatively, if prolactin levels are sufficiently high, perhaps at a level even exceeding the secretory capacity of the *in situ* pituitary, these steroid hormones may not be essential for chemical carcinogenesis of the rat mammary gland. It has not been shown that chemical carcinogenesis in the rat mammary gland can occur in animals free of pituitary hormones, because hypophysectomized rats are generally intolerant of carcinogen treatment. The sole exception to this was a study conducted a number of years ago by Young (139) that demonstrated successful chemical (MCA) induction of mammary cancers in hypophysectomized Sprague-Dawley rats chronically treated with estrogen, progesterone, and large doses of bovine GH. However, the purity of the GH was not indicated in the report, and it may have contained some prolactin.

Growth of *established* carcinogen-induced rat mammary cancers also appears to be regulated by steroid and pituitary hormonal interactions. Ovariectomy of rats bearing these neoplasms resulted in prompt and prolonged regression of these cancers (47,110). Concurrent enhancement of prolactin secretion by placement of median eminence hypothalamic lesions in these rats prevented this regression; cancer growth actually was stimulated by this experimental procedure (119). However, this enhanced mammary cancer growth did not persist for long periods unless ovaries were reimplanted into these animals (102). In agreement with these findings, daily injection of ovine prolactin or human placental lactogen into ovariectomized-adrenalectomized or ovariectomized-adrenalectomized-hypophysectomized rats bearing carcinogen-induced mammary cancers also resulted, at least initially, in increased growth of these cancers (85,87,93). These results suggest that prolactin can stimulate growth of carcinogen-induced rat mammary cancers in animals lacking ovarian steroids, but for persistent optimal growth of these neoplasms, despite hyperprolactinemia, ovarian steroids may still be essential. Further evidence for significant prolactin and ovarian hormone interaction in growth of carcinogen-induced rat mammary carcinomas is the observation that the combination of drug-induced prolactin suppression and ovariectomy caused greater cancer regression than either treatment alone (96). It is probable that the growth dependency of carcinogen-induced rat mammary cancers for prolactin and ovarian hormones can vary from cancer to cancer, i.e., some cancers will require substantially greater or lesser amounts of prolactin and/or ovarian hormones for optimal growth processes (9). This may be related to the different availabilities of estrogen and prolactin receptors in mammary cancers.

Whether or not estrogens can influence growth of carcinogen-induced rat mammary cancers in hypophysectomized animals was investigated by Pearson and colleagues (93,106). Hypophysectomy caused rapid regression of mammary cancers. Administration of estrogens to the cancer-bearing hypophysectomized rats did not cause resumption of cancer growth, which clearly demonstrates a pituitary dependency of steroid action for this experimental cancer model. It is probable that there are variants of rodent mammary cancers that can be stimulated by prolactin in the absence of ovarian secretions or, on rare occasions, by ovarian hormones in the absence of prolactin, but most hormone-responsive mammary cancers in rodents appear to require participation of both prolactin and ovarian hormones for optimal growth processes.

Prolactin can influence development and growth of normal and cancerous rodent mammary tissue by direct action on the mammary epithelium or by an indirect mechanism, i.e., via the ovary. It has been known for many years that prolactin is luteotrophic and, under certain conditions, luteolytic in rodents (74,136). Prolactin is known to stimulate progesterone secretion by the ovaries of rats and mice, and progesterone can increase growth of established mammary cancers in rats (47). However, the primary action of prolactin on growth of the carcinogen-induced rat mammary cancer model appears to be direct, i.e., this hormone appears to have a direct mitogenic effect on this neoplastic tissue. For example, the administration of prolactin to ovariectomized, ovariectomized-adrenalectomized, or ovariectomized-adrenalectomized-hypophysectomized rats bearing these neoplasms resulted in initial increases in growth of these cancers (85,93,119). Furthermore, administration of this hormone to organ cultures of these cancers resulted in increased DNA synthesis of these tissues (132). Although these studies provide evidence indicating that prolactin alone can directly stimulate growth of carcinogen-induced rat mammary cancers, a distinct synergistic effect of optimal levels of ovarian hormones in the growth process does appear to occur (96,102,111).

Although physiological doses of estrogen may enhance the action of prolactin (86), larger doses *in vitro* (132) and *in vivo* (72) may actually inhibit the direct stimulatory effect of prolactin on normal and cancerous rodent mammary tissues. In ovariectomized and intact rats the injection of large doses of estrogen into rats bearing carcinogen-induced mammary cancers resulted in regression of these cancers, despite relatively high levels of blood prolactin. This cancer regression was prevented by concurrent treatment with high doses of prolactin (72). An inhibitory effect of large doses of estrogen (counteracted by prolactin) has also been demonstrated *in vitro* in cultures of carcinogen-induced rat mammary carcinomas. Prolactin stimulates DNA synthesis of these neoplasms *in vitro,* an effect that can be suppressed by the addition of a relatively high level of estrogen to the culture medium (132). These results therefore suggest that relatively high doses of estrogen may interfere with the action of prolactin at the site of the neoplasm, but lower levels of the steroid may enhance the action of prolactin at these sites. Recent evidence shows that high doses of estrogen that suppress growth of DMBA-induced mammary cancers in rats also reduce the number of prolactin receptors in mammary cancer tissue (53). Thus, although serum prolactin levels are increased by the high-estrogen treatment, the prolactin presumably cannot exert its full effects because of a deficiency of prolactin receptors.

A number of recent studies have indicated that the ability of prolactin to promote mammary cancer growth in rats depends to a considerable extent on the number of prolactin receptors in the tumor tissue. Similarly, the action of estrogen on growth of mammary cancers appears to depend largely on the number of estrogen receptors in the tumor tissue. The first action of a hormone on a tissue is to bind with specific receptors in that tissue, and in the case of prolactin it has been shown that it binds to specific receptors in plasma membranes of the cells of the mammary cancers.

In a collaborative study (50), rats with DMBA-induced mammary cancers were injected subcutaneously daily for 12 days with 1 mg NIH ovine prolactin (26 IU/mg). Cancer size was measured for each of the 34 cancers present; 6 days after the last injection of prolactin the rats were sacrificed and the cancers were excised, weighed, frozen, and subsequently measured for prolactin receptors. The results are shown in Table 4. It can be seen that on the average the mammary cancers that responded the most to prolactin by exhibiting the greatest growth responses had the highest number of prolactin receptors, whereas those cancers showing the least growth response to prolactin had smaller numbers of prolactin receptors. Not every mammary cancer exhibited this direct relationship to growth response by prolactin, which suggests that factors other than prolactin receptors may influence the growth response to prolactin. In a subse-

TABLE 4. *Carcinogen-induced mammary cancer growth in female rats and specific binding of ^{125}I-labeled ovine prolactin (oPRL)*

Rank	Final cancer size (1 + w + d) (cm)	Growth index (cm)	Specific binding[a] of ^{125}I-oPRL (%)
1–8	6.1 ± 1.1	2.2 ± 0.2	22.1 ± 2.4
9–17	5.0 ± 0.6	1.0 ± 0.6	12.7 ± 2.6
18–26	3.3 ± 0.5	0.5 ± 0.0	10.0 ± 2.4
27–34	2.8 ± 0.2	0.0 ± 0.0	7.3 ± 1.5

[a] Total cpm minus nonspecific counts bound to membrane (counts in presence of excess unlabeled hormone) expressed as percentage of total cpm added to tube. Nonspecific binding was usually 5–8% of total radioactivity added to incubation tube.

From Kelly et al. (50), with permission.

quent study (27) it was shown that estrogen as well as prolactin receptors influenced the response of DMBA-induced mammary cancers to ovariectomy. The concentrations of prolactin and estrogen receptors tended to be lower in the cancers that responded least to endocrine ablation, and a better correlation of response was seen when both estrogen and prolactin receptors were considered. Again, not every cancer response could be related to the absolute number of prolactin or estrogen receptors present in the cancerous tissue. Other investigators have made similar observations (45).

There are more experimental examples of a stimulatory effect of prolactin in rodent mammary cancerigenesis (123,130,131) than there are examples of inhibition. Nevertheless, there are certain endocrine conditions in which increased secretion of this protein in mice and rats is consistently inhibitory to this neoplastic process. Perhaps the most striking example of this phenomenon is the carcinogen-induced rat mammary cancer model. When prolactin secretion was increased by pregnancy (23), pituitary homografts (118), ether stress (38, 101), reserpine (128), estrogens (54), oral contraceptives (127), or hypothalamic lesions (119) prior to carcinogen treatment, mammary cancer incidence was sharply reduced as compared with controls. As previously indicated, these treatments consistently enhance the growth of existing carcinogen-induced rat mammary cancers. These treatments also elicit intense stimulation of growth of the normal mammary gland, resulting in a predominant lobuloalveolar morphology, in contrast to a predominant ductal system seen in nontreated controls. Therefore it appears that a predominant lobuloalveolar system in the rat is refractory to the action of the carcinogen. Carcinogen-induced mammary cancers in the rat appear to arise from the ductal or end-bud elements of the mammary gland (76) rather than from alveoli, which may explain this phenomenon, at least in part.

Another example in which a sustained increase in secretion of prolactin is inhibitory to chemical carcinogenesis of the rodent mammary gland is during lactation. Lactating rats and mice are relatively refractory to the action of chemical carcinogens, as compared with nonlactating controls (23,67). It is conceivable that this inhibition may be accounted for by an increased elimination of the carcinogen by the secretory mammary epithelium (23,67) and/or the low rate of DNA synthesis that is characteristic of the lactating mammary gland (39). It has been reported that the frequency of cell division at the time of carcinogen treatment may be an important limiting factor in chemical carcinogenesis of the rodent mammary gland (88).

Increased secretion of prolactin during lactation not only inhibits the induction of chemical-induced carcinogenesis of the rat mammary gland but also causes regression of existing carcinogen-induced rat mammary cancers (24,69). It is conceivable that the deficiency of estrogen secretion during lactation is responsible for this growth inhibition. Alternatively, lactation may induce a degree of differentiation in the carcinomatous epithelium that opposes cancer cell proliferation (112).

PROLACTIN AND HUMAN BREAST CANCERIGENESIS

A number of *in vivo* studies have been designed to determine if patients with breast cancer have higher mean serum prolactin levels than disease-free controls. The results have been conflicting, i.e., a few groups (81,97) have shown a positive correlation between elevated serum prolactin levels and the presence of breast cancer, whereas a number of other groups (8,32,99,135) have not been able to observe such correlation. Another group has reported that although no correlation could be found between serum prolactin and the presence or absence of this disease, a high prolactin level could be found in patients with a family history of breast cancer (56). A greater pituitary reserve of prolactin in women with advanced breast cancer, as compared with women without the disease, has been reported (79), although no correlation between serum prolactin and the presence or absence of the disease was noted in these patients. In patients with benign breast disease, increases in serum prolactin were observed, as compared with women without this disease (22).

Administration of prolactin-suppressing drugs (e.g., CB-154, L-DOPA) to patients with breast cancer also has yielded conflicting results. A few groups (78,81,98,107) have induced remissions in breast cancer patients by using these drugs, whereas other groups have been unable to observe any beneficial anticancer activities of these drugs (42). Furthermore, pituitary stalk section, a surgical procedure that increases prolactin secretion, induces regression, not stimulation, in a significant fraction of patients with advanced breast cancer (1,29). However, stalk section may also result in loss of ovarian function. Provocative reports by three independent laboratories (2,41,49) provided statistical evidence suggesting that women treated chronically with the tranquilizer reserpine, a potent stimulator of prolactin secretion, were in a twofold to sixfold breast cancer risk group. However, these reports have not been confirmed (51,58,66,91).

In vitro studies also have been used to evaluate the rôle of prolactin in human breast cancerigenesis. Ovine-prolactin-treated cell or organ cultures of human breast carcinomas responded to the hormone by increased cellular proliferation (55,77). It was also reported (3,43) that human breast carcinomas grown in organ culture responded positively to the stimulatory effects of ovine prolactin by increased pentose shunt activity. However, the results of these latter studies have not been confirmed (4,68). In our laboratory, addition of ovine prolactin to organ cultures of human breast carcinoma slices resulted in marked stimulation of incorporation of [^{3}H]thymidine into DNA in only a small fraction ($<15\%$) of the biopsy specimens (116). In agreement with this, a recent study indicated that only about 20% of human breast cancer biopsy specimens showed specific prolactin binding greater than 1% (46). A stimulatory effect of ovine or bovine prolactin on growth of organ cultures of human benign breast dysplasias and normal ductal tissues obtained from biopsies or mastectomies also was reported (17,31). A more recent report (28), confirmed and extended by our laboratory (126), showed that normal and benign human breast tissues grown in organ culture were not significantly stimulated by ovine prolactin but were stimulated by human prolactin or human placental lactogen. Most recently, we also observed that normal and benign human breast tissues maintained in the athymic nude mouse responded to injected human placental lactogen with significantly increased mitotic activity (70). From the foregoing it is clear that any role for prolactin in the development and growth of human breast cancers has yet to be clearly established. Nevertheless, the results derived from a number of the aforementioned human studies and the unequivocal key role for prolactin in rodent mammary cancerigenesis should provide sufficient impetus for vigorous efforts toward defining the role of this pituitary protein hormone in human breast cancerigenesis.

SUMMARY

A number of laboratories have provided a substantial volume of data demonstrating a crucial role for pituitary prolactin in the development and growth of rodent mammary cancers. In certain endocrinological conditions, chronic hyperprolactinemia in susceptible strains of mice and rats can invariably enhance mammary cancerigenesis. In other endocrinological states, hyperprolactinemia can actually inhibit this cancerigenic process in both mice and rats. Chronic hypoprolactinemia, on the other hand, can cause regression of existing rat mammary cancers; under certain conditions, in mice, it can suppress or virtually totally prevent development of these neoplasms. Therefore it is clear that prolactin is a key hormone during cancerigenesis in the rodent mammary gland.

Whether or not prolactin is of significant importance in human breast cancerigenesis remains to be determined. This is an extremely important area of research that is receiving increasing attention. If prolactin can be shown to influence human breast epithelium in a manner similar to its effect on rodent mammary tissue, then prophylactic and/or chemotherapeutic control of human breast cancerigenesis may be feasible by appropriate drug-mediated prolactin suppression.

ACKNOWLEDGMENTS

This research was supported in part by U.S. Public Health Service research grant CA-13777 and American Cancer Society research grant ET-59 to C.W.W. and U.S. Public Health Service research grants CA-10771, AM-04784, and AG-00416 to J.M.

REFERENCES

1. Antony, G. J., Van Wyk, J. J., French, F. S., Weaver, R. P., Dugger, G. S., Timmons, R. L., and Newsome, J. F. (1969): Influence of pituitary stalk section on growth hormone, insulin and TSH secretion in women with metastatic breast cancer. *J. Clin. Endocrinol. Metab.*, 29:1238–1250.

2. Armstrong, B., Stevens, N., and Doll, R. (1974): Retrospective study of the association between use of rauwolfia derivatives and breast cancer in English women. *Lancet,* 2:672–675.
3. Bapat, C. V., and Kesava-Rao, K. V. (1976): An "in vitro" method for the prediction of hormone dependency of human breast tumours by succinic dehydrogenase activity. *Indian J. Cancer,* 13:57–63.
4. Beeby, D. I., Easty, G. C., Gazet, J. C., Grigor, K., and Neville, A. M. (1975): An assessment of the effects of hormones on short term organ cultures of human breast carcinomata. *Br. J. Cancer,* 31:317–328.
5. Bern, H. A., and Nandi, S. (1961): Recent studies of the hormonal influence in mouse mammary tumorigenesis. *Prog. Exp. Tumor Res.,* 2:90–144.
6. Bittner, J. J., and Cole, H. L. (1961): Induction of mammary cancer in agent-free mice bearing pituitary isografts correlated with inherited hormonal mechanisms. *J. Natl. Cancer Inst.,* 27:1273–1284.
7. Boot, L. M., Mühlbock, O., and Röpcke, G. (1962): Prolactin and the induction of mammary tumors in mice. *Gen. Comp. Endocrinol.,* 2:601–603.
8. Boyns, A. R., Cole, E. N., Griffiths, K., Roberts, M. M., Buchan, R., Wilson, R. G., and Forrest, A. P. M. (1973): Plasma prolactin in breast cancer. *Eur. J. Cancer,* 9:99–102.
9. Bradley, C., Kledzik, G. S., and Meites, J. (1976): Prolactin and estrogen dependency of rat mammary cancers at early and late stages of development. *Cancer Res.,* 36:319–324.
10. Brooks, C. L., and Welsch, C. W. (1974): Inhibition of mammary dysplasia in estrogen-treated C3H/HeJ female mice by treatment with 2-bromo-α-ergocryptine. *Proc. Soc. Exp. Biol. Med.,* 145:484–487.
11. Brooks, C. L., and Welsch, C. W. (1974): Reduction of serum prolactin in rats by 2 ergot alkaloids and 2 ergoline derivatives: A comparison. *Proc. Soc. Exp. Biol. Med.,* 146:863–867.
12. Bruni, J. E., and Montemurro, D. G. (1971): Effect of hypothalamic lesions on the genesis of spontaneous mammary gland tumors in the mouse. *Cancer Res.,* 31:854–863.
13. Burns, E. L., and Schenken, J. R. (1940): Quantitative studies on relationship between estrogen and mammary gland carcinoma in strain C3H mice. *Proc. Soc. Exp. Biol. Med.,* 43:608–610.
14. Campbell, G. A., Kurcz, M., Marshall, S., and Meites, J. (1977). Effects of starvation in rats on serum levels of follicle stimulating hormone, luteinizing hormone, thyrotropin, growth hormone and prolactin; response to LH-releasing hormone and thyrotropin-releasing hormone. *Endocrinology,* 100:580–587.
15. Carroll, K. K., and Khor, H. T. (1970): Effects of dietary fat and dose level of 7,12-dimethylbenzanthracene on mammary tumor incidence in rats. *Cancer Res.,* 30:2260–2264.
16. Cassell, E. E., Meites, J., and Welsch, C. W. (1971): Effects of ergocornine and ergocryptine on growth of 7,12-dimethylbenzanthracene-induced mammary tumors in rats. *Cancer Res.,* 31:1051–1053.
17. Ceriani, R. L., Contesso, G. P., and Natof, B. M. (1972): Hormone requirement for growth and differentiation of the human mammary gland in organ culture. *Cancer Res.,* 32:2190–2196.
18. Chan, P., Didato, F., and Cohen, L. A. (1975): High dietary fat, elevation of rat serum prolactin and mammary cancer. *Proc. Soc. Exp. Biol. Med.,* 149:133–135.
19. Chen, H. J., Bradley, C. J., and Meites, J. (1976): Stimulation of carcinogen-induced mammary tumor growth in rats by adrenalectomy. *Cancer Res.,* 36:1414–1417.
20. Clemens, J. A., and Meites, J. (1974): Hypothalamic control of prolactin secretion. In: *Mammary Cancer and Neuroendocrine Therapy,* edited by B. A. Stoll, pp. 160–178. Butterworth, London.
21. Clemens, J. A., and Shaar, C. J. (1972): Inhibition by ergocornine of initiation and growth of 7,12-dimethylbenzanthracene-induced mammary tumors in rats. Effect of tumor size. *Proc. Soc. Exp. Biol. Med.,* 139:659–662.
22. Cole, E. N., Sellwood, R. A., England, P. C., and Griffiths, K. (1977): Serum prolactin concentrations in benign breast disease throughout the menstrual cycle. *Eur. J. Cancer,* 13:597–603.
23. Dao, T. L., Bock, F. G., and Greiner, M. J. (1960): Mammary carcinogenesis by 3-methylcholanthrene. II. Inhibitory effect of pregnancy and lactation on tumor induction. *J. Natl. Cancer Inst.,* 25:991–1003.
24. Dao, T. L., and Sunderland, H. (1959): Mammary carcinogenesis by 3-methylcholanthrene. I. Hormonal aspects in tumor induction and growth. *J. Natl. Cancer Inst.,* 23:567–585.

25. DeOme, K. B., Faulkin, L. J., Bern, H. A., and Blair, P. B. (1959): Development of mammary tumors from hyperplastic alveolar nodules transplanted into gland-free mammary fat pads of female C3H mice. *Cancer Res.,* 19:515–520.
26. Desclin, L. (1950): A propos du mécanisme d'action des oestrogènes sur le lobe anterieur de l'hypophyse chez la rat. *Annee Endocrinol.,* 11:656–659.
27. DeSombre, E. R., Kledzik, G., Marshall, S., and Meites, J. (1976): Estrogen and prolactin receptor concentrations in rat mammary tumors and response to endocrine ablation. *Cancer Res.,* 36:354–358.
28. Dilley, W. G., and Kister, S. J. (1975): In vitro stimulation of human breast tissue by human prolactin. *J. Natl. Cancer Inst.,* 55:35–36.
29. Ehni, G., and Eckles, N. E. (1959): Interruption of the pituitary stalk in the patient with mammary cancer. *J. Neurosurg.,* 16:628–652.
30. Everett, J. W. (1954): Luteotrophic function of autografts of the rat hypophysis. *Endocrinology,* 54:685–690.
31. Flaxman, B. A., and Lasfargues, E. Y. (1973): Hormone-independent DNA synthesis by epithelial cells of adult human mammary gland in organ culture. *Proc. Soc. Exp. Biol. Med.,* 143:371–374.
32. Franks, S., Ralphs, D. N. L., Seagroatt, V., and Jacobs, H. S. (1974): Prolactin concentrations in patients with breast cancer. *Br. Med. J.,* 4:320–321.
33. Frantz, A. G., Kleinberg, D. L., and Noel, G. L. (1972): Studies on prolactin in man. *Recent Prog. Horm. Res.,* 28:527–590.
34. Frantz, W. L., MacIndoe, J. H., and Turkington, R. W. (1974): Prolactin receptors: Characteristics of the particulate fraction binding activity. *J. Endocrinol.,* 60:485–497.
35. Frantz, W. L., Mann, L. C., and Welsch, C. W. (1977): Induction of specific binding sites for prolactin in the livers of Dw/J dwarf mice by injected prolactin. *I.R.C.S. Med. Sci.,* 5:32.
36. Friesen, H., Hwang, P., Guyda, H., Tolis, G., Tyson, J., and Myers, R. A. (1972): Radioimmunoassay for human prolactin. In: *Prolactin and Carcinogenesis,* edited by A. R. Boyns and K. Griffiths, pp. 64–80. Alpha Omega Alpha Publishing, Cardiff, Wales.
37. Furth, J. (1973): The role of prolactin in mammary carcinogenesis. In: *Human Prolactin,* edited by J. L. Pasteels and C. Robyn, pp. 233–248. Excerpta Medica/American Elsevier, New York.
38. Gala, R. R., and Loginsky, S. J. (1973): Correlation between serum prolactin levels and incidence of mammary tumors induced by 7,12-dimethylbenzanthracene in the rat. *J. Natl. Cancer Inst.,* 51:593–597.
39. Grahame, R. E., and Bertalanffy, F. D. (1972): Cell division in normal and neoplastic mammary gland tissue in the rat. *Anat. Rec.,* 174:1–8.
40. Hagen, E. O., and Rawlinson, H. E. (1964): The induction of mammary cancer in male mice by isologous pituitary implants. *Cancer Res.,* 24:59–60.
41. Heinonen, O. P., Shapiro, S., Tuominen, L., and Turunen, M. I. (1974): Reserpine use in relation to breast cancer. *Lancet,* 2:675–677.
42. Heuson, J. C., Coune, A., and Staquet, M. (1972): Clinical trial of 2-Br-α-ergocryptine (CB-154) in advanced breast cancer. *Eur. J. Cancer,* 8:155–156.
43. Hobbs, J. R., DeSouza, I., Salih, H., and Raggott, P. (1974): Selection of hormone-dependent breast cancers. *Br. J. Surg.,* 61:785–786.
44. Hodson, C. A., Mioduszewski, R., and Meites, J. (1978): Effects of catecholaminergic and anti-catecholaminergic drugs on growth of carcinogen-induced mammary tumors in rats. *Proc. Soc. Exp. Biol. Med., (in press).*
45. Holdaway, I. M., and Friesen, H. G. (1976): Correlation between hormone binding and growth response of rat mammary tumor. *Cancer Res.,* 36:1562–1567.
46. Holdaway, I. M., and Friesen, H. G. (1977): Hormone binding by human mammary carcinoma. *Cancer Res.,* 37:1946–1952.
47. Huggins, C., Briziarelli, G., and Sutton, H. (1959): Rapid induction of mammary carcinoma in the rat and the influence of hormones on the tumors. *J. Exp. Med.,* 109:25–42.
48. Iturri, G., and Welsch, C. W. (1976): Effects of prolactin and growth hormone on DNA synthesis of rat mammary carcinomas *in vitro. Experientia,* 32:1045–1046.
49. Jick, H., Sloan, D., Shapiro, S., Heinonen, O. P., Hartz, S. C., Miettinen, O. S., Vessey, M. P., Lawson, D. H., and Miller, R. R. (1974): Reserpine and breast cancer. *Lancet,* 2:669–671.

50. Kelly, P. A., Bradley, C., Shiro, R. P. C., Meites, J., and Friesen, H. G. (1974): Prolactin binding to rat mammary tumor tissues. *Proc. Soc. Exp. Biol. Med.,* 146:816–819.
51. Kewitz, H., Jesdinsky, H. J., Schröter, P. M., and Lindtner, E. (1977): Reserpine and breast cancer in women in Germany. *Eur. J. Clin. Pharmacol.,* 11:79–83.
52. Kim, U., Furth, J., and Clifton, K. H. (1960): Relation of mammary tumors to mammotropes. II. Hormone responsiveness of 3-methylcholanthrene induced mammary carcinomas. *Proc. Soc. Exp. Biol. Med.,* 103:646–650.
53. Kledzik, G. G., Bradley, C. J., Marshall, S., Campbell, G. A., and Meites, J. (1976): Effects of high doses of estrogen on prolactin-binding activity and growth of carcinogen-induced mammary cancers in rats. *Cancer Res.,* 36:3265–3268.
54. Kledzik, G. S., Bradley, C. J., and Meites, J. (1974): Reduction of carcinogen-induced mammary cancer incidence in rats by early treatment with hormones or drugs. *Cancer Res.,* 34:2953–2956.
55. Klevjer-Anderson, P., and Buehring, G. C. (1976): Hormone responsiveness of human mammary epithelium. *Proc. Am. Assoc. Cancer Res.,* 17:87.
56. Kwa, H. G., Cleton, F., DeJong-Bakker, M., Bulbrook, R. D., Hayward, J. L., and Wang, D. Y. (1976): Plasma prolactin and its relationship to risk factors in human breast cancer. *Int. J. Cancer,* 17:441–447.
57. Lacassagne, A., and Duplan, J. F. (1959): Le mécanisme de la cancérisation de la mamelle chez la souris, considéré d'après les résultats d'experiences au mojen de la réserpine. *C. R. Acad. Sci. [D] (Paris),* 249:810–812.
58. Laska, E. M., Siegel, C., Meisner, M., Fischer, S., and Wanderlang, J. (1975): Matched-pair study of reserpine use and breast cancer. *Lancet,* 2:296–300.
59. Lathrop, A. E. C., and Loeb, L. (1916): Further investigations on the origin of tumors in mice. III. On the part played by internal secretion in the spontaneous development of tumors. *J. Cancer Res.,* 1:1–19.
60. Liebelt, R. A. (1959): Effects of gold-thioglucose-induced hypothalamic lesions in mammary tumorigenesis in RIII × CBA mice. *Proc. Am. Assoc. Cancer Res.,* 3:37.
61. Liebelt, A. G., and Liebelt, R. A. (1961): Effects of a single pituitary isograft on mammary tumorigenesis in mice. *Cancer Res.,* 21:86–91.
62. Loeb, L., and Kirtz, M. M. (1939): The effects of transplants of anterior lobes of the hypophysis in the growth of the mammary gland and on the development of mammary gland carcinoma in various strains of mice. *Am. J. Cancer,* 36:56–82.
63. Lu, K. H., Amenomori, Y., Chen, C. L., and Meites, J. (1970): Effects of central acting drugs on serum and pituitary prolactin levels in rats. *Endocrinology,* 87:667–672.
64. Lu, K. H., Koch, Y., and Meites, J. (1971): Direct inhibition by ergocornine of pituitary prolactin release. *Endocrinology,* 89:229–233.
65. Lutterbeck, P. M., Pryor, J. S., Varga, L., and Wenner, R. (1971): Treatment of non-puerperal galactorrhoea with an ergot alkaloid. *Br. Med. J.,* 3:228–229.
66. Mack, T. M., Henderson, B. E., Gerkins, V. R., Arthur, M., Baptista, J., and Pike, M. C. (1975): Reserpine and breast cancer in a retirement community. *N. Engl. J. Med.,* 292:1366–1371.
67. Marchant, J. (1959): Local inhibition by lactation of chemically induced breast tumours in mice of the IF strain. *Nature,* 183:629–631.
68. Masters, J. R. W., Sangster, K., and Smith, I. I. (1977): Hormonal sensitivity of human breast tumors in vitro: Pentose-shunt activity. *Cancer,* 39:1978–1980.
69. McCormick, G. M., and Moon, R. C. (1965): Effect of pregnancy and lactation on growth of mammary tumours induced by 7,12-dimethylbenzanthracene (DMBA). *Br. J. Cancer,* 19:160–166.
70. McManus, M. J., Patten, S. E., Pienkowski, M. M., and Welsch, C. W. (1977): Treatment of athymic "nude" mice with human placental lactogen (HPL) enhanced DNA synthesis of grafted human breast tissues. *Physiologist,* 20:62.
71. Medina, D. (1976): Preneoplastic lesions in murine mammary cancer. *Cancer Res.,* 36:2589–2595.
72. Meites, J., Cassell, E., and Clark, J. (1971): Estrogen inhibition of mammary tumor growth in rats; counteraction by prolactin. *Proc. Soc. Exp. Biol. Med.,* 137:1225–1227.
73. Meites, J., and Kragt, C. L. (1964): Effects of a pituitary homotransplant and thyroxine on body and mammary growth in immature hypophysectomized rats. *Endocrinology,* 75:565–570.

74. Meites, J., and Nicoll, C. S. (1966): Adenohypophysis: Prolactin. *Annu. Rev. Physiol.,* 28:57–88.
75. Meites, J., Simpkins, J., Bruni, J., and Advis, J. (1977): Role of biogenic amines in control of anterior pituitary hormones. *I.R.C.S. J. Med. Sci.,* 5:1–7.
76. Middleton, P. J. (1965): The histogenesis of mammary tumours induced in the rat by chemical carcinogens. *Br. J. Cancer,* 19:830–839.
77. Mioduszewska, O., Koszarowski, T., and Gorski, C. (1968): The influence of hormones on breast cancer in vitro in relation to the clinical course of the disease. In: *Prognostic Factors in Breast Cancer,* edited by A. P. M. Forrest and P. P. Kunkler, pp. 347–353. Williams & Wilkins, Baltimore.
78. Minton, J. P. (1974): Prolactin and human breast cancer. *Am. J. Surg.,* 128:628–630.
79. Mittra, I., Hayward, J. L., and McNeilly, A. S. (1974): Hypothalamic-pituitary-prolactin axis in breast cancer. *Lancet,* 1:889–891.
80. Mühlbock, O., and Boot, L. M. (1959): Induction of mammary cancer in mice without the mammary tumor agent by isografts of hypophysis. *Cancer Res.,* 19:402–412.
81. Murray, R. M. L., Mozaffarian, G., and Pearson, O. H. (1972): Prolactin levels with L-dopa treatment in metastatic breast carcinoma. In: *Prolactin and Carcinogenesis,* edited by A. R. Boyns and K. Griffiths, pp. 158–161. Alpha Omega Alpha Publishing, Cardiff, Wales.
82. Nagasawa, H., Kuretani, K., and Kanzawa, F. (1966): Effect of prolactin on the growth of spontaneous mammary tumor in mice. *Gann,* 57:637–640.
83. Nagasawa, H., and Meites, J. (1970): Effect of a hypothalamic estrogen implant on growth of carcinogen-induced mammary tumors in rats. *Cancer Res.,* 30:1327–1329.
84. Nagasawa, H., and Meites, J. (1970): Suppression by ergocornine and iproniazid of carcinogen-induced mammary tumors in rats: Effect on serum and pituitary prolactin levels. *Proc. Soc. Exp. Biol. Med.,* 135:469–472.
85. Nagasawa, H., and Yanai, R. (1970): Effects of prolactin or growth hormone on growth of carcinogen-induced mammary tumors of adreno-ovariectomized rats. *Int. J. Cancer,* 6:488–495.
86. Nagasawa, H., and Yanai, R. (1971): Increased mammary gland response to pituitary mammotropic hormones by estrogen in rats. *Endocrinol. Jpn.,* 18:53–56.
87. Nagasawa, H., and Yanai, R. (1973): Effect of human placental lactogen on growth of carcinogen-induced mammary tumors in rats. *Int. J. Cancer,* 11:131–137.
88. Nagasawa, H., and Yanai, R. (1974): Frequency of mammary cell division in relation to age: Its significance in the induction of mammary tumors by carcinogen in rats. *J. Natl. Cancer Inst.,* 52:609–610.
89. Nagasawa, H., Yanai, R., Iwahashi, H., Fujimoto, M., and Kuretani, K. (1967): Effect of pituitary isografts on the growth of spontaneous mammary tumor in mice. *Gann,* 58:337–342.
90. Nagasawa, H., Yanai, R., Taneguchi, H., Tokuzen, R., and Nakahara, W. (1976): Two-way selection of a stock of Swiss-albino mice of mammary tumorigenesis: Establishment of two new strains (SHN and SLN). *J. Natl. Cancer Inst.,* 57:425–430.
91. O'Fallon, W. M., Labarthe, D. R., and Kurland, L. T. (1975): Rauwolfia derivatives and breast cancer. *Lancet,* 2:292–296.
92. Pass, K. A., and Meites, J. (1977): Enhanced growth of carcinogen-induced mammary tumors in rats by sulpiride. *I.R.C.S. J. Med. Sci.,* 5:241.
93. Pearson, O. H., Llerena, O., Llerena, L., Molina, A., and Butler, T. (1969): Prolactin-dependent rat mammary cancer: A model for man? *Trans. Assoc. Am. Physicians,* 82:225–238.
94. Quadri, S. K., Clark, J. L., and Meites, J. (1973): Effects of LSD, pargyline and haloperidol on mammary tumor growth in rats. *Proc. Soc. Exp. Biol. Med.,* 142:22–26.
95. Quadri, S. K., Kledzik, G. S., and Meites, J. (1973): Effects of L-dopa and methyl-dopa on growth of mammary cancers in rats. *Proc. Soc. Exp. Biol. Med.,* 142:759–761.
96. Quadri, S. K., Kledzik, G. S., and Meites, J. (1974): Enhanced regression of DMBA-induced mammary cancers in rats by combination of ergocornine with ovariectomy or high doses of estrogen. *Cancer Res.,* 34:499–501.
97. Rolandi, E., Barreca, T., Masturzo, P., Polleri, A., Indiveri, F., and Barabino, A. (1974): Plasma prolactin in breast cancer. *Lancet,* 2:845–846.
98. Schulz, K. D., Czygan, P. J., del Pozo, E., and Friesen, H. G. (1973): Varying response of human metastasizing breast cancer to the treatment with 2-Br-α-ergocryptine (CB-154). Case report. In: *Human Prolactin,* edited by C. Robyn and J. L. Pasteels, pp. 268–271. Excerpta Medica/American Elsevier, New York.

99. Sheth, N. A., Ranadive, K. J., Suraiya, J. N., and Sheth, A. R. (1975): Circulating levels of prolactin in human breast cancer. *Br. J. Cancer,* 32:160–167.
100. Shiu, R. P. C., Kelly, P. A., and Friesen, H. G. (1973): Radioreceptor assay for prolactin and other lactogenic hormones. *Science,* 180:968–971.
101. Simonel, C. E., Brooks, C. L., and Welsch, C. W. (1975): Effects of ether anesthesia on plasma prolactin sampling. *Experientia,* 31:688–689.
102. Sinha, D., Cooper, D., and Dao, T. L. (1973): The nature of estrogen and prolactin effect on mammary tumorigenesis. *Cancer Res.,* 33:411–414.
103. Sinha, Y. N., Salocks, C. B., Lewis, U. J., and Vanderlaan, W. P. (1974): Influence of nursing on the release of prolactin and GH in mice with high and low incidence of mammary tumors. *Endocrinology,* 95:947–954.
104. Sinha, Y. N., Selby, F. W., and Vanderlaan, W. P. (1974): The natural history of prolactin and GH secretion in mice with high and low incidence of mammary tumors. *Endocrinology,* 94:757–764.
105. Sluyser, M., and Van Nie, R. (1974): Estrogen receptor content and hormone responsive growth of mouse mammary tumors. *Cancer Res.,* 34:3253–3257.
106. Sterental, A., Dominguez, J. M., Weissman, C., and Pearson, O. H. (1963): Pituitary role in the estrogen dependency of experimental mammary cancer. *Cancer Res.,* 23:481–484.
107. Stoll, B. A. (1972): Brain catecholamines and breast cancer. A hypothesis. *Lancet,* 1:431–432.
108. Sweeney, M. J., Poore, G. A., Kornfeld, E. C., Bach, N. J., Owen, N. V., and Clemens, J. A. (1975): Activity of 6-methyl-8-substituted ergolines against the 7,12-dimethylbenzanthracene-induced mammary carcinoma. *Cancer Res.,* 35:106–109.
109. Talwalker, P. K., Meites, J., and Mizuno, H. (1964): Mammary tumor induction by estrogen or anterior pituitary hormones in ovariectomized rats given 7,12-dimethylbenzanthracene. *Proc. Soc. Exp. Biol. Med.,* 116:531–534.
110. Welsch, C. W. (1971): Growth inhibition of rat mammary carcinoma induced by cis-platinum diammino-dichloride-II. *J. Natl. Cancer Inst.,* 47:1071–1078.
111. Welsch, C. W. (1972): Effect of brain lesions on mammary tumorigenesis. In: *Estrogen Target Tissues and Neoplasia,* edited by T. L. Dao, pp. 317–331. University of Chicago Press, Chicago.
112. Welsch, C. W. (1975): The role of the neuroendocrine system in murine mammary tumorigenesis. In: *Host Defense against Cancer and Its Potentiation,* edited by D. Mizuno, G. Chihara, F. Fukuoka, T. Yamamoto, and Y. Yamamura, pp. 281–301. University Park Press, Baltimore.
113. Welsch, C. W. (1976): Interaction of estrogen and prolactin in spontaneous mammary tumorigenesis of the mouse. *J. Toxicol. Environ. Health* [*Suppl.*], 1:161–175.
114. Welsch, C. W. (1976): Prophylaxis of early preneoplastic lesions of the mammary gland. *Cancer Res.,* 36:2621–2625.
115. Welsch, C. W., Adams, C., Lambrecht, L. K., Hassett, C. C., and Brooks, C. L. (1977): 17β-Oestradiol and enovid mammary tumorigenesis in C3H/HeJ female mice: Counteraction by concurrent 2-bromo-α-ergocryptine. *Br. J. Cancer,* 35:322–328.
116. Welsch, C. W., Calaf de Iturri, G., and Brennan, M. J. (1976): DNA synthesis of human, mouse and rat mammary carcinomas in vitro: Influence of insulin and prolactin. *Cancer,* 38:1272–1281.
117. Welsch, C. W., and Clemens, J. A. (1973): 6-methyl-8-β-ergoline-acetonitrile-induced inhibition of mammary hyperplastic alveolar nodular development and growth in C3H/HeJ female mice. *Proc. Soc. Exp. Biol. Med.,* 142:1067–1071.
118. Welsch, C. W., Clemens, J. A., and Meites, J. (1968): Effects of multiple pituitary homografts or progesterone on 7,12-dimethylbenzanthracene-induced mammary tumors in rats. *J. Natl. Cancer Inst.,* 41:465–471.
119. Welsch, C. W., Clemens, J. A., and Meites, J. (1969): Effects of hypothalamic and amygdaloid lesions on development and growth of carcinogen-induced mammary tumors in the female rat. *Cancer Res.,* 29:1541–1549.
120. Welsch, C. W., and Gribler, C. (1973): Prophylaxis of spontaneously developing mammary carcinoma in C3H/HeJ female mice by suppression of prolactin. *Cancer Res.,* 33:2939–2946.
121. Welsch, C. W., Gribler, C., and Clemens, J. A. (1974): 6-methyl-8-β-ergoline-acetonitrile (MEA)-induced suppression of mammary tumorigenesis in C3H/HeJ female mice. *Eur. J. Cancer,* 10:595–600.
122. Welsch, C. W., Iturri, G., and Meites, J. (1973): Comparative effects of hypophysectomy, ergocornine and ergocornine-reserpine treatments on rat mammary carcinoma. *Int. J. Cancer,* 12:206–212.

123. Welsch, C. W., Jenkins, T. W., and Meites, J. (1970): Increased incidence of mammary tumors in the female rat grafted with multiple pituitaries. *Cancer Res.,* 30:1024–1029.
124. Welsch, C. W., Lambrecht, L. K., and Hassett, C. C. (1977): Suppression of mammary tumorigenesis in C3H/He mice by ovariectomy or treatment with 2-bromo-α-ergocryptine: A comparison. *J. Natl. Cancer Inst.,* 58:1135–1138.
125. Welsch, C. W., Louks, G., Fox, D., and Brooks, C. (1975): Enhancement by prolactin of carcinogen induced mammary cancerigenesis in the male rat. *Br. J. Cancer,* 32:427–431.
126. Welsch, C. W., and McManus, M. J. (1977): Stimulation of DNA synthesis by human placental lactogen or insulin in organ cultures of benign human breast tumors. *Cancer Res.,* 37:2257–2261.
127. Welsch, C. W., and Meites, J. (1969): Effects of a norethynodrel-mestranol combination (enovid) on development and growth of carcinogen-induced mammary tumors in female rats. *Cancer,* 23:601–607.
128. Welsch, C. W., and Meites, J. (1970): Effects of reserpine on development of 7,12-dimethylbenzanthracene-induced mammary tumors in female rats. *Experientia,* 26:1133–1134.
129. Welsch, C. W., and Morford, L. K. (1974): Influence of chronic treatment with 2-bromo-α-ergocryptine (CB-154) on the reproductive and lactational performance of the C3H/HeJ mouse. *Experientia,* 30:1353–1355.
130. Welsch, C. W., Nagasawa, H., and Meites, J. (1970): Increased incidence of spontaneous mammary tumors in female rats with induced hypothalamic lesions. *Cancer Res.,* 30:2310–2313.
131. Welsch, C. W., and Nagasawa, H. (1977): Prolactin and murine mammary tumorigenesis: A review. *Cancer Res.,* 37:951–963.
132. Welsch, C. W., and Rivera, E. M. (1972): Differential effects of estrogen and prolactin on DNA synthesis in organ cultures of DMBA-induced rat mammary carcinoma. *Proc. Soc. Exp. Biol. Med.,* 139:623–626.
133. Welsch, C. W., Squiers, M. D., Cassell, E., Chen, C. L., and Meites, J. (1971): Median eminence lesions and serum prolactin: Influence of ovariectomy and ergocornine. *Am. J. Physiol.,* 221:1714–1717.
134. White, F. R. (1961): The relationship between underfeeding and tumor formation, transplantation, and growth in rats and mice. *Cancer Res.,* 21:281–290.
135. Wilson, R. G., Buchan, R., Roberts, M. M., Forrest, A. P. M., Boyns, A. R., Cole, E. N., and Griffiths, K. (1974): Plasma prolactin and breast cancer. *Cancer,* 33:1325–1327.
136. Wuttke, W., and Meites, J. (1971): Luteolytic role of prolactin during the estrous cycle of the rat. *Proc. Soc. Exp. Biol. Med.,* 137:988–991.
137. Yanai, R., and Nagasawa, H. (1971): Mammary growth and placental mammotropin during pregnancy in mice with high or low lactational performance. *J. Dairy Sci.,* 54:906–910.
138. Yanai, R., and Nagasawa, H. (1972): Inhibition of mammary tumorigenesis by ergot alkaloids and promotion of mammary tumorigenesis by pituitary isografts in adreno-ovariectomized mice. *J. Natl. Cancer Inst.,* 48:715–719.
139. Young, S. (1961): Induction of mammary carcinoma in hypophysectomized rats treated with 3-methylcholanthrene, oestradiol-17β, progesterone and growth hormone. *Nature,* 190:356–357.

Endocrine Control in Neoplasia, edited by
R. K. Sharma and W. E. Criss.
Raven Press, New York © 1978.

Hormonal Control in Animal Breast Cancer

V. P. Hollander and E. J. Diamond

Research Institute for Skeletomuscular Diseases, Hospital for Joint Diseases and Medical Center, New York, New York 10035

Endocrine support of normal and neoplastic mammary tissue has been the subject of several excellent reviews (33,42). This chapter will attempt to place the work carried out in our laboratory over recent years into the framework sketched by these reviews. Our recent studies have been concerned with generation of sublines of transplantable rat tumors that differ in hormone receptor content and ovariectomy-induced regression. Evidence will be presented for the existence of a humoral factor (as yet uncharacterized) that inhibits ovariectomy-induced regression. These findings will be discussed with respect to the suitability of this tumor system as a model for human disease; they will also be discussed in terms of how they relate to the known endocrine factors that influence mammary tumor growth, regression, and viability. It is suggested that tumor receptor content is not a genetic marker and that it may be altered by changing the endocrine environment, with consequent alteration in therapeutic response.

RODENT MODELS FOR MAMMARY TUMORS

Selection of an optimal model for biochemical study of endocrine control of the growth of mammary cancer depends on the resemblance of the model to human mammary cancer and on the particular focus of the investigator. We were concerned with determining why certain mammary tumors that contained both prolactin and estradiol receptor failed to regress after ovariectomy. For this study we required a model that would provide reproducible tumors that were both ovariectomy-responsive and -resistant. Thus it was possible to restrict our review of useful models to carcinogen-induced and transplantable tumors in mice and rats.

Mouse Mammary Tumors

The development of spontaneous tumors in mice depends on viral, genetic, and hormonal factors. These factors were reviewed by Foulds who presented an excellent bibliography of the older literature (25). Unfortunately, the endocrine factors required for tumorigenesis ceased to operate once tumors developed within hyperplastic mammary nodules. Neither administration of steroids nor ovariectomy influenced the behavior of most mouse tumors once they had developed. However, there were some interesting exceptions described by Foulds. These involved tumors arising in BR mice (C57 ♀ × RIII ♂) that were transplantable to female mice but not to male mice. Ovariectomy prevented prompt outgrowth of transplants, and insertion of diethylstilbestrol (DES), pellets in castrates allowed for growth. The refractory state of the male was overcome by an increase in transplant inoculum size. In some hosts, pregnancy increased the growth of transplants, which then regressed after parturition, only to recur with subsequent pregnancy. This murine system is very interesting, but it is difficult to maintain, and it is not sufficiently reproducible for the studies that are our major theme (23,24). An excellent review surveying the role of prolactin in murine mammary tumorigenesis has recently appeared (98). A reproducible transplantable mouse mammary tumor has been described that is ovarian-dependent, but it will grow in the ovariectomized mouse treated with estradiol benzoate. The tumor is induced by administration of urethane to (C57BL × DBAf) F_1 mice. It is readily transplantable, and it should be convenient for many biochemical studies (96).

Rat Mammary Tumors

If one were to select the model that has had the most profound effect on our understanding of endocrine effects in mammary cancer, carcinogen-induced cancer in the rat would be the choice. Shay demonstrated that intragastric administration of methylcholanthrene (MCA)[1] to rats resulted in frequent development of mammary cancer (8). Huggins described production of mammary cancers in all Sprague-Dawley rats given intragastric dimethylbenzanthracene (DMBA) according to a definite technique (36). Hilf provided an excellent description of many biochemical studies using DMBA-induced tumors (32). Studies of hormone receptors, growth stimulation, and regression in these tumors will be discussed elsewhere in this review. The advantages of DMBA tumors are their ready availability and the high frequency with which hormone dependency is found. However, tumors arising in Sprague-Dawley rats are not transplantable, and DMBA tumor induction in inbred rats is not as reproducible as in Sprague-Dawley rats. For this reason and other reasons that will become apparent, we chose to study the mechanism of ovariectomy regression in transplantable rat tumors.

---

[1] The abbreviations used in this chapter include the following: MCA, methylcholanthrene; DMBA, dimethylbenanthracene; W/Fu, Wistar-Furth rats; MTW9, a transplantable mammary carcinoma grown in female W/Fu rats; MtT, a mammosomatotropic tumor; MTW9-MtT, MTW9 supported by coimplantation with a mammosomatotropic tumor; MtTW5 and MtTW10, mammosomatotropic tumors; MtTW5-OM, a growth-hormone-secreting variant of MtTW5; MTW9-P, a variant of MTW9 obtained by daily perphenazine administration; MTW9-PD, MTW9-P after cessation of perphenazine administration.

Transplantable Rat Mammary Carcinomas

Huggins's discovery that all Sprague-Dawley rats given intragastric MCA or DMBA develop mammary cancer gave investigators a large supply of primary tumors, each presumably different from the others. Because Sprague-Dawley rats are not inbred, the resulting tumors are not transplantable. For many biochemical investigations it is highly desirable to have a stable transplantable tumor line. Mammary tumors do not occur in W/Fu rats after a single dose of intragastric MCA unless the mammary glands are stimulated by growth of a transplantable mammosomatotropic tumor. Furth developed dose schedules that would allow all W/Fu rats treated over a period of time with intragastric carcinogen to develop mammary cancers. Most of these tumors were only partially endocrine-dependent in that they would regress after ovariectomy or hypophysectomy but would grow in normal hosts of both sexes. The tumors were readily transplantable, and many strains developed in Furth's laboratory maintained their biological behavior for many years. The strain that we have used in most of our studies, MTW9, was developed by giving a subcarcinogenic dose (10 mg) of intragastric 3-MCA to a W/Fu rat bearing a mammosomatotropic tumor. Furth perpetuated MTW9 by transplant because it failed to grow in normal females, but grew in both male and female rats bearing MtT. Because of the exceptional stability of this strain and the ease of transplantation of the mammary and mammosomatotropic tumors, it was selected as the tumor of choice in most of our studies (47–50).

HORMONAL REQUIREMENTS FOR GROWTH OF MTW9

Effect of Ovariectomy on Rats Bearing MTW9-MtT

MacLeod et al. (61) studied the hormonal requirements for growth of MTW9. The purpose of the study was to determine whether ovarian hormones played a role in the growth of this mammary tumor. When growth of MTW9 was supported by MtTW5 or MtTW10, mammosomatotropic tumors developed by Furth ovariectomy (46,101) produced no tumor regression (21,67). Furth had suggested that a mammotropic hormone secreted by a cell of pituitary origin was the primary stimulus for the growth of normal and neoplastic mammary cells (47). Estrogen was relegated to a secondary role, i.e., the stimulation of prolactin secretion. However, Lyons had demonstrated direct estrogen stimulation of lobuloalveolar development in rat mammary tissue. The local effects of estrogen pellets on mammary tissue were clearly demonstrated with hormone doses that gave no systemic effects (60). It was soon learned that when ovariectomy was performed at the time of implantation of MTW9 and MtTW5, MTW9 did not grow. MtTW5 grew as well in ovariectomized rats as in intact animals (61). When ovariectomy was delayed after implantation of MTW9 and MtT, the inhibition of MTW9 growth became less, so that rats spayed 30 days after both tumors were inoculated had large mammary tumors 14 days later. MTW9 grew perfectly well in ovariectomized rats if both estradiol and progesterone were administered daily. Although administration of either estradiol or progesterone allowed some tumor growth, the latent period of MTW9 growth was long, and the tumors were quite small. The combination of 10 μg estradiol and 3 mg progesterone daily resulted in growth of MTW9 supported by MtTW5 in spayed rats that was equal to the growth in intact animals. This result demonstrated that progesterone was an important growth factor in the early development of MTW9, and it raised a question regarding the relatively high dose of estradiol. Did estradiol administration allow MTW9 to develop because MtT produced insufficient prolactin in the absence of ovarian hormones, or did estrogen have some direct stimulatory effect on the mammary tumor cell? Estrogen administration was known to increase serum prolactin in normal animals, and ovariectomy was known to reduce serum prolactin (1). Perhaps ovariectomy prevented MtTW5 from secreting sufficient prolactin for the support of MTW9. The question was resolved by Murota and Hollander (72). Figure 1 shows the sizes of MTW9 and MtTW5 at different times after both tumors were inoculated into W/Fu rats weighing 160 to 170 g. In the same figure, serum prolactin as determined by radioimmunoassay is plotted. MtT was palpable 1 month after implantation, but it required another month to attain measurable size, at which

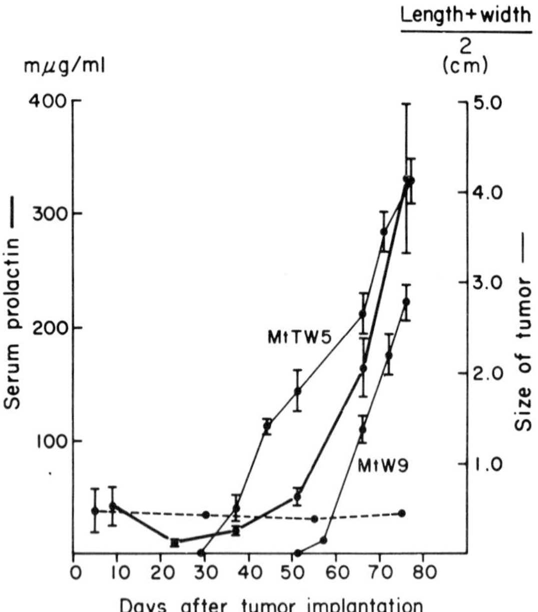

FIG. 1. Growth of two implanted tumors is illustrated by labeled thinner lines. Mean value of serum prolactin in 6 intact female control rats is illustrated by dashed line. Heavy line illustrates changes in serum prolactin that accompany growth of MtT. (From Murota and Hollander, ref. 72, with permission.)

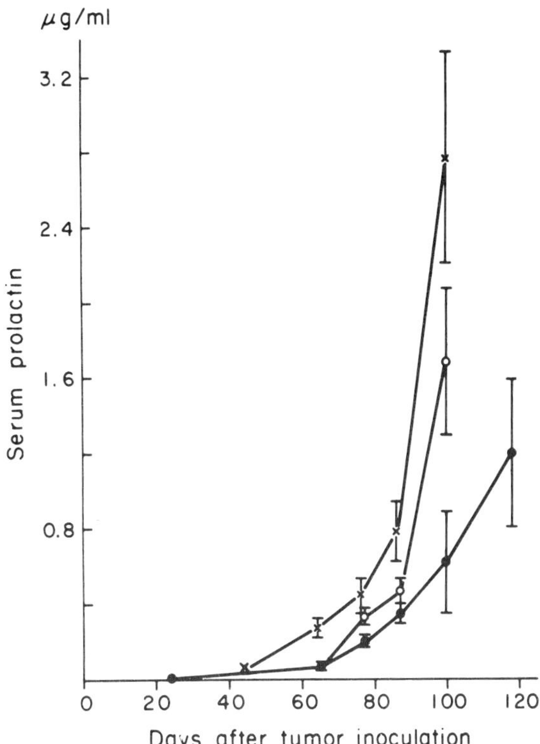

FIG. 2. Rises in serum prolactin levels in control *(crosses)*, ovariectomized *(filled circles)* and oophorectomized steroid-treated *(open circles)* rats. The three groups of 6 rats each were implanted with MtT and MTW9 at day 0. Oophorectomy was performed on following day. In the steroid-treated group, 10 μg of estradiol 17β and 3 mg of progesterone were injected daily, starting on day 65. (From Murota and Hollander, ref. 72, with permission.)

time serum prolactin was much higher than in control rats. Growth of MTW9 coincided with increased serum prolactin and was rapid when the latter reached 200 ng/ml. Figure 2 shows that although ovariectomized rats bearing MtT had lower serum prolactin concentrations than did comparable animals with intact ovarian function, diminished serum prolactin concentration was always well above normal and was in a range that should have supported growth of MTW9. The late restoration of the depressed serum prolactin concentration by ovarian steroids is also shown. The study shows that the failure of MTW9 to grow in the spayed rat bearing MtTW5 is not a result of insufficient prolactin concentration but results directly from a deficiency of ovarian steroids.

MtT Stimulation of MTW9

Mammosomatotropic tumors MtTW5 and MtTW10 are known to secrete large amounts of prolactin and growth hormone (38,46). Various lines of evidence support the belief that prolactin is the hormone secreted by MtT that is responsible for growth of MTW9.

When MTW9 is transplanted into W/Fu rats bearing no MtT but having pituitary isografts beneath the renal capsule, the mammary tumor grows. Animals bearing pituitary isografts have high levels of serum prolactin; other pituitary hormones are secreted at a minimal rate. In our studies MTW9 grew well in hypophysectomized rats transplanted with two pituitary isografts beneath the renal capsule and maintained by injection of 6 U ACTH every 10 days (61). These experiments demonstrated that MtT could be replaced by pituitary transplants, which gave rise to high levels of serum prolactin and presumably to low concentrations of other known pituitary hormones. Adrenal steroid hormones may have played a role in allowing growth. When MTW9 is coimplanted with MtTW5-OM, a transplantable variant of MtTW5 that secretes little prolactin and large amounts of growth hormone (35), the mammary tumor fails to grow (unpublished observation). MTW9 grows in rats subjected to chronic perphenazine administration (MTW9-P) without coimplantation of MtT. In such animals serum prolactin is increased (21). However, phenothiazine administration results in decreased secretion of gonadotropins and growth hormone (90,91). When perphenazine administration is stopped, most tumors (MTW9-PD) neither grow nor regress; only 20% show even limited growth. When ovine prolactin is administered to such rats bearing MTW9-PD, the tumors resume rapid growth coincident with a sharp increase in serum prolactin. Administration of growth hormone shows only slight stimulation of MTW9. These studies indicate that prolactin, rather than growth hormone, is the peptide hormone secreted by MtT that is responsible for the growth of MTW9. The roles of the steroid hormones are complex; ovarian hormones are required for initial growth of MTW9 in rats bearing MtT, but after ovariectomy no tumor regression occurs. The roles of ovarian hormones will be discussed in detail along with the mechanism of ovariectomy-induced regression.

MTW9 in Perphenazine-treated Rats

When MTW9 is transplanted into hosts bearing mammosomatotropic tumors, the mammary tumors grow rapidly. We call this mammary tumor MTW9-MtT. Coimplantation of MTW9 with MtTW10 is a convenient method for routine maintenance of MTW9, but it exposes the tumor not only to the required high concentration of serum prolactin but also to high levels of serum growth hormone and other abnormalities to be discussed later. We have shown that MTW9 can be grown in rats with high levels of serum prolactin produced by transplantation of pituitaries beneath the renal capsule or by administration of prolactin (61). Chronic administration of perphenazine appears to be a convenient method for maintenance of a high level of serum prolactin without an increase in other pituitary hormones (5). Pearson et al. (74) and Bogden et al. (7) have shown that chronic perphenazine administration increases serum prolactin and stimulates growth of DMBA-induced and transplantable rat mammary tumors. Our study demonstrates that MTW9 can be conveniently grown in rats given chronic perphenazine treatment (MTW9-P) and that important differences between the parent MTW9-MtT and MTW9-P can be shown.

MTW9 obtained from rats in which the mammary tumor was supported by MtTW10 was finely minced with an equal volume of medium 199 containing penicillin and streptomycin; 0.6 ml was injected subcutaneously into the right flank of each 150-g W/Fu female rat. Perphenazine (4 mg/kg) was injected daily. Animals receiving perphenazine were maintained at 27 to 28°C because the drug deranges body temperature control (W. McGuire gave us helpful advice on the care of perphenazine-treated rats). No effect on growth or on other biological behavior was observed when rats bearing MTW9-MtT were maintained at 27 to 28°C or the usual 22 to 23°C. Tumors implanted in rats given chronic perphenazine treatment were palpable between 26 and 40 days, and they achieved an average diameter of 1 to 1.5 cm in 50 days. MTW9-MtT grows faster than MTW9-P; MTW9-MtT-bearing rats have much higher serum prolactin concentrations (500–7,000 ng/ml) than those with MTW9-P (250–600 ng/ml). However, MTW9-P proved a convenient source of tumor for chemical study. MTW9-P cannot be distinguished by light microscopy from MTW9-MtT. The high serum prolactin concentrations of perphenazine-treated animals (250–600 ng/ml) declined to normal values within 24 hr after stopping perphenazine. When perphenazine treatment was discontinued, the mammary tumor (now referred to as MTW9-PD) did not regress but remained stationary for months. The most interesting difference between MTW9-MtT and MTW9-P is observed after ovariectomy. MTW9-MtT does not regress after ovariectomy, MTW9-P does regress. MTW9-PD, the tumor that remains after perphenazine administration is stopped, also regresses after ovariectomy. When ovariectomy is carried out in rats bearing MTW9-P and perphenazine administration is continued, serum prolactin decreases, presumably as a result of lowered serum estradiol concentration, but it remains above the 200 ng/ml previously established as the limiting requirement for growth of MTW9. In spite of the fact that there is a concentration of serum prolactin adequate for growth, the mammary tumor invariably shows significant or complete regression after ovariectomy. When MTW9-P has completely regressed after ovariectomy, the tumor recurs and grows well if 5 to 10 μg of estradiol are administered daily.

Study of MTW9 growth in perphenazine-treated rats shows that an ovariectomy-responsive tumor (MTW9-P) can be derived from a nonresponsive tumor (MTW9-MtT). Estradiol and prolactin receptors have been measured in the two tumors in an effort to explain the appearance of ovariectomy response.

TUMOR RECEPTORS

The first step in hormonal action involves recognition of the effector by specific receptors that bind the ligand with a tight but noncovalent linkage. Different mechanisms then transmit the hormonal stimulus to appropriate loci. Steroid hormones are bound by specific cytosol receptor; the hormone-receptor complex is then activated, transported to the nucleus, and bound to genomic material, where it interacts to modulate gene activity. Peptide hormones are bound by membrane receptors; hormone-receptor complex activates intermediate processes usually involving cyclic nucleotides, and gene modulation is accomplished through activation of appropriate protein kinases. Receptor studies have already contributed to our knowledge of the neoplastic state and to the practical management of patients with breast cancer (18,66).

Growth of the mammary gland is influenced by a number of hormones: insulin, estradiol, prolactin, growth hormone, progesterone, and thyroid hormones (2,17). Of these, estradiol and prolactin have been subjected to the most study; we shall consider them together in the next section because our laboratory has been concerned with their interaction.

Estradiol Receptors

The early studies of Jensen were responsible for our concepts about specific hormonal binding to target organs in general and the interactions of estrogens with receptors in particular (41,42). Estrogen enters the cell by diffusion and binds to a specific cytosol receptor. Such interaction can be studied by sucrose gradient centrifugation, which readily distinguishes an ionic-strength-dependent interconversion of 8S and 4S cytosol receptors. The latter undergoes a temperature-dependent conversion to a 5S receptor that can enter the nucleus, where it is bound to chromatin material. Nuclear-bound hormone-receptor complex is dissociated by 0.3 M KCl, and 5S hormone-receptor complex is extracted. These observations were repeated with lactating mammary gland, and substantial 8S estradiol receptor was found that also underwent conversion to a 5S nuclear-bound form (26,85). These studies suggested that some human mammary cancers might contain estradiol receptor. It was soon found that about one-half of human breast tumors contain receptor and that tumors that lack estradiol receptor almost never respond to hormonal therapy. These human studies are of great theoretical importance and practical utility. They have been well reviewed (42,66) and will not be discussed further here; this review will concentrate on animal models with emphasis on our studies using MTW9.

Specific estradiol receptors have been found in DMBA-induced mammary tumors (43,51,70). McGuire and associates (69,71) studied estradiol receptors in R3230AC, a transplantable mammary tumor described by Hilf and associates (34). Although injected ^{3}H-estradiol did not localize in R3230AC nuclei as it did in the nuclei of most DMBA-induced tumors, these nuclei were able to bind estradiol receptor complex from rat uterus. This experiment attributed the failure of *in vivo* localization to lack of estradiol cytosol receptor in the tumor, and showed that tumor chromatin from nonresponsive cells could not be distinguished from nuclei of tumors that show excellent regression after ovariectomy (67,68).

Since binding of estradiol receptor complex to target cell nuclei shows neither specificity nor saturation (11,12), it is unlikely that nuclear binding studies in tumor will be helpful unless a method is found to distinguish specific sites. For this reason we have confined our own studies to estradiol cytosol receptors.

Since it soon became apparent that MTW9-P derived from MTW9-MtT had much more cytosol estradiol receptor than the original tumor, prolactin binding studies were also made on these tumors.

Prolactin Receptors

In contrast to the cytoplasmic and nuclear binding of estradiol, prolactin acts at the cell surface (6,93). There is evidence that binding of ^{125}I-prolactin to several tissues is related to dependence on the hormone (76,92).

DeSombre and associates (19) studied the binding of estradiol and prolactin to receptors in 24 DMBA-induced mammary tumors in Sprague-Dawley rats. The hormone receptor concentration was correlated with tumor regression after ovariectomy or hypophysectomy. Estradiol receptor was present in all tumors; values ranged from barely detectable (18 fmoles/g tumor) to extremely high (2,875 fmoles/g tumor). Prolactin receptor was detected in all but three tumors, and the range of concentration was also very great. All tumors with high content of both receptors proved hormone-dependent; only one tumor with low content of both receptors proved dependent. In the group with one receptor content low and the other high, there were both dependent and independent tumors. These studies demonstrated that both receptors are important for the growth of DMBA-induced tumors. They showed the variation that may be expected in receptor content of primary carcinogen-induced tumors. However, the relevance of both estradiol binding and prolactin binding in tumor growth was clearly shown by these studies.

Estradiol Binding Methods

Estradiol binding for total and occupied sites was measured in tumor cytosol by a modification of the method of Katzenellenbogen and associates (45). Tumor cytosols were diluted with 10 mM MOPS, 1.5 mM EDTA, 1 mM dithiothreitol, and 0.02% NaN_3 (pH 7.5) to a protein concentration between 1.5 and 5.0 mg/ml and incubated with a saturating concentration (8.5–12 nM of ^{3}H-estradiol). For the assay of empty binding sites, incubation was carried out at 0° C for 1 hr, but binding remained constant at this temperature for 18 hr. Total binding sites (empty sites plus sites filled by endogenous hormone) were measured by exchange at 25° C for an additional 3 hr. Specific binding was estimated as the difference between the levels of binding in the absence and presence of a

100-fold excess of nonradioactive estradiol. Bound and free hormones were separated by dextran-coated charcoal (20).

When K_a (approximately 10^{10} M^{-1}) was measured by Scatchard analysis of binding to cytosols, no significant differences between tumors were found, but there were striking differences in numbers of sites between MTW9 supported by MtT and MTW9 supported by perphenazine.

Prolactin Binding Methods

Tumor membrane suspensions were prepared by the method of Shiu et al. (84). They were incubated for 24 hr at 4°C with ^{125}I-prolactin (125 μCi/μg) in 0.025 M Tris-HCl (pH 7.6), 10 mM $CaCl_2$, and 1% BSA. The incubation mixture was then diluted and centrifuged, and the pellet was washed before measurement of bound radioactivity. Nonspecific binding was measured as the binding that occurred in a similar incubation to which a 2,000-fold excess of nonradioactive prolactin was added. Tumor membrane preparations gave linear Scatchard plots when studied at different hormone concentrations. The K_a values (approximately 1.2×10^9 M^{-1}) were similar for membrane preparations from different tumors, but the numbers of sites were quite different.

Receptor Studies on MTW9

Table 1 summarizes the estradiol and prolactin binding studies carried out on MTW9-MtT and MTW9-P. The two tumors had very different receptor contents; both ligands showed fourfold more binding to MTW9-P than to MTW9-MtT. When perphenazine administration was stopped, no change in tumor size occurred in MTW9-P, but estradiol binding decreased. When the mammosomatotropic tumor MtTW10 that supported the growth of MTW9 was surgically resected, the prolactin receptor content of tumor membranes doubled, but the estradiol receptor showed no apparent change. In view of the strikingly different effects of ovariectomy on the two tumors, it was surprising that this procedure did not produce more of an effect on hormone receptor

TABLE 1. *Effect of endocrine environment on hormonal receptors*

	MTW9-P		MTW9-MtT	
	Prolactin[a]	Estradiol[a]	Prolactin[a]	Estradiol[a]
Control	12.2 ± 1.3[b,c]	196 ± 29	2.9 ± 0.3	48 ± 3.6
Stop perphenazine	12.2 ± 1.7	86 ± 6	—	—
Resect MtT	—	—	7.5 ± 0.3	41 ± 5.5
Ovariectomy	11.3 ± 1.5	271 ± 63	3.7 ± 0.8	34 ± 0.78

[a] No changes in K_a for either hormone.
[b] Mean ± SE.
[c] Hormone (fmoles) bound specifically per milligram of protein.

content. These results must be examined from the standpoint of receptor occupancy by endogenous hormone and from the standpoint of regulation of hormone receptor content by alteration in the endocrine environment.

The effect of endogenous hormone occupation of receptor sites must always be evaluated when such sites are measured. If binding sites are occupied at the time of assay by nonradioactive hormones, the sites will not be detected unless exchange with radioactive hormone occurs under the conditions of the assay. The possibility that the difference in estradiol receptor contents between MTW9-MtT and MTW9-P could be attributed to a large number of cytosol binding sites occupied by nonradioactive hormone in MTW9-MtT was critically examined. The possibility was considered unlikely because serum estradiol[2] was lower in hosts bearing MTW9-MtT (11.4 ± 4.0 pg/ml) than in hosts bearing MTW9-P[2] (28.9 ± 6.4 pg/ml). Such a difference in hormone concentrations would tend to fill more sites in the perphenazine-supported tumor and would give a result opposite from that observed. Ovariectomy of MTW9-MtT-bearing rats either had no effect or caused a small decrease in estradiol binding sites. The fall in serum estradiol that occurs after ovariectomy would be expected to increase the observed binding sites if endogenous hormone played a role in the measurement. Finally, estradiol binding was measured under conditions that allowed exchange of occupied sites with tracer hormone. No significant differences were found in estradiol receptor content before and after exchange. Sakai and Saez (79) studied human mammary cancers by an exchange assay and also concluded that differences in receptor content of tumors could not be explained on the basis of receptor sites initially filled with endogenous hormone.

It is unlikely that the difference in prolactin binding between MTW9-MtT and MTW9-P can be attributed to cold occupancy that results from the higher levels of serum prolactin of MtT-bearing animals. MtT resection of animals bearing MTW9-MtT results in a rise in prolactin receptor content (Table 1) consistent with such an explanation. However, when perphenazine administration is stopped in animals bearing MTW9-P, serum prolactin falls, but the receptor content is unchanged. This finding is inconsistent with the concept of cold occupancy, but further study is required to correlate serum prolactin levels at different times after perphenazine administration with estradiol and prolactin binding in perphenazine-treated rats.

Insulin Binding Studies in MTW9

The role of insulin in the growth of experimental mammary tumors has recently been reviewed (33); it will be discussed by Dr. J. Heuson, a fellow contributor to this volume. We will briefly review preliminary studies that were carried

[2] Serum estradiol was measured by radioimmunoassay in the laboratory of Neena Schwartz, Northwestern University.

out in our laboratory to determine whether or not insulin is an important gorwth factor for MTW9.

MTW9-MtT grows in rats chronically exposed to elevated levels of serum insulin. Coimplantation with a mammosomatotropic tumor increases serum insulin (64,89), and growth hormone is known to increase serum insulin (3,15). For these reasons we believed it important to evaluate the role of insulin. We predicted that insulin receptor sites would be found in MTW9 cells and that their characteristics would change as a function of endocrine environment. In preliminary experiments, we found no differences in insulin binding to MTW9 membranes prepared from hosts bearing mammosomatotropic tumors as compared to those receiving daily injections of perphenazine. Alterations of the hormonal environment of MTW9-MtT by MtT resection, by induction of streptozotocin diabetes, or by administration of estradiol (20 μg/day) did not elicit any differences in insulin binding. At present, the techniques available may not be sensitive enough to detect differences in insulin binding sites that may result from hormonal manipulation. We hope that further studies will be able to delineate chemical differences in total insulin binding sites.

Regulation of Tumor Receptor Sites

If tumor hormone receptors can be regulated in the same way as normal cell receptors, receptor content cannot be regarded as a marker for particular cells. There is considerable evidence for regulation of estradiol and prolactin receptors in mammary tumor.

Vignon and Rochefort (94,95) observed that DMBA-induced tumor regression in ovariectomized rats was associated with a 90% fall in the level of cytosol estradiol receptor. Partial restoration of the lost activity occurred on treatment with estradiol (2 μg/day) or prolactin (1 mg/day). However, estradiol administration failed to restore cytosol receptor in spayed rats if prolactin release was blocked by CB-154. It was suggested that prolactin specifically stimulates mammary tumor growth by sensitization toward estrogen through an increase in estradiol receptor sites. Leung and Sasaki (56) came to similar conclusions in studies on stimulation of DMBA-induced tumor growth with prolactin administration. Estradiol receptor depletion after ovariectomy was restored by administration of prolactin but not by administration of prolactin plus nafoxidine. This observation is consistent with an obligatory role for estrogen in the mechanism of prolactin stimulation of growth and estradiol receptor restoration. Gibson and Hilf (27) observed that the decrease in cytosol estradiol receptor in DMBA tumors after ovariectomy occurred only in regressing tumors and not in static tumors. The regulatory action of prolactin on tumor cell estradiol cytosol receptor is direct. Shafie and Brooks (80) studied the effect of prolactin on estradiol receptor content of MCF-7 cells in culture. MCF-7 is a human tumor line (87) that contains estradiol receptor (9) and that increases its growth rate in low concentrations of estradiol (58). Both ovine prolactin and human prolactin added to cultures were capable of doubling the estradiol receptor content; the latter was effective at lower concentrations, although neither hormone stimulated growth even when stimulation of estradiol receptor was maximal.

Prolactin receptor in DMBA tumors can also be regulated. Kledzik et al. (52) showed a reduction in specific prolactin binding sites that accompanied tumor regression caused by administration of high doses of estrogen. This experiment is important because it suggests that the beneficial effects of high-dose estrogen treatment of some patients with breast cancer may result from regulation of prolactin receptors. However, further study of the effects that increased serum prolactin concentrations caused by estrogen treatment have on prolactin binding assays must be undertaken.

Current knowledge of hormonal regulation of receptors cannot explain the different receptor contents of our two models, MTW9-MtT and MTW9-P.

Table 2 shows the endocrine environments of hosts bearing MTW9-MtT, MTW9-P, and MTW9-PD. From what is known regarding prolactin stimulation of cytosol estradiol receptor, one would predict that MTW9-MtT should have a higher estradiol receptor content than either MTW9-P or MTW9-PD; serum prolactin is much higher in hosts bearing the mammosomatotropic tumor than in the other tumor-bearing rats. The prediction is based not only on the work cited earlier regarding regulation of estradiol receptor by prolactin in mammary tumor (56,80,94,95), but also on similar *in vitro* stimulation of estradiol receptor by prolactin in uterine and mammary tissue (55). The prediction for MTW9-MtT is wrong; although it is exposed to the highest levels of serum prolactin, it has the lowest cytosol estradiol receptor content of the tumors studied.

TABLE 2. *Endocrine environment of mammary tumors*

	MTW9-MtT	MTW9-P	MTW9-PD
Serum prolactin	very high[a]	high[a]	N[b]
Serum growth hormone	very high[c]	low[d]	N
Serum insulin	very high[e]	N	N
Serum gonadotropins	low	low[d]	N
Serum estrogen	low[f]	low[f]	N
Serum progesterone	high[g]	high[g]	N
Estrus cycle	no (pseudo-pregnant)	no (pseudo-pregnant)	yes
Tumor estradiol receptor[f]	present	high	high
Tumor prolactin receptor[h]	present	high	high

[a] Diamond et al. (21).
[b] No change expected from normal.
[c] Ito et al. (38).
[d] Sulman and Winnik (91).
[e] Martin et al. (64) and Stewart et al. (89).
[f] Diamond et al. (20).
[g] MTW9-MtT = 33.5 ± 3.1 ng/ml (n = 9); MTW9-P = 36.5 ± 9.7 ng/ml (n = 9); non-tumor-bearing W/Fu female rats = 12.0 ± 1.3 ng/ml (n = 9).
[h] Powell et al. (77).

Progesterone is known to decrease estradiol cytosol receptor in uterus (14,99). However, there is no evidence that increased serum progesterone is responsible for the low receptor content of MTW9-MtT; animals bearing MTW9-P have equally high serum progesterone values (see Table 2), presumably as a result of high serum prolactin.

Posner found that chronic high levels of serum prolactin induced specific prolactin binding sites in rat liver. Animals bearing prolactin-secreting mammo-somatotropic tumors have very high liver membrane binding capacity (75). Djiane and Durand (22) showed that administration of prolactin to pseudopregnant rabbits increased prolactin receptor in mammary gland. However, in our studies the extremely high serum prolactin concentrations in MtT-bearing rats were again associated with the lowest prolactin receptor capacity in mammary tumor membranes (Table 2). Progesterone administration to the rabbits studied by Djiane and Durand blocked prolactin-induced increases in prolactin receptor. Sherman et al. (82) showed that medroxyprogesterone acetate reduces membrane receptor sites for prolactin in rat liver. However, MtT-bearing animals have progesterone concentrations equivalent to those of perphenazine-treated animals; thus we are unable to explain the low prolactin receptor content of MTW9-MtT membranes on the basis of progesterone effects.

We were surprised to learn that MTW9 showed little change in estradiol cytosol receptor after ovariectomy (Table 1). Other convincing studies have shown a significant fall in estradiol receptor in DMBA-induced tumors after ovariectomy (27,56,94,95). Ovariectomy produced no significant change in estradiol receptor in MTW9, MTW9–MtT, or MTW9–PD in spite of obvious tumor regression.

Although the effects of some hormones that are present at abnormal serum concentrations in MtT-bearing rats (growth hormone, insulin, and gonadotropins) have not been studied from the standpoint of regulation of receptor, there is no reason to suspect that they cause the low receptor content of MTW9-MtT by some regulatory mechanism. Since we were unable to explain the differences in estradiol and prolactin receptors between the tumors studied in terms of receptor occupancy by endogenous hormone or by regulation of receptor content by known hormones, we looked for endocrine host factors that would explain the striking response to ovariectomy by MTW9-P and MTW9-PD and the lack of response by MTW9-MtT.

Why Does MTW9-MtT Not Regress after Ovariectomy?

MTW9-MtT contains definite estradiol receptor, but it does not regress after ovariectomy. The tumor is a model for an important clinical problem. Patients with mammary cancers that lack estradiol receptor have little chance for remission after ovariectomy. But only a little over one-half of premenopausal patients with tumors that contain estrogen-binding protein will benefit from ovariectomy. If we understood the reason for failure of response in such patients, current therapy might be significantly improved.

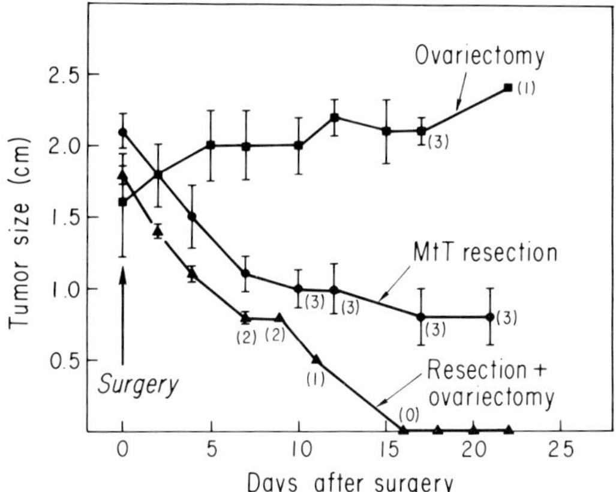

FIG. 3. Effects of resection, ovariectomy, and resection plus ovariectomy on growth of MTW9-MtT. Rats bearing MTW9-MtT were subjected to MtT resection *(filled circles)*, ovariectomy *(squares)*, or ovariectomy + MtT resection *(triangles)* on day 0. Four animals were subjected to each surgical procedure. Tumors were measured at intervals noted. Numbers in parentheses indicate number of animals remaining with palpable tumor. In the ovariectomized group, 1 animal died by day 17 and 3 died by day 24. Tumor size is expressed as average diameter [(length + width)/2] (mean ± SE). (From Diamond et al., ref. 21, with permission.)

Tumors with estradiol cytosol receptor might be resistant to ovariectomy for a variety of reasons based on some genetic defect. Defective cytosol receptor with inability to transform, inability to bind to chromatin, or inability to initiate a translational response can easily be envisaged. How often such factors occur in our mammary tumors is currently under study. However, MTW9-MtT possesses the genetic information for ovariectomy-induced regression. When MtT is resected from such hosts, MTW9 regresses. However, regression is faster and more complete when ovariectomy is combined with MtT resection (Fig. 3). This result could not be obtained if there were genetic inability to respond to estrogen withdrawal.

Accordingly, we investigated the possibility that MTW9-MtT failed to regress after ovariectomy not because it lacked the genetic machinery but because the mammosomatotropic tumor MtTW10 secreted a factor that inhibited ovariectomy-induced regression. MTW9-PD, which regresses after ovariectomy, has a significantly different endocrine environment than MTW9-MtT (Table 2). The experimental design consisted of simulating the known endocrine abnormalities of MtT-bearing animals in MTW9-PD hosts and testing the response to subsequent ovariectomy. This approach required that we exclude estrogen production (direct or indirect) by the MtT. Sufficient estrogen secretion from an extra-ovarian source would readily explain the lack of ovariectomy-induced regression of MTW9-MtT. No evidence for this was found. Rats bearing mammosomatotropic tumors do not manifest a normal estrus cycle; they are pseudopregnant (62), their uteri are small, and serum estradiol is low (20). Hence in rats bearing

TABLE 3. *Effects of various endocrine treatments on responses of MTW9-PD to ovariectomy*

Treatment to hosts of MTW9-PD	Days of treatment at time of ovariectomy[a]	Ovariectomy response
ACTH (2–9 U/day)	10–30	+
17-hydroxyprogesterone caproate (4 mg/day)	29	+
Bovine growth hormone (4 mg/day)	21	+
Implantation of MtTW50M[b]	24	+
Ovine prolactin (2 and 4 mg/day)[c]	20–24	+
Bovine prolactin (12 mg/day[c] (slow-release preparation)	7	+
Implantation of MtTW10	27	−

[a]Treatments were continued after ovariectomy.
[b]A growth-hormone-secreting pituitary tumor.
[c]Administered in multiple doses.

MTW9-PD we directed our attention to simulation of the high progestational, adrenotropic, somatotropic, and lactogenic activities characteristic of hosts of MTW9-MtT.

Table 3 shows how the endocrine environment of the MtT bearer was simulated in hosts of MTW9-PD. Administrations of ACTH, the long-acting progestin hydroxyprogesterone caproate, growth hormone, and prolactin, as well as implantation of the growth-hormone-secreting tumor MtTW5-OM (35), all failed to inhibit ovariectomy-induced regression of MTW9-PD. Table 3 also shows that only implantation of MtTW10 prevented mammary tumor regression. Implantation of MtTW10 greatly stimulated growth of MTW9-PD; in contrast to the results with all other treatments, the tumors continued to grow after ovariectomy, and no regression occurred. Administrations of ACTH, growth hormone, and prolactin, as well as implantation of MtTW5-OM, all showed the expected biological responses. ACTH-treated rats had enlarged adrenals, and growth hormone administration and MtTW5-OM implantation caused increases in body weight. All three doses of prolactin administered stimulated growth of mammary glands and tumors, indicating that the injected prolactin was biologically active.

The failure of prolactin (4–12 mg/day administered in multiple daily doses) to inhibit ovariectomy-induced tumor regression was explored further. Injected prolactin has a very short half-life (28,53); hence it is possible that even large doses of prolactin may not have been sufficient to achieve serum prolactin concentrations as high as those measured in rats bearing mammosomatotropic tumors (500–7,000 ng/ml). Since administered ovine and bovine prolactins could not be detected by radioimmunoassay for rat prolactin, elevated levels of exogenous prolactin in the sera of tumor-bearing prolactin-treated rats were measured using a radioreceptor assay adapted from the procedure of Shiu and Friesen (83). The assay used female rat liver membranes as a source of receptor, and it measured exogenous ovine prolactin and any biologically inactive but competing

TABLE 4. *Serum prolactin concentrations after a single injection of ovine prolactin (2 mg) in MTW9-PD-bearing rats*[a]

Rat number	Time after injection 2 hr (ng/ml)	6 hr (ng/ml)	8 hr (ng/ml)
1	54,000	15,500	5,900
2	25,000	12,800	3,500
3	42,000	27,700	10,000

[a] Tumor-bearing rats received injections of prolactin (4 mg/day) administered in two daily doses. After 13 days of treatment a test dose of prolactin (2 mg) was administered, and the animals were tailbled at the times indicated.

metabolite. The presence of competing inactive hormone in sera of rats receiving injections of prolactin could not be excluded. However, in rats so treated, we observed extreme mammary gland hyperplasia comparable to that seen in rats bearing mammosomatotropic tumors.

Table 4 shows that the concentration of serum ovine prolactin after a single subcutaneous injection of ovine prolactin (2 mg) was within the range of that produced by most mammosomatotropic tumors and that the high serum concentration persisted over an 8-hr period. In experiments where the total daily dose of prolactin was administered to hosts of MTW9-PD in multiple doses, the elevated serum concentrations would be expected to persist for about 16 to 18 hr. It seems clear that sustained levels of serum prolactin as high as those achieved by MtT growth are obtained in rats bearing MTW9-PD and that MTW9-PD regresses after ovariectomy in this high-prolactin environment.

None of the known products of MtT growth (prolactin, growth hormone, and ACTH) can explain the inhibition of ovariectomy-induced regression in MTW9-MtT. Only implantation of the mammosomatotropic tumor itself prevented regression after ovariectomy. Either MtTW10 secretes some factor(s) that inhibit ovariectomy-induced regression or some combination of hormones present in MtT bearers acts as an inhibitor. This last possibility is difficult to test. Such experiments involve large amounts of expensive hormones and take considerable time. There are also many possible hormone combinations that should be tested. We chose to administer a high-dose mixture of prolactin (10 mg/day), growth hormone (10 mg/day), and ACTH (8 U/day) to a limited number of rats bearing MTW9-PD. A similar treatment regimen was used by Bates and associates (4) to obtain highly stimulated mammary glands. We found this combination to be quite toxic, but in spite of the poor condition of the animals, it stimulated growth of MTW9-PD in several rats, although tumor regression still occurred after ovariectomy.

All our efforts to simulate the endocrine environment of the MtT bearer in MTW9-PD-bearing rats, except actual MtT implantation, failed to inhibit ovariectomy-induced mammary tumor regression. We have not yet evaluated the effect of insulin, but it is presumed that animals receiving daily injections of growth hormone and those bearing the growth-hormone-secreting tumor MtTW5-OM also have high serum insulin concentrations (3,15,64,89). We cannot rule out insulin as the inhibitor, but ovariectomy-induced regression of mammary tumors of growth-hormone-treated rats makes it unlikely.

We have not excluded the possibility that some combination of hormones not tested prevents ovariectomy-induced mammary tumor regression; however, our studies to date suggest that MtTW10 secretes some factor(s) that are responsible for this inhibition. Efforts are being made to find factors that control ovariectomy-induced regression. MTW9 is a good model for the study of such factors.

Roles of Estradiol and Prolactin in Growth of Mammary Cancer

It is probable that both estradiol and prolactin are required for growth of mammary tumors. Estradiol has little effect on growth of rat mammary gland or mammary tumor in hypophysectomized rats (60,88). Estradiol cannot stimulate *in vivo* growth of mammary gland or tumor in the absence of prolactin, but Lippman et al. (59) have reported that estradiol can stimulate some human mammary tumors in cell culture in the absence of prolactin. However, the mechanism of estrogen stimulation requires further study, since the estrogen inhibitor tamoxifen inhibits these cells in the apparent absence of estrogen. The statement that prolactin cannot act on growth of mammary tissue without estradiol is more difficult to justify. Pituitary preparations alone can stimulate limited mammary duct formation in hypophysectomized, ovariectomized, and adrenalectomized rats (60). Pituitary isografts only incompletely prevented mammary gland involution in ovariectomized-adrenalectomized rodents (100). Pearson and associates (74) were the first to point out the primary role of prolactin in stimulating the growth of rat mammary cancer. Their most recent evidence is concerned with the observation that perphenazine administration to rats after ovariectomy-induced regression of DMBA-induced tumors produced regrowth of tumor even when tamoxifen was also given. Perphenazine administration increases serum prolactin, and tamoxifen, a potent antiestrogen, should have prevented the action of residual estrogen from the adrenal or from other sources (63).

However, a number of reports are consistent with the existence of an estrogen-induced effect persisting for weeks after ovariectomy that is required for prolactin stimulation of mammary tumor growth. Although prolactin stimulation enhances growth of DMBA-induced tumors in ovariectomized rats, the stimulation lasts only for a few weeks; the tumor then regresses (13,57,73,97). This behavior is typical of at least most primary carcinogen-induced tumors and is consistent with the observations of Sinha et al. (86) on DMBA-induced tumors with hyperprolactinemia induced by median eminence lesions. The mammary tumors in such rats continued to grow after removal of both ovaries and adrenals; but after several weeks the tumors regressed, although serum prolactin remained high. MTW9-P also regressed after ovariectomy, although serum prolactin remained high (21); as in the tumors described by Sinha, estrogen seems to be required for long-term stimulation of host mammary cancer in rats.

Bradley et al. (8) attempted to classify DMBA-induced tumors as estrogen- or prolactin-dependent in the sense that the presence of the hormone caused growth stimulation and its absence caused regression. These criteria allowed about 30% of the tumors to be designated prolactin-dependent and 40% estrogen-dependent. However, when serum prolactin concentrations were maintained at presumably normal levels after ovariectomy, less than 10% of tumors were classified as estrogen-dependent. From this study the authors concluded that most DMBA tumors are dependent on both estrogen and prolactin. Until individual cells in tumors can be examined by autoradiography for hormone receptors and the tumors can be cloned, it is probably premature to seek hormonal classifications that imply dependence on a single hormone. Leung et al. (57) also stressed the interaction of prolactin and estradiol for the growth of DMBA tumors. They found that DMBA tumors that had regressed after combined ovariectomy-adrenalectomy showed excellent growth during administration of prolactin and the antiestrogen nafoxidine. However, after prolactin withdrawal and subsequent tumor regression, further treatment with prolactin failed to cause tumor regrowth. Manni et al. (63) were able to stimulate growth with perphenazine in ovariectomized rats bearing DMBA tumors that had been stimulated by treatment with perphenazine and the antiestrogen tamoxifen and then allowed to regress. It is important to resolve the differences between these experiments. The experiments of Manni and associates suggested stimulation of tumor growth by prolactin in the absence of estradiol cytosol receptor. Perhaps the adrenal in this study made enough estrogen to permit prolactin stimulation in the ovariectomized rat, or perhaps nuclear receptor filled with tamoxifen-receptor complex satisfied an estrogen requirement. Such explanations, although speculative, are consistent with regression of mammary tumors in hosts deprived of estrogen either by ovariectomy or by ovariectomy plus adrenalectomy, but with high serum prolactin concentrations (13,21,73,86,97).

Progesterone and Mammary Cancer

There is little doubt that progesterone enhances tumorigenesis in the DMBA-injected animal (16,37,39,40,65). Under appropriate experimental conditions, stimulation of mammary tumor growth by progesterone can be demonstrated. MTW9 does not usually grow in rats unless a high level of serum prolactin exists in the host. A high level of serum prolactin is not the only hormonal requirement for growth of MTW9 after transplantation; ovarian hormones are also required. When MTW9 is coimplanted with MtTW5 into ovariectomized rats or into intact rats that are ovariectomized shortly thereafter, growth of MtTW5 produces high levels of serum prolactin, but MTW9 will not grow

(61,72). Administration of 10 μg estradiol 17β and 3 mg progesterone daily resulted in growth of MTW9 equal to that obtained when MTW9 was transplanted into control animals bearing MtTW5. When progesterone or estradiol was administered alone, much less growth occurred, and the latent period for growth was considerably longer. These effects are particularly interesting when it is recalled *(vide supra)* that ovariectomy in animals bearing MTW9 supported by MtT does not result in regression of mammary tumor. Current efforts in our laboratory to explain the roles of progesterone and estradiol in the early growth of tumor are concerned with the idea that ovarian hormones may be required for the development of angiogenesis in the implant. Perhaps progesterone acts as an immunosuppressive agent that allows early growth of implant material.

Regression of MTW9

Gullino and associates showed that regression of MTW9 after resection of MtT and ovariectomy could not be explained by alteration of metabolic rate, by alteration of blood flow, by alteration of oxygen or glucose consumption per unit of tumor weight, by cell loss into the circulation, or by homograft rejection (10,29,30). They also demonstrated that the increase in lysosomal enzymes that occurs in MTW9 after MtT resection and during tumor regression is not the immediate cause of regression. Lysosomal enzyme activity was increased in regressing MTW9 on the third day after hormone withdrawal, a time at which a 50% decrease in tumor size had already occurred (54). Increased lysosomal enzymes are not found in the interstitial fluid of regressing MTW9 in spite of a significant increase in intracellular lysosomal activity (31). The ratio between free and inactive (bound) lysosomal enzymes did not change during 72 hr after hormone withdrawal, a time when tumor regression was very significant. Gullino and associates made an important observation on the cytosol proteins of MTW9 during tumor regression after hormone withdrawal: the proteins are more easily digested by several proteolytic enzymes. The increased susceptibility to proteolysis during tumor regression cannot be explained by disulfide reduction or by the presence of various hormones. The effect is significant, but it is small enough that it could actually be explained by the susceptibility of only a few of the protein constituents of tumor cytosol. However, no difference in proteolytic activity of cytosols between regressing and growing tumors was noted. Çytosol from growing tumors did not contain an inhibitor to proteolytic action, nor was the electrophoretic pattern of tumor cytosol in growing tumors different from that in regressing tumors. Finally, it is of interest that heat denaturation of cytosol proteins removed the enhanced susceptibility of tumor cytosol protein (78).

The exact mechanism by which mammary tumors regress after hormonal treatment is of considerable importance. Our own observations suggest that cessation of growth and tumor regression are separate mechanisms. When

MTW9-P is actively growing in animals receiving chronic perphenazine treatment, growth can be stopped in most tumors by cessation of drug administration. Serum prolactin becomes normal. Most tumors simply stop growing; they do not regress. Such tumors regress after ovariectomy. The regression process merits detailed biochemical study. If the biochemical events that occur after ovariectomy were understood, we might be able to reproduce the same events by means of more effective agents.

Tumors may be resistant to hormonal effectors because some portion of the genetic machinery necessary for response is missing or because some factor in the cell environment prevents a portion of this machinery from responding. Such a factor may be subject to external control. Every effort to demonstrate this type of resistance should be made; such resistance is presumably reversible. Normal tissues may be resistant to response on such a reversible basis; metabolic acidosis may cause insulin resistance, whereas chronic high serum concentrations of insulin may reduce sensitivity to insulin by reducing the number of specific receptor sites (44).

Androgens and estrogens may inhibit each other's function. Androgens may inhibit the catabolic influence of glucocorticoid on skeletal muscle. Perhaps an undetected metabolic abnormality in rats bearing MTW9-MtT would prevent tumor regression in response to the fall in serum estradiol observed after ovariectomy. An alternative explanation may also explain the lack of response of MTW9-MtT to ovariectomy. It is possible that MTW9-MtT consists of (at least) two populations of cells, cells that are destroyed after ovariectomy (S) and cells that are destroyed after MtT resection but not after ovariectomy (R). If we assume that the MtT-supported tumor consists of at least 90% R cells and the perphenazine- supported MTW9 consists of at least 90% S cells, we can attempt to explain the apparent resistance of MTW9-MtT and the response of MTW9-P to ovariectomy. After ovariectomy of rats bearing MTW9-MtT there is either cessation of growth or decreased growth of the mammary tumor, but no regression. For tumors (MTW9-MtT) that maintain a constant volume after ovariectomy, it would be difficult to imagine maintenance of volume by the constant disappearance of S cells exactly balanced by the rate of growth of the major R cell population. It is obvious that the hypothetical R cell population cannot be stimulated by prolactin alone to anywhere near the extent possible with intact ovarian function; it is not truly resistant to the effect of estrogen. For those MTW9-MtT tumors that show greatly reduced growth after ovariectomy, the reduced growth cannot be explained in terms of regression of a minor population. If the population of S cells in MTW9-MtT were not minor, their regression after ovariectomy could not be masked by growth of R cells, which are either absent or greatly reduced after estrogen withdrawal. The hypothetical division of MTW9-MtT into S and R cells is not consistent with the behavior after ovariectomy.

The R and S bimodal hypothesis is not consistent with our observations on estradiol receptor in MTW9. MTW9-MtT cytosol contains 48 fmoles/mg protein; MTW9-P contains 196 fmoles/mg protein (Table 1). Assume that the receptor content of the MtT-supported tumor represents $0.9(X) + 0.1(196) = 48$,[3] so that the major population of R cells has a binding capacity of 31 fmoles. When MtT is resected and MTW9-MtT shrinks to 40% of the initial average diameter, the volume ($4\pi r^3/3$) has shrunk to over 90% of the former volume and should represent nothing but S cells. However, instead of the binding capacity rising to 196 fmoles/mg protein, no significant change in estradiol binding was observed (Table 1) (20). This kind of reasoning suggests that MTW9-MtT does not consist of a major cell population with low estradiol receptor content that responds to lowered serum prolactin plus a minor cell population with high estradiol receptor content that does not regress after serum prolactin is lowered by MtT resection.

Effect of Steroid Hormones on Viability of MTW9

It is well known that women may show recurrence of mammary cancer decades after removal of the primary tumor. Experimental models for the study of tumor viability in the dormant state should improve our knowledge of how such dormant cells survive and the mechanism by which they are reactivated. Most rats inoculated with MTW9 and given no treatment to produce a high level of serum prolactin fail to develop mammary tumors. However, MTW9 remains viable for long periods of time when the tumor is transplanted into intact female rats. We have demonstrated outgrowth of MTW9 a year after the original implantation of mammary tumor by inoculation of MtT. The tumor that develops seems to grow with the usual latent period, and it has the expected morphological appearance. Ovarian hormones are involved in the viability of MTW9 in the dormant state. When MTW9 and MtTW5 were inoculated into ovariectomized rats, only the mammosomatotropic tumor grew. Treatment of spayed rats with estradiol and progesterone allowed mammary tumors to grow (61). Figure 4 shows that when steroid treatment to ovariectomized animals bearing implants of MTW9 and MtTW5 was delayed by 65 days, no growth of mammary tumor occurred. When a second MTW9 was implanted on day 85, there was prompt growth of the mammary tumor in animals given ovarian hormones from the time of ovariectomy. This experiment shows that the ovariectomized rats in which MTW9 could not be reactivated by late administration of ovarian hormones are not immune to the growth of tumor when it is kept viable by prompt administration of estradiol and progesterone (72). Further study is necessary to elucidate the exact relationship between viability and the presence of steroid hormones. The long dormancy of MTW9 in the absence of high levels of serum prolactin but adequate steroid hormone may relate to the acquisition of a suitable blood supply by the implant, even though the inoculum is not stimulated to grow. In view of current studies on prophylactic chemotherapy in women after mastectomy, the effect of hormonal environment on the efficacy of such chemical agents should be studied.

---

[3] Where X represents the receptor content of R cells.

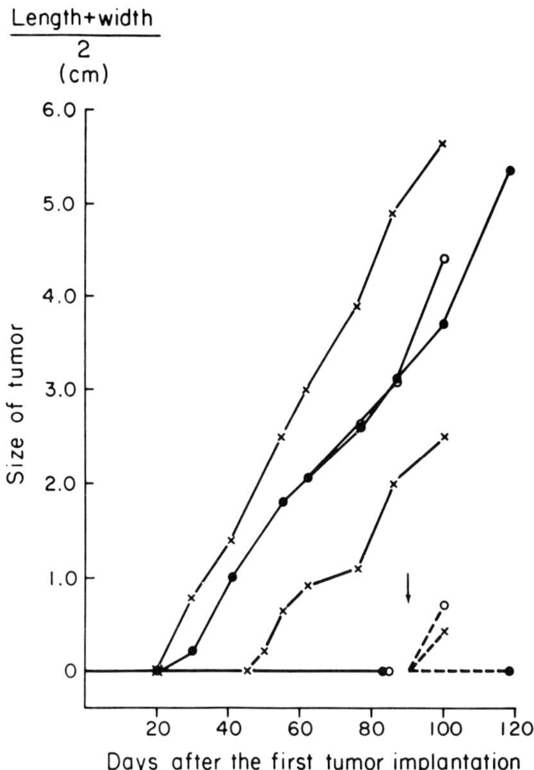

FIG. 4. Growth of MtTW5 (the three curves to the left starting at day 20) and MTW9 (all other points on the figure) in control *(crosses)*, oophorectomized *(filled circles)*, and oophorectomized steroid-treatment rats *(open circles)*. Steroid treatment consisted of daily injections of 10 μg of estradiol 17β and 3 mg progesterone. Three groups of 6 rats each were implanted with both MtT and MTW9 on day 0. Oophorectomy was done on day 1. Steroid treatment began on day 65. MTW9 showed no growth on day 85 in either oophorectomized group. On day 85 (indicated by arrow) a second MTW9 was implanted in each rat. The prompt growth of this tumor in control and oophorectomized steroid-treated rats is shown by the dashed lines. The second implants failed to grow in the oophorectomized group that did not receive steroid treatment. (From Murota and Hollander, ref. 72, with permission.)

ACKNOWLEDGMENTS

The authors wish to thank Samuel Koprak, Annie Miller, and Sukur Khan for their excellent technical assistance. This article was supported by U.S. Public Health Service grants P30 CA-14194, CA-10064, and CA-5215.

REFERENCES

1. Amenomori, Y., Chen, C. L., and Meites, J. (1970): Serum prolactin levels in rats during different reproductive states. *Endocrinology,* 86:506–510.

2. Anderson, R. R. (1974): Endocrinological control in lactation. In: *Lactation, Vol. I,* edited by B. L. Larson and V. R. Smith, pp. 97–140. Academic Press, New York.
3. Bates, R. W., and Garrison, M. M. (1973): Synergism among growth hormone, ACTH, cortisol and dexamethasone in the hormonal induction of diabetes in rats and the diabetogenic effect of tolbutamide. *Endocrinology,* 93:1109–1118.
4. Bates, R. W., Milkovic, S., and Garrison, M. M. (1964): Effects of prolactin, growth hormone and ACTH, alone and in combination upon organ weights and adrenal function in normal rats. *Endocrinology,* 74:714–723.
5. Ben-David, M. (1968): Mechanism of induction of mammary differentiation of Sprague Dawley female rats by perphenazine. *Endocrinology,* 83:1212–1223.
6. Birkinshaw, M., and Falconer, I. R. (1972): The localization of prolactin labeled with radioactive iodine in rabbit mammary tissue. *J. Endocrinol.,* 55:323–334.
7. Bogden, A. E., Taylor, D. J., Kor, E. Y. H., Mason, M. M., and Speropoulos, A. (1974): The effect of perphenazine induced serum prolactin response on estrogen-primed mammary tumor host systems 13762 and R35 mammary adenocarcinomas. *Cancer Res.,* 34:3018–3025.
8. Bradley, C. J., Kledzik, G. S., and Meites, J. (1976): Prolactin and estrogen dependency of rat mammary cancers at early and late stages of development. *Cancer Res.,* 36:319–324.
9. Brooks, S. C., Locke, E. R., and Soule, H. D. (1973): Estrogen receptor in a human cell line (MCF-7) from breast carcinoma. *J. Biol. Chem.,* 248:6251–6253.
10. Butler, T. P., and Gullino, P. M. (1975): Quantitation of cell shedding into efferent blood of mammary adenocarcinoma. *Cancer Res.,* 35:512–516.
11. Chamness, G. C., Jennings, A. W., and McGuire, W. L. (1974): Estrogen receptor binding to isolated nuclei. A nonsaturable process. *Biochemistry,* 13:327–331.
12. Chamness, G. C., Jennings, A. W., and McGuire, W. L. (1973): Oestrogen receptor binding is not restricted to target nuclei. *Nature,* 241:248.
13. Clemens, J. A., Welsch, C. W., and Meites, J. (1968): Effects of hypothalamic lesions on incidence and growth of mammary tumors in carcinogen-treated rats. *Proc. Soc. Exp. Biol. Med.,* 127:969–972.
14. Coulson, P. B., and Pavlik, E. J. (1977): Effects of estogen and progesterone on cytoplasmic estrogen receptor and rates of protein synthesis in rat uterus. *J. Steroid Biochem.,* 8:205–212.
15. Curry, D. L., and Bennett, L. L. (1973): Dynamics of insulin release by perfused rat pancreas: Effects of hypophysectomy, growth hormone, adrenocorticotropic hormone and hydrocortisone. *Endocrinology,* 93:602–609.
16. Dao, T. L. (1964): Carcinogenesis of mammary gland in rat. *Prog. Exp. Tumor Res.,* 5:157–216.
17. Denamur, R. (1971): Hormonal control of lactogenesis. *J. Dairy Res.,* 38:237–264.
18. DeSombre, E. R., and Jensen, E. V. (1976): Steroid receptors in breast neoplasia. In: *Control Mechanisms in Cancer,* edited by W. E. Criss, T. Ono, and J. R. Sabine, pp. 67–97. Raven Press, New York.
19. DeSombre, E. R., Kledzik, G., Marshall, S., and Meites, J. (1976): Estrogen and prolactin receptor concentrations in rat mammary tumors and response to endocrine ablation. *Cancer Res.,* 36:354–358.
20. Diamond, E. J., Giladi, M., Khan, S., and Hollander, V. P. (1977): Estradiol binding in ovariectomy-responsive and -nonresponsive rat mammary carcinoma. *Cancer Res.,* 37:1852–1856.
21. Diamond, E. J., Koprak, S., Shen, S. K., and Hollander, V. P. (1976): The conversion of an ovariectomy-nonresponsive to an ovariectomy-responsive mammary tumor strain. *Cancer Res.,* 36:77–80.
22. Djiane, J., and Durand, P. (1977): Prolactin-progesterone antagonism in self regulation of prolactin receptors in the mammary gland. *Nature,* 266:641–643.
23. Foulds, L. (1949): Mammary tumors in hybrid mice: Hormone responses of transplanted tumors. *Br. J. Cancer,* 3:240–246.
24. Foulds, L. (1949): Mammary tumors in hybrid mice: Progression of spontaneous tumors. *Br. J. Cancer,* 3:345–375.
25. Foulds, L. (1969): *Neoplastic Development, Vol. 1,* pp. 3–27. Academic Press, New York.
26. Gardner, D. G., and Witliff, J. L. (1973): Specific estrogen receptors in the lactating mammary gland of the rat. *Biochemistry,* 12:3090–3096.
27. Gibson, S. L., and Hilf, R. (1976): Influence of hormonal alteration of host on estrogen-

binding capacity in 7,12-dimethylbenz*(a)*anthracene-induced mammary tumors. *Cancer Res.,* 36:3736–3741.

28. Grosvenor, C. E. (1967): Disappearance rate of exogenous prolactin from serum of female rats. *Endocrinology,* 80:195–200.
29. Gullino, P. M., Grantham, F. H., Losonczy, I., and Berghoffer, B. (1972): Mammary tumor regression. I. Physiopathologic characteristics of hormone-dependent tissue. *J. Natl. Cancer Inst.,* 49:1333–1348.
30. Gullino, P. M., Grantham, F. H., Losonczy, I., and Berghoffer, B. (1972): Mammary tumor regression. III. Uptake and loss of substrates by regressing tumors. *J. Natl. Cancer Inst.,* 49:1675–1684.
31. Gullino, P. M., and Lanzerotti, R. H. (1972): Mammary tumor regression. II. Autophagy of neoplastic cells. *J. Natl. Cancer Inst.,* 49:1349–1356.
32. Hilf, R. (1973): Biochemical studies on experimental mammary tumors as related to human breast cancer. In: *Methods in Cancer Research, Vol. VII,* edited by Harris Busch, pp. 55–114. Academic Press, New York.
33. Hilf, R., Harmon, J. T., Matusik, R. J., and Rengler, M. B. (1976): In: *Control Mechanisms in Cancer,* edited by W. E. Criss, T. Ono, and J. R. Sabine, pp. 1–24. Raven Press, New York.
34. Hilf, R., Michel, I., and Bell, C. (1967): Biochemical responses of normal and neoplastic mammary tissue to hormonal treatment. *Recent Prog. Horm. Res.,* 23:229–295.
35. Hollander, N., and Hollander, V. P. (1971): Development of a somatotropic variant of the mammosomatotropic tumor MtT/W5. *Proc. Soc. Exp. Biol. Med.,* 137:1157–1162.
36. Huggins, C., Briziarelli, G., and Sutton, H., Jr. (1976): Rapid induction of mammary carcinoma in the rat and the influence of hormones on the tumors. *J. Exp. Med.,* 109:25–41.
37. Huggins, C., Moon, R. C., and Morii, S. (1962): Extinction of experimental mammary cancer. I. Estradiol-17β and progesterone. *Proc. Natl. Acad. Sci. U.S.A.,* 48:379–386.
38. Ito, A., Martin, J. M., Grindeland, R. W., Takizawa, S., and Furth, J. (1971): Mammotropic and somatotropic hormones in sera of normal rats and in rats bearing primary and grafted pituitary tumors. *Int. J. Cancer,* 7:416–429.
39. Jabara, A. G. (1967): Effects of progesterone on 9,10-dimethyl-1,2-benzanthracene-induced mammary tumors in Sprague-Dawley rats. *Br. J. Cancer,* 21:418–429.
40. Jabara, A. G., and Hartcourt, A. G. (1970): The effects of progesterone and ovariectomy on mammary tumors induced by 7,12-dimethylbenz*(a)*anthracene in Sprague-Dawley rats. *Pathology,* 2:115–123.
41. Jensen, E. V., and DeSombre, E. R. (1972): Mechanism of action of the female sex hormones. *Annu. Rev. Biochem.,* 41:203–230.
42. Jensen, E. V., and DeSombre, E. R. (1977): Steroid hormone receptors in breast cancer. In: *Receptors and Mechanism of Action of Steroid Hormones,* edited by J. R. Pasqualini, pp. 569–594. Marcel Dekker, New York.
43. Jensen, E. V., DeSombre, E. R., and Jungblut, P. W. (1967): Estrogen receptors in hormone responsive tissues and tumors. In: *Endogenous Factors Influencing Host-Tumor Balance,* edited by R. W. Wissler, T. L. Dao, and S. Wood, Jr., pp. 15–30. University of Chicago Press, Chicago.
44. Kahn, C. R., and Roth, J. (1976): Insulin receptors in disease states. In: *Hormone-Receptor Interaction: Molecular Aspects,* edited by G. S. Levey, pp. 1–29. Marcel Dekker, New York.
45. Katzenellenbogen, J. A., Johnson, H. J., and Carlson, K. E. (1973): Studies on the uterine cytoplasmic estogen binding protein. Thermal stability and ligand dissociation rate. An assay of empty and filled sites by exchange. *Biochemistry,* 12:4092–4099.
46. Kim, U. (1963): Pituitary function and hormonal therapy of experimental breast cancer. *Cancer Res.,* 25:1146–1156.
47. Kim, U., and Furth, J. (1960): Relation of mammary tumors to mammotropes. I. Induction of mammary tumors in rats. *Proc. Soc. Exp. Biol. Med.,* 103:640–642.
48. Kim, U., and Furth, J. (1960): Relation of mammary tumors to mammotropes. II. Hormone responsiveness of 3-methylcholanthrene induced mammary carcinomas. *Proc. Soc. Exp. Biol. Med.,* 103:643–645.
49. Kim, U., and Furth, J. (1960): Relation of mammotropes to mammary tumors. IV. Development of highly hormone dependent mammary tumors. *Proc. Soc. Exp. Biol. Med.,* 105:490–492.
50. Kim, U., Furth, J., and Clifton, K. H. (1960): Relation of mammary tumors to mammotropes. *Proc. Soc. Exp. Biol. Med.,* 103:646–650.

51. King, R. J. B., Cowan, D., and Inman, D. R. (1965): The uptake of (6,7-^{3}H) oestradiol by dimethylbanzanthracene-induced rat mammary tumors. *J. Endocrinol.,* 32:83–90.
52. Kledzik, G. S., Bradley, C. J., Marshall, S., Campbell, G. A., and Meites, J. (1976): Effects of high doses of estrogen on prolactin-binding activity and growth of carcinogen-induced mammary cancers in rats. *Cancer Res.,* 36:3265–3268.
53. Koch, Y., Chow, Y. F., and Meites, J. (1971): Metabolic clearance and secretion rates of prolactin in the rat. *Endocrinology,* 89:1303–1308.
54. Lanzerotti, R. H., and Gullino, P. M. (1972): Activities and quantities of lysosomal enzymes during mammary tumor regression. *Cancer Res.,* 32:2679–2685.
55. Leung, B. S., and Sasaki, G. H. (1973): Prolactin and progesterone effect on specific estradiol binding in uterine and mammary tissues *in vitro. Biochem. Biophys. Res. Commun.,* 55:1180–1187.
56. Leung, B. S., and Sasaki, G. H. (1975): On the mechanism of prolactin and estrogen action in 7,12-dimethylbenz*(a)*anthracene-induced mammary carcinoma in the rat. II. *In vivo* tumor responses and estrogen receptor. *Endocrinology,* 97:564–572.
57. Leung, B. S., Sasaki, G. H., and Leung, J. S. (1975): Estrogen-prolactin dependency in 7,12-dimethylbenz*(a)*anthracene-induced tumors. *Cancer Res.,* 35:621–627.
58. Lippman, M. E., and Bolan, G. (1975): Oestrogen-responsive human breast cancer in long term tissue culture. *Nature,* 256:592–593.
59. Lippman, M. E., Osborne, C. K., Knazek, R., and Young, N. (1977): *In vitro* model systems for the study of hormone-dependent human breast cancer. *N. Engl. J. Med.,* 296:154–159.
60. Lyons, W. R., Li, C. H., and Johnson, R. W. (1958): The hormonal control of mammary growth and lactation. *Recent Prog. Horm. Res.,* 14:219–248.
61. MacLeod, R. M., Allen, M. S., and Hollander, V. P. (1964): Hormonal requirements for the growth of mammary adenocarcinoma (MTW9) in rats. *Endocrinology,* 75:249–258.
62. MacLeod, R. M., Smith, M. C., and DeWitt, G. W. (1966): Hormonal properties of transplanted pituitary tumors and their relation to the pituitary gland. *Endocrinology,* 79:1149–1156.
63. Manni, A., Trujilli, J. E., and Pearson, O. H. (1977): Predominant role of prolactin in stimulating the growth of 7,12-dimethylbenz*(a)*anthracene-induced rat mammary tumor. *Cancer Res.,* 37:1216–1219.
64. Martin, J. M., Akerblom, H. K., and Garay, G. (1968): Insulin secretion in rats with elevated levels of circulating growth hormone due to MtT-W15. *Diabetes,* 17:661–667.
65. McCormick, G. M., and Moon, R. C. (1967): Effect of nursing and litter size on growth of 7,12-dimethylbenz*(a)*anthracene (DMBA)-induced mammary tumors. *Br. J. Cancer,* 21:586–591.
66. McGuire, W. L., Carbone, P. P., and Vollmer, E. P. (1975): *Estrogen Receptors in Human Breast Cancer.* Raven Press, New York.
67. McGuire, W. L., and Chamness, G. C. (1973): Studies on the estrogen receptor in breast cancer. *Adv. Exp. Med. Biol.,* 36:113–136.
68. McGuire, W. L., Huff, K., and Chamness, G. C. (1972): Temperature-dependent binding of estrogen receptor to chromatin. *Biochemistry,* 11:4562–4565.
69. McGuire, W. L., Huff, K., Jennings, A., and Chamness, G. C. (1972): Mammary carcinoma: A specific biochemical defect in autonomous tumors. *Science,* 175:335–336.
70. McGuire, W. L., and Julian, J. A. (1971): Comparison of macromolecular binding of estradiol in hormone-dependent and hormone-independent rat mammary carcinoma. *Cancer Res.,* 31:1440–1445.
71. McGuire, W. L., Julian, J. A., and Chamness, G. C. (1971): A dissociation between ovarian dependent growth and estrogen sensitivity in mammary carcinoma. *Endocrinology,* 89:969–973.
72. Murota, S., and Hollander, V. P. (1971): Role of ovarian hormones in the growth of transplantable mammary carcinoma. *Endocrinology,* 89:560–564.
73. Nagasawa, H., and Yanai, R. (1970): Effects of prolactin or growth hormone on growth of carcinogen-induced mammary tumors of adreno-ovariectomized rats. *Int. J. Cancer,* 6:488–495.
74. Pearson, O. H., Llerena, O., Llerena, L., Molina, A., and Butler, T. (1969): Prolactin-dependent rat mammary cancer: A model for man? *Trans. Assoc. Am. Physicians,* 82:225–238.
75. Posner, B. I. (1976): Regulation of lactogen specific binding sites in rat liver: Studies on the role of lactogens and estrogen. *Endocrinology,* 99:1168–1177.
76. Posner, B. I., Kelly, P. A., Shiu, P. C., and Friesen, H. G. (1974): Studies of insulin, growth

hormone and prolactin binding: Tissue distribution, species variation and characterization. *Endocrinology,* 95:521–530.
77. Powell, B. L., Diamond, E. J., Koprak, S., and Hollander, V. P. (1977): Prolactin binding in ovariectomy-responsive and ovariectomy-nonresponsive rat mammary carcinoma. *Cancer Res.,* 37:1328–1332.
78. Rouleau, M., and Gullino, P. M. (1977): Increased susceptibility of cytosol proteins to proteolytic digestion during regression of a hormone-dependent mammary tumor. *Cancer Res.,* 37:670–677.
79. Sakai, F., and Saez, S. (1976): Existence of receptors bound to endogenous estradiol in breast cancers of premenopausal and postmenopausal women. *Steroids,* 27:99–110.
80. Shafie, S., and Brooks, S. C. (1977): Effect of prolactin on growth and the estrogen receptor level of human breast cancer cells (MCF-7). *Cancer Res.,* 37:792–799.
81. Shay, H., Aegerter, E. A., Gruensterin, M., and Komsrov, S. A. (1949): Development of adenocarcinoma of the breast in the Wistar rat following the gastric instillation of methylcholanthrene. *J. Natl. Cancer Inst.,* 10:255–266.
82. Sherman, B. M., Stagner, J. I., and Zamudio, R. (1977): Regulation of lactogenic hormone binding in rat liver by steroid hormones. *Endocrinology,* 100:101–107.
83. Shiu, R. P. C., and Friesen, H. G. (1976): Prolactin receptors. In: *Methods in Receptor Research, Vol. 9,* edited by M. Blecher, pp. 565–598. Marcel Dekker, New York.
84. Shiu, R. P. C., Kelly, P. A., and Friesen, H. G. (1973): Radioreceptor assay for prolactin and other lactogenic hormones. *Science,* 180:968–970.
85. Shymala, G., and Nandi, S. (1972): Interactions of 6,7-^{3}H-17β-estradiol with the mouse lactating mammary tissue in vivo and in vitro. *Endocrinology,* 91:861–877.
86. Sinha, D., Cooper, D., and Dao, T. L. (1973): The nature of estrogen and prolactin effect on mammary tumorigenesis. *Cancer Res.,* 33:411–414.
87. Soule, H. D., Vazquez, J., Long, A., Albert, S., and Brennan, M. (1973): A human cell line from a pleural effusion derived from a breast carcinoma. *J. Natl. Cancer Inst.,* 51:1409–1416.
88. Sterental, A., Dominguez, J. M., Weissman, C., and Pearson, O. H. (1963): Pituitary role in the estrogen dependency of experimental mammary cancer. *Cancer Res.,* 23:481–485.
89. Stewart, J. K., Reagan, C. R., and Kostyo, J. L. (1977): Correlation between the biological and immunological activities of growth hormone circulating in rats bearing MtTW15 tumors. *Endocrinology,* 100:1376–1383.
90. Sulman, F. G. (1970): Pharmacological regulation of lactation. In: *Hypothalamic Control of Lactation,* edited by F. G. Sulman, pp. 60–102. Springer-Verlag, New York.
91. Sulman, F. G., and Winnik, H. Z. (1956): Hormonal depression due to treatment of animals with chlorpromazine. *Nature,* 178:365.
92. Turkington, R. W. (1974): Prolactin receptors in mammary carcinoma cells. *Cancer Res.,* 34:758–763.
93. Turkington, R. W. (1970): Stimulation of RNA synthesis in isolated mammary cells by insulin and prolactin bound to sepharose. *Biochem. Biophys. Res. Commun.,* 41:1362–1367.
94. Vignon, F., and Rochefort, H. (1976): Regulation of estrogen receptors in ovarian-dependent rat mammary tumors. I. Effects of castration and prolactin. *Endocrinology,* 98:722–729.
95. Vignon, F., and Rochefort, H. (1974): Regulation des "recepteurs" des oestrogines dans les tumeurs mammaires: Effect de la prolactin *in vivo. C. R. Acad. Sci.* [*D*] *(Paris),* 278:103–106.
96. Watson, C., Medina, D., and Clark, J. H. (1977): Estrogen receptor characterization in a transplantable mouse mammary tumor. *Cancer Res.,* 37:3344–3348.
97. Welsch, C. W., Clemens, J. A., and Meites, J. (1969): Effects of hypothalamic and amygdaloid lesions on development and growth of carcinogen-induced mammary tumors in the female rat. *Cancer Res.,* 29:1541–1549.
98. Welsch, C. W., and Nagasawa, H. (1977): Prolactin and murine mammary tumorigenesis: A review. *Cancer Res.,* 37:951–963.
99. West, N. B., Verhage, H. G., and Brenner, R. M. (1976): Suppression of the estradiol receptor system by progesterone in the oviduct and uterus of the cat. *Endocrinology,* 99:1010–1016.
100. Yanai, R., and Nagasawa, H. (1971): Enhancement by pituitary isografts of mammary hyperplastic nodules in adreno-ovariectomized mice. *J. Natl. Cancer Inst.,* 46:1251–1255.
101. Yokoro, K., Furth, J., and Haran-Ghera, N. (1961): Induction of mammotropic pituitary tumors by X-rays in rats and mice: The role of mammotropes in development of mammary tumors. *Cancer Res.,* 21:178–186.

Endocrine Control in Neoplasia, edited by
R. K. Sharma and W. E. Criss.
Raven Press, New York © 1978.

Prolactin Receptors and Hormone Dependence in Mammary Carcinoma

*Mark E. Costlow and **William L. McGuire

**Department of Biochemistry, St. Jude Children's Research Hospital, Memphis, Tennessee 38101; and **Department of Medicine, University of Texas Health Science Center at San Antonio, San Antonio, Texas 78284*

1. The hormone prolactin provides a major support, but not the sole support, for hormone-dependent mammary tumor growth.

2. Prolactin receptors can be either maintained or lost in the process of malignant transformation of mammary tissue.

3. A loss of prolactin receptors can be correlated with loss of hormone-dependent growth characteristics in some experimental models but not in others.

4. Although the numbers of prolactin receptors in mammary tumors can vary widely, their specificity or binding affinity does not appear to change.

5. In some tumors, variations in receptor number might stem from a heterogeneous cell population, some cells containing receptors and others having few receptors or none at all.

6. The number of prolactin receptors in a mammary tumor is partly controlled by the hormonal environment.

7. Human mammary tumors contain binding sites for prolactin, which suggests that the hormone has a direct effect on this tissue.

8. Prolactin receptors are important components of the complex hormonal control mechanisms that regulate the growth of mammary carcinoma.

INTRODUCTION

The use of endocrine therapy in the treatment of breast cancer is based on the possibility that a tumor is hormone-dependent. Unfortunately, we are not yet able to predict with certainty the 30% of human breast tumors that will respond, and our knowledge of which hormones actually regulate a particular dependent tumor is still meager. In experimental mammary tumor models, prolactin, a polypeptide hormone secreted by the pituitary, has a major role in the regulation of tumor growth (76,174). Although the exact mechanisms by which prolactin affects mammary tissue are largely unknown, the first and requisite step in its action is interaction with a cell-surface receptor. With the increasing availability of techniques to identify and quantitate prolactin receptors, considerable information has accumulated on the relationship of these receptors to hormone dependence. In this chapter we shall survey major contributions toward defining prolactin and prolactin receptor involvement in the control of mammary tumor growth. We stress the possible interrelationships of prolactin and its receptor with other hormones and receptors that participate in endocrine regulation of breast tissue. By necessity, emphasis is placed on information obtained with experimental animal tumor models, but reference to experiments performed on human breast tumors will be made where appropriate.

HORMONE DEPENDENCE *IN VIVO*

Prolactin

Lactogenic hormones have two main functions in normal mammary tissues: stimulation of cell proliferation and modulation of cell function. During pregnancy the proliferation of mammary tissue is stimulated by placental lactogen. Prolactin can mimic this effect on mammary cell growth (41,158), and administration of tranquilizers such as perphenazine that increase the circulating level of prolactin (5) also stimulates mammary gland development (3). Late in pregnancy, placental lactogen levels (149) and cellular proliferation decrease (52); following parturition, lactation is controlled by prolactin, which in turn is modulated by suckling. If suckling is prevented, lactation subsides and the gland involutes (30).

When exposed to chemical carcinogens such as 7,12-dimethylbenzanthracene (DMBA), mammary tissue undergoes malignant transformation (69). The induced tumors can be placed in two categories, based on loss or retention of hormonal control mechanisms normally present in mammary tissue. If the controls are retained, the tumors are considered to be hormone-dependent; that is, growth and, in some cases, function can be modulated by hormones that influence normal mammary tissue. If these controls are lost, tumors are considered to be autonomous; that is, growth is not influenced by hormones.

In hormone-dependent mammary tumors, one of prolactin's "normal" functions, the proliferative stimulus, predominates; but unlike the normal mammary cell, the hormone-dependent tumor cell is committed to proliferate even at low physiological levels of circulating hormones (99).

There is compelling evidence that prolactin is the single most important hormone controlling hormone-dependent tumor growth. Prolactin injection stimulates tumor growth in intact animals (74) and reactivates tumor growth for brief periods in animals whose ovaries, adrenals, and pituitary glands have been removed (119). Prolactin, but not growth hormone, increases the numbers and sizes of tumors in adrenalectomized-ovariectomized rats in a dose-related manner (110). Perphenazine, haloperiodol, thyrotropin-releasing hormone, and adrenalectomy, all of which increase circulating prolactin concentrations, increase the numbers and sizes of DMBA-induced rat mammary tumors (15,16,119,128). Pituitary homographs placed under the renal capsule likewise increase serum levels of prolactin, leading to stimulation of mammary tumor growth (54,170). The presence of lesions in the median eminence of the tuber cinereum increases prolactin release but causes a decrease in levels of all other pituitary hormones (102); implanting estrogen in the median eminence also causes a rise in circulating prolactin levels. Both of these procedures, when performed on tumor-bearing rats, produce an increase in numbers and sizes of mammary tumors (18,77,109).

When endogenous levels of prolactin are reduced by drugs such as ergocornine, lysergic acid diethylamide, pargyline, or L-DOPA, by administration of antiprolactin antiserum, or by hypophysectomy, mammary tumors regress (10,11, 63,101,119,128,172). Ovariectomy of tumor-bearing rats can also cause mammary tumors to regress, and subsequent estradiol injection stimulates regrowth. However, the effect of estrogen has been considered by some to be indirect, since reductions in circulating estrogen are associated with decreased serum levels of prolactin, and estrogen administration causes an increase in circulating prolactin concentrations (101). Estrogen will not reactivate tumor growth in the absence of a pituitary gland (154).

The breast tumors of some patients have regressed after hypophysectomy (89), but regression as a result of suppression of circulating prolactin with L-DOPA or ergot drugs has been rare (35,40,44,45,53,57,103,104,108,144,155). Reports of the effects of human prolactin, human growth hormone, and ovine prolactin on progression of osteolytic metastases have been conflicting (88, 118,120,121); in two studies (38,166) tumor regression occurred in patients with high prolactin levels after pituitary stalk section.

Estrogen

Although findings in experimental systems have suggested that prolactin is solely responsible for hormone-dependent tumor growth, more recent investigations have indicated that estrogen may have more than an indirect involvement. Sinha et al. (150) have shown that the presence of lesions in the median eminence not only increases circulating prolactin levels but also stimulates tumor growth. However, subsequent removal of the ovaries results in tumor regression; tumor growth is stimulated when ovaries are implanted into these same animals. In another study, some mammary tumors that had regressed after ovariectomy and adrenalectomy could be only slightly reactivated by prolactin injection. Administration of prolactin with as little as 0.01 μg of estradiol per day (which by itself could not reactivate growth) caused the regressed tumors to reinitiate growth (83). If hormone dependence is determined on the basis of regression in the absence of one hormone and resumption of growth following its replacement, approximately one-third of DMBA-induced rat mammary tumors can be classified as either estrogen- or prolactin-dependent. However, the percentage of strictly estrogen-dependent tumors is small if prolactin levels are maintained after ovariectomy (9). These results suggest that both estrogen and prolactin are necessary to support mammary tumor growth. However, it is not clear if estrogen is necessary for prolactin to exert its effects or, conversely, if prolactin is "permissive" to the action of estrogen.

Insulin

Some mammary tumors can be classified as insulin-dependent as well as prolactin- and estrogen-dependent (19,20,58,60,62). Induction of diabetes in tumor-bearing rats with streptozotocin (20) or alloxan (58,60,62) caused 60 to 90% of tumors to regress, and administration of insulin to intact rats decreased tumor size (60). However, these tumors were not solely insulin-dependent. Insulin cannot overcome tumor regression due to ovariectomy (60), and estrogen injection does not prevent tumor regression in diabetic rats (62). Whether insulin alone is capable of reactivating tumor growth following hypophysectomy is not known, but in hypophysectomized rats prolactin plus insulin clearly stimulates tumors more than prolactin alone (60).

Progesterone

Although progesterone alone will not maintain DMBA-induced rat mammary tumor growth, the same tumors are stimulated by a combination of estradiol and progesterone or estradiol alone (68). By contrast, Heuson *et al.* (61) reported that progesterone stimulates tumor growth in ovariectomized rats nearly as much as estradiol. However, the hormone dependence of the individual tumors that responded to progesterone was not tested directly. The transplantable MTW9 rat mammary tumor does not grow in ovariectomized rats unless a prolactin-secreting pituitary tumor is coimplanted. Optimal growth requires co-administration of progesterone and estradiol; progesterone or estradiol given singly is less effective (90). Progesterone clearly enhances induction of DMBA-induced rat mammary tumors and may be necessary to prevent regression of established tumors following parturition (70,71,94). In GR mice with estrone-progesterone-induced mammary tumors, progesterone increases DNA synthesis (143,178), and in DDD mice with pregnancy-dependent TPD MT-4 mammary tumors, progesterone together with estradiol and prolactin is necessary for growth (91–93). Thus prolactin and estrogen appear to have closely linked roles as primary determinants of hormone-dependent tumor growth. Insulin has profound effects on tumor growth, but its relationship to estrogen and prolactin is not understood. Results with progesterone, although conflicting in rat mammary tumors, indicate that this hormone together with estrogen and prolactin may be involved in supporting growth of hormone-dependent murine tumors. Table 1 summarizes the reported effects of endocrine manipulation on mammary tumor growth *in vivo.*

TABLE 1. *Hormone-dependent mammary tumor growth* in vivo

Tumor	Experimental conditions promoting: Progression	Experimental conditions promoting: Regression
DMBA-induced, Sprague-Dawley rat	Intact + prolactin, E_2,[a] insulin, or prolactin-stimulating drugs	Intact + prolactin-suppressing drugs
	Hx-Ovex-Adx + prolactin (short term)	Hx-Ovex-Adx (long term)
	Ovex-Adx + prolactin and/or E_2	Ovex; Hx + E_2
	Diabetic + insulin	Diabetic
	Median eminence lesions + Ovex (short term) + transplanted ovaries (long term)	Median eminence lesions + Ovex (long term)
MTW9, Wistar-Furth rat	Intact + prolactin-secreting pituitary tumor	Intact
MTW9-MD, MTW9-A, MTW9-P, Wistar-Furth rat	Intact	Ovex
Primary estrone-progesterone-induced in GR mice	Castrated + E_2 + Pg	Castrated
TPD MT-4 in DDD mice	Pregnant	Intact
	Intact + E_2 + Pg	Intact + E_2 or Pg
	Pituitary isographs	Pituitary isographs + Ovex
	Pituitary isographs + Ovex + E_2 + Pg	Hx + E_2 + Pg
	Ovex-Adx + E_2 + Pg	

[a] Abbreviations: E_2, estradiol; Pg, progesterone; Hx, hypophysectomy; Ovex, ovariectomy; Adx, adrenalectomy.

HORMONE DEPENDENCE *IN VITRO*

In vitro methods have been used extensively to define the relative roles of ovarian, adrenal, pituitary, and pancreatic hormones in mammary tumor growth and metabolism. The intent has been to use a precisely controlled hormonal environment to confirm and extend observations originally made *in vivo.* Such experiments have been based on previously published work concerned with elucidation of the hormone requirements for growth and differentiation of normal mammary tissue. A number of comprehensive reviews on this subject are available (43,81).

The principal vehicle for *in vitro* studies of hormone dependence are organ cultures of tumor tissue freshly excised from the animal. Various hormones are then added to a chemically defined culture medium in concentrations ranging from physiologic to pharmacologic. At intervals of up to 4 days after hormone addition, the proliferative response is assessed by measuring the incorporation of radioactive thymidine into DNA, counting the number of cells engaged in DNA synthesis by autoradiography, or by determining the mitotic index.

Prolactin

When added to cultures of some mammary tumors, prolactin plus insulin stimulates growth or DNA synthesis more than in controls incubated with insulin alone (36,85,117) or with insulin plus glucocorticoids (85,175). Serum from rats bearing prolactin-secreting pituitary tumors also stimulates DNA synthesis in organ cultures of hormone-responsive mammary tumors, but not autonomous mammary tumors, in medium containing insulin (157).

Rudland et al. (137) recently reported methods for preparation of hormone-sensitive primary and secondary monolayer cultures of normal and neoplastic rat mammary tissue, thus avoiding the problems of tissue damage, degradation, and hormone penetration inherent in organ culture experiments. Tumors or mammary glands from perphenazine-treated rats were dispersed by gentle enzymatic digestion and grown in medium containing serum. Prolactin in the presence of 5% fetal calf serum stimulated DNA synthesis twofold to threefold in primary tumor cultures. The numbers of ^{3}H-thymidine-labeled nuclei were increased approximately 30-fold when prolactin was added to insulin and cortisol containing medium, but insulin and/or cortisol were without effect in the absence of prolactin. In contrast, as in organ culture (114,162), insulin and cortisol appeared to be necessary for prolactin to stimulate DNA synthesis in monolayers of normal mammary tissue.

Insulin

Insulin added to a defined culture medium will increase DNA synthesis in some rodent (56,117,164,171) and human (36,171,173) mammary tumors, in mammary gland organ cultures (43,127,162), and in a continuous cell line derived from a human breast cancer (115,132). In other mammary tumors, the rate of DNA synthesis in the presence of insulin is no different from that measured when the tumor is removed (59,85,156), whereas some tumors do not maintain DNA synthesis in the presence of insulin (117,156). The degree of tumor stimulation by insulin is highest in cultures of virgin mammary gland (43,114), and it appears to be maximal at 24 to 48 hr after addition (43,114,162).

The relative importance of prolactin and insulin in stimulating DNA synthesis in mammary tissue is not clear. Prolactin has been reported to sensitize normal mammary cells to the stimulating action of insulin (114), which suggests that insulin is the mitogenic stimulus. However, it was recently found that prolactin with insulin, but not insulin or prolactin alone, is capable of initiating a new round of cell division. Thus insulin may be necessary for mammary cells to complete DNA synthesis, but prolactin may be required to initiate a new round of cell division (107). Such experiments have not been carried out with either rodent or human mammary tumor tissue.

Estrogen

Although estrogen appears to stimulate the growth of experimental mammary tumors *in vivo,* it inhibits DNA synthesis in rat mammary tumors *in vitro* (2,137,164,175), and it can limit a prolactin-induced increase (85,117,175). However, when combined with insulin, estrogen causes a slight increase in labeling index and mitotic index in normal mammary tissue (80). In organ cultures of human breast tumors, estrogen prolongs the survival of some tumors (14) and increases DNA synthesis if the medium contains 20% male calf serum (42). In another experiment, estradiol inhibited DNA synthesis in short-term human breast tumor cultures (131). Recently a human mammary tumor cell line (MCF-7) was shown to respond to estradiol with a twofold to fourfold increase in DNA synthesis. The same line was inhibited by high doses of estradiol (86,87).

Glucocorticoids and Progesterone

Glucocorticoids have been used in organ cultures of normal mammary tissue, and they appear to be necessary for the expression of differentiated function (31,39,165), most likely because they maintain rough endoplasmic reticulum (113). However, they do not appear to be necessary for maintenance of DNA synthesis in normal mammary tissue or tumors in organ culture (2,39,80,85); high concentrations have been shown to be deleterious (80,133). Maximum effects of prolactin on DNA synthesis in DMBA-induced mammary tumors in organ cultures are seen when glucocorticoids are added to an insulin-containing medium (85).

Information on the effect of progesterone on mammary tumor growth *in vitro* is limited. Pasteels et al. (117) recently showed that in 9 of 12 organ cultures of insulin-responsive DMBA-induced rat mammary tumors, a combination of progesterone and prolactin stimulated DNA synthesis more than in

TABLE 2. *Effect of hormones on DNA synthesis in DMBA-induced rat mammary tumors* in vitro

Culture type	Stimulation	Maintenance	Inhibition
Organ culture	Insulin Prolactin + insulin Prolactin + insulin + glucocorticoid Prolactin + insulin + progesterone	Insulin Insulin + glucocorticoid	Estrogen Glucocorticoid (high levels)
Primary monolayer	Prolactin + 0.5% fetal calf serum	Insulin + glucocorticoid + 0.5% fetal calf serum	—

controls incubated with insulin alone. Given singly, progesterone or prolactin was effective in only 25% of the tumors tested. Similar results have been obtained in organ cultures of normal rat mammary tissue (80), but in secondary monolayer cultures of DMBA-induced rat mammary tumors, progesterone added to a medium containing insulin and prolactin in 0.5% fetal calf serum had no discernible effect (137).

Thus prolactin can stimulate DNA synthesis in mammary tumors cultured *in vitro* (Table 2). Insulin and possibly glucocorticoids appear to be necessary for prolactin to exert its effects in monolayers of normal rat mammary tissue and to maximize prolactin responses in tumors. Prolactin alone can stimulate DNA synthesis in primary cultures derived from DMBA-induced mammary tumors. Reports of the effects of estradiol on DNA synthesis in human breast tissue *in vitro* are conflicting, but in cultured rat mammary tumors the hormone appears to inhibit DNA synthesis.

It is clear from the preceding discussion that prolactin is probably the most important hormone, but not the only hormone, controlling hormone-dependent mammary tumor growth both *in vivo* and *in vitro.* Estrogen as well as prolactin appears to maintain tumor growth *in vivo,* but this effect has not been conclusively shown *in vitro.* Much less is known about the involvement of insulin and progesterone. However, it is clear that these studies do not clarify the mechanism of hormone dependence, nor do they indicate why some tumors respond to hormones and others do not.

MECHANISMS OF PROLACTIN DEPENDENCE

It is now generally accepted that the actions of hormones are mediated by specific interactions with receptor proteins—cytoplasmic receptors for steroids and cell-surface membrane receptors for polypeptide hormones. In mammary tumors these receptors might be either retained or lost during malignant transformation. On the one hand, the presence of receptors in certain tumors might reflect retention of hormonal control mechanisms present in normal cells, so that the tumors were rendered hormone-dependent. A loss of receptors would indicate that a tumor cell had lost the ability to recognize (and hence be regulated by) hormones. Over the past few years much attention has been directed toward identification and quantitation of receptors for estrogen and determination of the relationships of these receptors to hormone-dependent mammary tumor growth. Estrogen binding is reportedly much lower in autonomous mammary tumors than in hormone-dependent mammary tumors (25,96,106,139,159). However, more recent investigations comparing estrogen receptors in ovarian-dependent and -independent DMBA-induced rat mammary tumors have disclosed a more complex situation. Although independent tumors tended to contain fewer estrogen receptors, the extent of overlap between receptor levels in autonomous versus dependent tumors did not allow accurate prediction of hormone dependence for individual tumors (8,32).

This finding does not alter the conclusion that tumors that lack estrogen receptors are autonomous, but it does indicate that tumors that do contain estrogen receptor are not always hormone-dependent. Similar conclusions have been reached by others in studies of the relationship between estrogen receptors and response to endocrine therapy in human breast cancer (95). Several explanations can be offered to account for these observations. First, an estrogen receptor may recognize estrogen but not be capable of initiating events beyond the binding step. Thus a product of estrogen action might be a more accurate indicator of the integrity of the estrogen response system than estrogen receptor alone. Since it is well established that synthesis of progesterone receptor in the uterus is dependent on the action of estrogen, it was possible that a similar relationship may exist in mammary tumors. Horwitz and McGuire (68) and others (98) recently demonstrated that estrogen does in fact induce progesterone receptors in DMBA-induced rat mammary tumors. In addition, the presence of progesterone receptors correlates with response to endocrine therapy in human breast cancer better than the presence of estrogen receptors alone, which suggests that the pathway of hormonal control can be altered after initial estrogen binding (97). This subject has been considered in detail elsewhere (98).

A second possibility is alteration in the control mechanisms for hormones (other than estrogen) that regulate hormone-dependent mammary tumor growth. Because of prolactin's key position in controlling the growth of hormone-dependent mammary tumors, it seemed essential to determine if prolactin receptors and hormone dependence were directly related. Earlier studies to test this possibility were hampered by lack of suitably labeled tracer, but in 1972, Frantz and Turkington (48) described a technique that produced ^{125}I-labeled prolactin of high specific activity without loss of biological activity. Using this material, they demonstrated the presence of specific high-affinity binding sites for prolactin in normal mammary gland. Subsequent reports confirmed and extended these initial observations to mammary tumors (Table 3) and other tissues and species (1,46,79,116,125,148).

TABLE 3. *Prolactin receptors in mammary tumors*[a]

Tumor type	Status of animal/tumor	Preparation assayed	Prolactin binding sites: fmoles/mg protein or μg DNA	Prolactin binding sites: Percentage specific binding per 100 μg protein	Prolactin binding sites: K_d ($\times 10^{10}$ M)	Reference
DMBA-induced	Intact, ↑, ↓ Pr[b]/responsive, nonresponsive, biopsy, treated tumor	Slice	—	1–3	—	66
	Intact, ↓ Pr, E_2 (2 μg/day)/variable	M	—	5–5.5	—	152
	Intact, ↑ Pr/variable		—	1.7	—	
	Intact, 20 μg/day E_2/variable		—	3.1	—	
	Intact/biopsy, Ov responsive	M	—	2.6	—	32
	Intact/biopsy, Ov nonresponsive		—	1.3	—	
	Intact, Ov/growing, responsive, nonresponsive	Slice	2.7–4.1[c]	—	10–30	23
	Intact, Hx/growing, regressing	M	—	13–83	—	
	Intact + Opr/response ranked	M	203–530	2.4–7.4	5–6	74
	Intact/growing	M	187	7.7–12	3	151
	Diabetic/regressing		46	4.6–7.9	—	
	Intact/growing	M	433	3.2	—	78
	Intact + E_2 (10–25 μg/day)/regressing		—	1.5–1.8	—	
	Intact/growing	M	260	—	1.1	21
	Intact + TP/regressing		95	—	1.1	
	Intact + TP/nonresponsive		138	—	1.3	
R3230AC	Intact, Ov/growing	Slice	0.61[c]	—	18	72
	Intact/growing	M	—	1.1	—	153
	Diabetic/growing		—	0.76	—	
MTW9-MD	Intact, Ov/Ov responsive	Slice	1.0[c]	—	19	25
MTW9-MA	Intact, Ov/Ov nonresponsive	Slice	0.15[c]	—	14	

MTW9-P	Intact, Ov/Ov responsive	M	12.2	—	7.9	126
MTW9-MtT	Intact, ↑ Opr/growing		2.9	—	—	
	Intact, ↓ Pr/responsive		7.5	—	—	
DMBA-induced	Intact/growing	M	—	0.6–2.6	71	161
R3230AC	Intact/growing	M	—	0.2–0.4	—	
C3H BA mouse	Intact/growing	M	—	0	—	
Estrone-progesterone-induced, GR mice	Intact, Ov/responsive to autonomous	M	2.8–16	9.6–0.24	1	29
Human	—	Slice	9.4	0.2–0.8	4	67
	—	M	14–192	0.4–2.2	11	146

[a] The results are, by necessity, simplified. More than one receptor value is given only when a particular manipulation results in a change. For comparative purposes, receptor values not reported as fmoles/mg protein or μg of DNA have been expressed as percentage specific binding per 100 μg protein.

[b] Abbreviations and symbols: M, crude membrane pellet; Pr, circulating prolactin; Opr, injected ovine prolactin; Ov, ovariectomy; Hx, hypophysectomy; E_2, estradiol; TP, testosterone propionate; ↑, increase; ↓, decrease.

[c] fmoles/μg DNA; —, not reported.

Prolactin Receptors

As was mentioned previously, receptors for prolactin, like those for other polypeptide hormones, are believed to be associated predominantly with the cell-surface membrane (136). Evidence for surface localization of prolactin receptors comes from several observations: (a) prolactin covalently linked to sepharose (which presumably does not enter cells) stimulates RNA synthesis in isolated mammary cells (163); (b) injected ^{125}I-labeled prolactin is localized predominantly at the mammary cell surface (4,130); (c) in several target tissues subcellular fractions containing the highest specific activity of prolactin binding also have the highest activity of 5′-nucleotidase, a plasma membrane marker (125,134, 148). However, recent evidence suggests that prolactin receptors may not be localized solely on the cell periphery. Witorsch and associates have shown that immunoreactive prolactin is present intracellularly in rat mammary gland (112) and in sex accessory glands in male rats (176,177). In addition, prolactin receptors have been demonstrated in the Golgi of female rat liver (122). Whether intracellular uptake of prolactin, the prolactin receptor complex, or intracellular prolactin binding is involved in prolactin action is not known, but a preliminary communication has shown that prolactin can stimulate RNA synthesis in partially purified mammary cell nuclei (17).

Nonetheless, in most studies of prolactin receptors the source of receptor has been a crude "microsomal membrane" fraction derived from centrifuged (15,000 × *g*) supernatant of 0.3 M sucrose homogenate (149). Frantz and Turkington (48,161), by contrast, have used a relatively low-speed (3,000 × *g*) pellet of mammary gland and mammary tumor homogenate as a source of receptor. The recovery of receptor has not been determined in many instances, and the localization of receptor in particulate subcellular fractions appears to vary from one target tissue to another. For instance, Rolland et al. (134) found that in porcine granulosa cells the specific activity of prolactin binding was highest in the 15,000 × *g* pellet; Shiu and Friesen (148), using rabbit mammary gland, found essentially no binding in the 15,000 × *g* pellet. A variable distribution of specific binding activity has also been found in liver from various other species (125). We have observed that when the percentage of total prolactin binding in homogenates is determined in subcellular fractions, most (60–80%) of the rat liver receptor is localized in a 20,000 × *g* pellet, whereas in DMBA-induced rat mammary tumors centrifugation at 100,000 × *g* is necessary to achieve a comparable and consistent recovery (21,24). Since marked changes in the distribution of prolactin receptors could seriously affect the interpretation of binding data, we determined the recovery of receptor in a subcellular fraction from DMBA-induced rat mammary tumors before and after biopsy and regrowth and after androgen-induced regression (21). Recovery, which averaged 68% of homogenate binding, was not significantly altered by any of the treatments. However, these results do not preclude the possibility of altered receptor distribution in tissues in other physiological states. Indeed, Keenan et al. (73) recently demonstrated a striking difference in receptor distributions during development and lactation in rat mammary gland.

A simple approach to eliminate receptor recovery as a potential source of variation has been to bind radiolabeled hormone directly to whole tissue as 0.5-mm tissue slices (22,25,65,138) or frozen ultrathin sections (66) or to dissociated cells (47,153). Although complete penetration of hormones to all areas of a tissue slice might be considered a disadvantage, especially in 0.5-mm sections, we have found that, except for dense tissues such as rat liver, ^{125}I-labeled prolactin equilibrates with intracellular spaces in the 3 to 4 hr required to achieve steady state (27,28). Dispersed cell suspensions, as well, avoid the problem of receptor recovery and accessibility, but precautions must be taken to prevent receptor degradation by enzymes commonly used to dislodge cells from the intracellular matrix. We recently found that including excess prolactin during dissociation of DMBA-induced rat mammary tumors effectively prevented substantial loss of receptor (or receptor-containing cells) in primary monolayer cultures prepared from these tumors (26).

Thus in studies designed to compare numbers of prolactin binding sites quantitatively, either care should be taken to process the tissue in a manner that minimizes receptor loss or recovery of receptor should be determined to eliminate potential artifacts due to receptor redistribution.

If the measure of prolactin binding to tumors is to be considered an interaction with a "receptor," ideally all of the following criteria should be met:

1. The labeled hormone should retain biologic activity.
2. Binding should be time- and temperature-dependent, pH-sensitive, and reversible.
3. Binding should be of limited capacity (saturable), and the affinity of the receptor for hormone should be in the range of circulating levels of the hormone in the species being studied.
4. Binding should be specific only for biologically related hormones and should be limited to cells that respond to the hormone.

Ovine prolactin is most often used in studies on prolactin binding because it is known to be biologically active in rats and mice—species in which hormone-dependent mammary tumor systems have been developed. In addition, ovine prolactin is available from the National Institute of Arthritis and Metabolic Diseases in a purified form of known biologic potency. If receptors are to be detected by direct *in vitro* binding, prolactin must be labeled to high specific activity, since binding sites are present in extremely small (fmoles/mg protein) quantities. Iodination catalyzed by lactoperoxidase is the method of choice (105,160) based on an observation that the more harsh chloramine T method used to label hormones with ^{125}I for radioimmunoassay frequently destroys prolactin's biologic activity (48) and its ability to bind specifically to target tissues (48,148). Determining the biologic activity of labeled prolactin is a tedious procedure (48); hence it is used only rarely. A satisfactory alternative has been to demonstrate a direct relationship between the biologic potency of various unlabeled hormones and their ability to displace ^{125}I-labeled prolactin from its receptor (135). A more elegant demonstration was recently reported by Shiu and Friesen (147). Using antibody to soluble purified prolactin receptors from rabbit mammary gland, they showed that the antibody not only blocked ^{125}I-labeled prolactin binding to receptor but also effectively prevented prolactin from stimulating casein production or α-aminoisobutyric acid uptake in organ cultures of normal mammary gland.

For binding studies on receptor-containing membrane fractions, the incubation medium should contain the following: ^{125}I-labeled prolactin (approximately 0.5 ng); calcium or magnesium ions (5–10 mM), which are required for binding (148); 0.1 to 4% bovine serum albumin (to reduce nonspecific binding to membranes and incubation vessels); buffer at a pH of 7.0 to 7.6, depending on the tissue. Excess unlabeled prolactin or other hormones are incubated in parallel assays to evaluate the hormone specificity of ^{125}I-labeled prolactin binding and nonspecific binding to glassware and membranes. Receptor-containing membranes are added last, and the incubation is allowed to proceed to a steady state. Bound and free hormones are then separated by centrifugation. The time to steady state and the incubation temperature vary widely from one study to another. For example, Frantz et al. (46) contended that 10 to 20 min at either 4° or 37° C is adequate, whereas most other groups find that 6 to 12 hr at 22 to 24° C are required. In our experience, binding to whole tissue slices equilibrates at 3 to 4 hr at 22° C, whereas subcellular fractions require a much longer period. In addition, many authors find that at 4° C binding is extremely slow, requiring 48 to 96 hr to reach a steady state (32,78,152). At 37° C, uptake is faster, but binding begins to decline before reaching values obtained at lower temperatures (78,126). Nonspecific binding also increases at high temperature (65). Because of the slow rate of association, the binding reaction may be a diffusion-dependent process or, alternatively, a more complex multistep reaction. This latter possibility has been considered in detail elsewhere (6,72). Although binding assays performed at low concentrations of prolactin can yield information on relative binding capacity, saturating amounts are required to quantitate the actual number of receptor sites. In practice, this is accomplished by incubating small amounts of ^{125}I-labeled prolactin in the presence of increasing concentrations of unlabeled hormone up to and exceeding saturation of specific binding sites. From a dose-displacement curve the binding affinity (K_a or K_d) and the number of sites at saturation can be ascertained by correcting for nonspecific binding (13) and plotting the data according to Scatchard (142). The rationale for this approach is a practical one. ^{125}I-labeled proteins tend to bind avidly to incubation vessels as well as to nonreceptor proteins present in crude membrane preparations. This binding is considered to be nonspecific (i.e., not limited to receptors), since it is not saturable and is nondisplacable, it occurs in nontarget tissues, and it is strictly proportional to the amount of labeled hormone added. At saturating concentrations of ^{125}I-labeled prolactin, nonspecific binding can range from 50 to 80% of total binding, making accurate determination of specific binding difficult. Lowering the amount of labeled hormone effectively reduces nonspecific interactions to an acceptable 5 to 20% of the total bound. Nonspecific binding can also be reduced by purifying iodinated prolactin on ion-exchange columns before use. This procedure probably removes labeled hormone that has been damaged during the radioiodination procedure (48,65,135). The purified product binds to receptors in a manner identical to that of the native hormone (21). Scatchard analysis of prolactin binding to mammary tumors results in a straight-line plot, indicating that binding is to a single class of receptor sites. The dissociation constant for prolactin binding to receptor measured in this manner varies from 1×10^{-10} M to 7×10^{-9} M at 22°C (Table 3). These values are equivalent to a concentration of 2.3 to 161 ng/ml at half saturation and are within the range of circulating levels of prolactin present in rats, mice, and rabbits.

Finally, interpretation of the significance of identification and quantitation of hormone receptors must be approached with caution. Although the first step in hormone action is interaction with a molecule or molecular complex that has all the characteristics outlined above, this is followed by a series of complex events that ultimately results in a biologic response characteristic for that hormone in a particular tissue. Thus, although binding to receptor is necessary, it is not of itself sufficient for the expression of a hormone response.

Prolactin Receptors in Mammary Tumors

The presence of prolactin receptors in rat mammary tumors was first demonstrated by Turkington (161), who found receptors in amounts ranging from 30 to 80% of that determined in normal mammary tissue. Less than 15% of the normal complement of receptors was present in an autonomous transplantable mammary tumor (R3230AC). Similarly, autonomous mouse mammary tumors bound far less prolactin than did normal mouse mammary gland. These results suggested a correlation between prolactin receptors and hormone-dependent growth; receptors could be present in hormone-dependent tumors but low or absent in autonomous tumors. However, hormone-dependent growth characteristics were not tested directly in all these tumors.

The MTW9 transplantable rat mammary tumor is clearly dependent on prolactin, since it does not grow unless circulating prolactin is maintained at supraphysiological levels by a prolactin-secreting pituitary tumor (90). Two distinct sublines of this tumor have been isolated and characterized. One subline, MTW9-MD, grows in intact rats but regresses promptly after ovariectomy; therefore it is clearly hormone-dependent. This tumor has the same growth characteristics as the MTW9-A tumor line described by Kim (76) and the MTW9-P line isolated by Diamond et al. (34). The other subline, MTW9-MA, originally obtained from U. Kim, grows equally well in intact, ovariectomized, and hypophysectomized rats and is therefore considered autonomous. We found that prolactin receptors are present in the MTW9-MD tumor in amounts equal to those previously measured in lactating rat mammary tissue (22,65). By contrast, the autonomous tumor contains only 15% of the number of sites seen in the MTW9-MD tumor. There are no changes in the affinity of the receptor for prolactin. The K_d was 2×10^{-9} M for both tumors (25).

We recently investigated the relationship of prolactin receptors to hormone-dependent tumor growth in estrone-progesterone-induced mammary tumors in GR mice. These tumors are initially hormone-dependent, since they do not grow in castrated untreated mice, but when transplanted they eventually lose their hormone-dependent growth characteristics (29). In this study, prolactin binding was highest (16 fmoles/mg homogenate protein) in primary hormone-dependent tumors and declined progressively in transplanted hormone-dependent and hormone-responsive tumors. In autonomous tumors, binding was approximately 5% of that found in primary tumors. The decrease in bound hormone was attributed to a loss in the number of receptor sites, since binding affinity of the receptor was the same for all types of tumors.

Although these observations support a causal relationship between loss of prolactin receptors and loss of hormone dependence in experimental breast cancer, this interpretation is complicated by the following observations. First, the R3230AC transplantable rat mammary carcinoma does not depend on estrogen or prolactin for growth, although it does respond to these hormones with distinct changes in enzyme activities (64). In contrast to the autonomous MTW9-MA tumor, the R3230AC tumor contains nearly the same number of prolactin receptors as found in normal rat mammary tissue. There are no differences in the affinity of the receptor for prolactin or in its specificity of binding (22). These results have been confirmed by Smith et al. (153). Second, in recent studies of the relationship of prolactin receptors to hormone-dependent growth in DMBA-induced rat mammary tumors, binding was measured after a response to ovariectomy and was found to be slightly lower in autonomous tumors. However, because dependent and autonomous tumors were characterized by wide variations in receptor, it was not possible to correlate the number of binding sites and the response to ovariectomy. Moreover, if receptor levels in ovariectomy-dependent and -independent tumors are compared with those in tumors growing in intact rats, the mean receptor level decreases approximately 30% after ovariectomy, regardless of response. This suggests that removal of the ovaries rather than response (regression) accounts for the receptor decrease (23). If hormone dependence is assessed by tumor response to drugs that either increase or decrease circulating levels of prolactin (66), receptor levels are higher in tumors that respond to prolactin by increased growth. Response could not be predicted by the level of prolactin receptor in pretreatment biopsies. However, when tumors are classified on the basis of response to decreased circulating prolactin, receptor levels are higher in the responsive tumors both before and after biopsy. Nonetheless, this correlation is not sufficient to predict growth behavior for individual tumors.

Finally, in studies to assay growing tumors for prolactin receptor content and subsequently to assess hormone dependence in transplanted tumors, all but 3 of 24 tumors examined contained some prolactin receptor, and on the average, binding was 50% lower in autonomous tumors. Again, because of the overlap in receptor concentrations, no correlation could be made between hormone-dependent growth and prolactin receptor levels (32).

Since the numbers of receptors in both hormone-dependent and autonomous DMBA-induced mammary tumors cover a broad spectrum, from very low to very high levels, it is possible that the degree of dependence is related to receptor content. Kelly et al. (74) approached this question by measuring the number of prolactin receptors in DMBA-induced rat mammary tumors after ranking them according to their relative growth rates in response to prolactin administration. They found that receptor levels were highest in tumors that showed the greatest increase in tumor mass in response to prolactin, which suggests that the number of receptor sites in a tumor might indeed indicate the degree of responsiveness to prolactin. Alternatively, tumors might consist of a heterogeneous cell population with respect to prolactin receptors, so that growth response would be directly related to the proportion of tumor cells that contained receptor sites. We attempted to distinguish between these alternatives by identifying prolactin receptor sites in DMBA-induced rat mammary tumors using autoradiography. In some tumors, all tumor cells contained receptors; in others, up to one-half remained unlabeled. These results suggest that reported variations in receptor content in DMBA-induced mammary tumors may be caused by the presence of two distinct populations of cells, one containing prolactin receptors and another containing very few receptor sites or none at all (27).

Despite the apparent lack of direct correlation between prolactin receptor levels and hormone dependence in these studies, it is important to note that a nearly 90% (22 of 24) prediction of hormone dependence can be obtained in DMBA-induced rat mammary tumors when both estrogen and prolactin receptor levels are taken into account. This observation emphasizes the fact that endocrine control of mammary tumor growth is a complex phenomenon and that accurate prediction of response will probably require a complete understanding of the mechanisms by which all hormones influence mammary tumor growth (32).

The first studies of prolactin binding in human breast cancer were published only recently (67,146). In these reports, the levels of binding assessed with ^{125}I-labeled human prolactin were, on the average, much lower than in rat mammary tumors; e.g., 8 of 41 tumors (20%) specifically bound 1% or more of the added label (67), and 20 of 36 primary tumors (55%) contained 1 to 5.4% of the specific binding (146). By comparison, DMBA-induced rat mammary tumors can specifically bind up to 22% of added labeled prolactin under similar conditions (74). Although these observations suggest that prolactin directly influences the growth of human tumors, they must be qualified because of technical problems. Nonspecific binding may account for up to 8% of added label (67), and the limited number and heterogeneity of patient specimens make extensive characterization of binding difficult. Moreover, to date there have been no studies correlating prolactin binding with response to endocrine therapy or with tumor growth *in vitro.*

Receptor Regulation in Mammary Tumors

It has become increasingly evident that target tissue function is regulated not only by circulating levels of hormones but also by the target cell itself, whose response to hormonal stimulation is controlled by hormone receptor content [see Table 4, ref. (82)]. Investigation of the mechanism of receptor regulation in mammary carcinoma is of importance in order to understand how a given hormone controls cell growth and also because such information may ultimately be used to design more rational approaches to endocrine therapy in human breast cancer. As was mentioned earlier, estrogen controls progesterone receptors in mammary tumors. Hilf and associates recently studied the effects of estrogen, prolactin, lergotrile mesylate (which lowers circulating prolactin), and streptozotocin-induced diabetes on prolactin receptors in DMBA-induced rat mammary tumors and the transplantable R3230AC rat mammary carcinoma (151–153). In agreement with our observations (22,23,65), they found that the level of prolactin receptors in R3230AC tumors is the same as in normal mammary gland in late pregnancy and early lactation (153); in DMBA-induced mammary tumors, by contrast, binding is three times higher than in normal tissue (152). Prolactin administration decreases prolactin binding in both tumor types but increases growth only in DMBA-induced tumors. Lergotrile mesylate, when used to reduce circulating prolactin levels in animals bearing DMBA-induced tumors, causes a decrease in tumor growth, whereas estradiol (2 μg/day) has the opposite effect; neither treatment alters prolactin binding. In diabetic rats the growth of R3230AC tumors is slightly enhanced, whereas up to 50% of DMBA-induced tumors regress. Prolactin binding decreases slightly in R3230AC tumors (30%), and in DMBA-induced tumors binding falls by approximately 50%. Because of insulin's important role in prolactin-induced lactogenesis in normal mammary tissue *in vitro* and growth of DMBA-induced mammary tumors *in vivo,* these findings suggest that insulin may, in part, control tissue responsiveness to prolactin by regulating the number of prolactin binding sites. It would also appear from these reports that the effect of estrogen on tumor growth may be direct, since prolactin receptors are unaffected by doses of estradiol that clearly stimulate DMBA-induced mammary tumors. The effect of prolactin on its own receptor is less clear. As was mentioned earlier, other investigations have shown that raising prolactin levels increases the number of receptors in DMBA-induced rat mammary tumors but that this effect may be indirect by increasing the number of prolactin-receptor-containing cells. The inhibition of binding observed in these experiments might reflect masking of sites or an actual reduction of receptors in response to homologous hormone, as is seen in other systems (82). This latter possibility is supported by the observation that in the R3230AC tumor the rate of tumor growth has no apparent effect on the apparent number of binding sites.

Our interest in receptor regulation was prompted by observations that in autonomous and hormone-dependent sublines of the MTW9 rat mammary tumor, both estrogen and prolactin receptors decline with a transition to autonomy (25). This raised the question of whether losses of prolactin and estradiol receptors are independent or related events. A relationship was suggested by the work of Vignon and Rochefort (167,168) and was recently confirmed by Hawkins et al. (55). These investigations demonstrated marked reduction in estrogen receptors in hormone-dependent DMBA-induced tumors after ovariectomy, and they showed that prolactin injection restores tumor estrogen receptor to previous levels within 1 to 2 days. Similar observations in organ cultures of normal and neoplastic mammary tissue, i.e., prolactin-stimulated uptake of radiolabeled estradiol (84,140,141), also support the notion that prolactin regulates estrogen receptor in mammary tumors (33,49,145).

Because these effects might be due to a reversal of tumor regression and not a specific prolactin-induced increase in estrogen receptor, we examined the relationship of estrogen and prolactin receptors in the female rat liver. This tissue is responsive to both hormones, but its growth is not radically affected by endocrine manipulation. When circulating prolactin is eliminated by hypophysectomy, liver estrogen receptor levels fall precipitously (90%). Administration of a single 2-mg dose of ovine prolactin stimulates estrogen receptor within 18 hr. Increasing the dose of prolactin or prolonging injections does not cause further stimulation (12). Although this indicates that liver estrogen receptor is regulated by circulating prolactin, interpretation of these results is complicated by the findings of Posner et al. (123,124), who have shown that hypophysectomy is followed by a substantial decline in receptors for prolactin. Since increasing the circulating prolactin with pituitary homografts markedly increases prolactin binding sites, we sought to determine if exogenous prolactin could stimulate prolactin receptors as it stimulated estrogen receptors. We found that an optimal dose of 2 mg ovine prolactin stimulated prolactin receptor approximately sevenfold within 18 hr after injection, indicating that prolactin itself can induce its own receptor (24). Subsequently Bohnet et al. (7) reported that a full complement of liver prolactin receptors could be induced if ACTH and growth hormone were administered with ovine prolactin. The exact mechanism for this augmentation of the prolactin effect is not known.

In normal mammary tissue, numbers of prolactin binding sites appear to be low during pregnancy, but increase sharply at the onset of lactation (65,152). In contrast, when hysterectomies are performed on pregnant rats during various stages of pregnancy, receptor levels rise progressively from day 8 of pregnancy to parturition. Since neither estrogen nor progesterone injection altered this increase, we inferred that placental lactogen might be inducing prolactin receptors but that excess placental lactogen released during pregnancy was occupying available binding sites, making them unavailable for assay in intact animals

(65). Recently, Djiane and Durand (37) further demonstrated that preventing the prolactin surge during late pregnancy with CB-154 effectively prevented a subsequent rise in prolactin receptors during lactation. In addition, in pseudo-pregnant rabbits it was possible to prevent prolactin stimulation of prolactin receptors by coadministration of progesterone. Despite their discrepancies resulting from differences in species tested, differences in physiological states of the animals, and differences in experimental design, these two reports offer suggestive evidence that in normal mammary tissue, prolactin (and/or placental lactogen) may increase prolactin receptors. Under certain circumstances progesterone may be capable of regulating the level of prolactin receptor, which may, in part, explain why progesterone prevents a prolactin-induced increase in estrogen uptake in rat mammary tumors and normal mammary tissue in organ culture (84,140). Whether or not prolactin regulates its own receptor in tumors is still undetermined, but it is clear that endocrine regulation of prolactin receptors is distinctly different in normal liver and neoplastic mammary tissue. Three days after hypophysectomy, liver receptors are reduced by 90%, whereas those in tumors from the same animals are only moderately affected, if at all (23).

Administration of pharmacologic doses of steroid hormones causes regression of certain breast cancers in rats (100,129,178) and man (50,51,169). In particular, high doses of androgen reduce the numbers and sizes of DMBA-induced rat mammary tumors, whereas coadministration of prolactin with the androgen prevents regression. Since androgen does not reduce serum prolactin levels, it has been proposed that androgen may block the peripheral effect of prolactin at the level of the tumor cell (129). Similarly, high doses of estrogen cause regression of DMBA-induced rat mammary tumors. Coadministration of prolactin with estrogen also overcomes steroid-induced regression, possibly by a mechanism similar to the one proposed for the effects of androgen (100). To determine if the effect of androgen was due to alteration in the ability of the tumor cell to bind and hence respond to prolactin, we quantitated prolactin receptors in androgen-responsive and -nonresponsive tumors (21). In androgen-responsive tumors (50% regression in 26 days) we found that prolactin receptor levels averaged 63% lower than in tissue biopsied before androgen treatment; however, receptor levels did not fall in all cases. Compared to biopsy samples, tumors that did not regress following androgen administration showed no change in numbers of receptor sites, indicating that the reduction in binding sites in responsive tumors was not due to increased circulating prolactin in response to testosterone propionate (111). Prolactin binding in pretreatment biopsies from both groups varied considerably and could not be used to predict which tumors were likely to respond. The affinity of the receptor for prolactin was unaltered regardless of treatment or response. These findings, as well as a recent report by Kelly et al. (75) showing that androgen can reduce prolactin binding in rat liver, tend to support the hypothesis that androgen directly affects the ability of tumors to respond to prolactin by reducing prolactin receptors. However, there may be alternative mechanisms, since not all tumors that regressed showed a reduction in binding sites. First, some tumors may not have been solely dependent on prolactin for growth. If estrogen was required in these instances, regression might have been mediated by an androgen-induced decrease in cytoplasmic estrogen receptors, as demonstrated by Zava and McGuire (180). Second, because receptors in responsive tumors were not completely abolished, one might hypothesize that a certain level of intracellular signal in response to prolactin is necessary to support tumor growth. If prolactin receptors were reduced so that a critical level of signal was not obtained, tumor growth would have been retarded. Our data can be used to support this notion, since prolactin injection could overcome an inadequate signal by increasing receptor occupancy. However, all tumors initially grew at physiologic levels of prolactin; so unless each tumor had a unique requirement of signal to support growth, this hypothesis would be inadequate. Finally, other mechanisms involving prolactin receptors indirectly are feasible. Since prolactin can stimulate estrogen receptors in regressed DMBA-induced mammary tumors, a loss of prolactin receptor might lead to a reduction in estrogen receptor, and regression might be mediated by the inability of estrogen to stimulate the tumor cell. Prolactin could overcome androgen-induced regression in this case by increasing estrogen receptor and consequently estrogen responsiveness.

The observation that tumor regression due to pharmacologic doses of estrogen is also reversed by prolactin prompted Kledzik et al. (78) and Smith et al. (152) to consider whether alterations in prolactin binding might account for these effects. Prolactin receptors were measured in DMBA-induced rat mammary tumors after injection of doses of estrogen that either stimulated or inhibited tumor growth. To eliminate possible interference of *in vitro* prolactin binding by high levels of circulating prolactin, ergocornine was injected prior to sacrifice (78). Stimulation of tumor growth by estradiol benzoate at 0.2 or 2 μg/day did not alter receptor levels, but dosages of 10, 20, or 25 μg/day resulted in tumor regression and a 26 to 44% decrease in prolactin binding. Since pretreatment receptor levels were not determined in these studies, it is not known if all tumors that regressed lost receptor. Because prolactin receptors were decreased and prolactin reversed the effect of either steroid on tumor growth, these findings suggest a similar mode of action. However, because prolactin receptors were not completely abolished in either case, many of the same alternatives presented to account for androgen-induced regression may also apply to estrogen-mediated regression.

CONCLUSIONS

A model for the control of hormone receptors and growth in hormone-dependent mammary carcinomas is depicted in Fig. 1. The model incorporates presumed relationships among prolactin and its receptors and other hormones and receptors. Insulin, via its receptor, increases (or maintains) prolactin receptor and participates directly or permissively in controlling growth. Prolactin (which

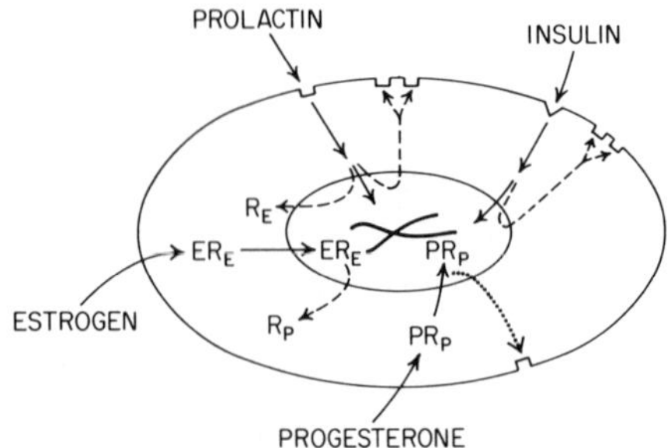

FIG. 1. Possible pathways for control of hormone receptors and growth in hormone-dependent mammary carcinoma. E, estrogen; P, progesterone; Re, estrogen receptor; Rp, progesterone receptor; dash line, increase; dotted line, decrease.

can be stimulated by estrogen) stimulates growth and estrogen receptor by acting through prolactin receptor. Estrogen directly participates in modulating growth and also increases progesterone receptor. Finally, interaction of progesterone with its receptor may affect tumor growth either directly (as in hormone-dependent mammary tumors in mice) or in a permissive fashion. Possible feedback controls may include prolactin regulation of its own receptor and progesterone-induced decreases in prolactin receptors. These controls may be operative in normal mammary tissue and in some mammary tumors. Since the transformation of mammary tissue probably occurs at more than one specific genetic locus, there could be a number of variations in this system. If, for instance, a single receptor is lost and its function in supporting growth is not maintained, then the cell will die (no tumor). On the other hand, if the receptor is lost but those biochemical events required to support growth by that hormone are maintained, then the cell is "autonomous" for that hormone. Obviously a receptor could also be retained in this situation, since the hormone's functions would be constituative. Thus, in order to predict hormone dependence in all possible situations, it will be necessary not only to determine if one or more receptors are retained in a given tumor but also to understand the biochemical events and complex hormonal interrelationships controlling mammary cell growth.

ACKNOWLEDGMENTS

The work described was supported in part by U.S. Public Health Service grants and contract (CA-11378 and CB-23862) and American Cancer Society grants IN 99C and BC-247.

Preparation of this manuscript was supported in part by grant BC-247 from the American Cancer Society, U.S. Public Health Service Medical Research Support grant RR-05584-12, and ALSAC. We thank Ms. Patricia Nicholas for typing the original manuscript, Mr. John Gilbert for editing the manuscript, and Drs. Paul Kelly, Russell Hilf, and Barry Sherman for preprints of manuscripts relevant to this review.

REFERENCES

1. Aragona, C., and Friesen, H. G. (1975): Specific prolactin binding sites in the prostate and testis of rats. *Endocrinology,* 97:677–684.
2. Aspegren, K. (1975): 7,12-DMBA-induced rat mammary tumour studied for hormonal responsiveness *in vitro. Acta Pathol. Microbiol. Scand. [A],* 83:37–50.
3. Ben-David, M. (1968): Mechanism of induction of mammary differentiation in Sprague-Dawley female rats by perphenazine. *Endocrinology,* 83:1217–1223.
4. Birkinshaw, M., and Falconer, I. R. (1972): The localization of prolactin labeled with radioactive iodine in rabbit mammary tissue. *J. Endocrinol.,* 55:323–334.
5. Blackwell, R., Vale, W., Rivier, C., and Guillemin, R. (1973): Effect of perphenazine on the secretion of prolactin *in vivo* and *in vitro. Proc. Soc. Exp. Biol. Med.,* 142:68–71.
6. Boeynaems, J. M., and Dumont, S. E. (1977): The two-step model of ligand-receptor interactions. *Mol. Cell. Endocrinol.,* 7:33–47.
7. Bohnet, H., Aragona, C., and Friesen, H. G. (1976): Induction of lactogenic receptors in male and female rat liver. *Fed. Proc.,* 35:219.
8. Boylan, E. S., and Wittliff, J. L. (1975): Specific estrogen binding in rat mammary tumors induced by 7,12-dimethylbenzanthracene. *Cancer Res.,* 35:506–511.
9. Bradley, C. J., Kledzik, G. S., and Meites, J. (1976): Prolactin and estrogen dependency of rat mammary cancers at early and late stages of development. *Cancer Res.,* 36:319–324.
10. Butler, T. P., and Pearson, O. H. (1971): Regression of prolactin-dependent rat mammary carcinoma in response to antihormone treatment. *Cancer Res.,* 31:817–820.
11. Cassell, E. E., Meites, J., and Welsch, C. W. (1971): Effects of ergocornine and ergocryptine on growth of 7,12-dimethylbenz*(a)*anthracene-induced mammary tumors in rats. *Cancer Res.,* 31:1051–1053.
12. Chamness, G. C., Costlow, M. E., and McGuire, W. L. (1975): Estrogen receptor in rat liver and its dependence on prolactin. *Steroids,* 26:363–371.
13. Chamness, G. C., and McGuire, W. L. (1975): Scatchard plots: Common errors in correction and interpretation. *Steroids,* 26:538–542.
14. Chayen, J., Altmaro, F. P., Bitensky, L., and Daley, J. R. (1970): Response of human breast cancer tissue to steroid hormones *in vitro. Lancet,* 1:868–870.
15. Chen, H. J., Bradley, C. J., and Meites, J. (1976): Stimulation of carcinogen-induced mammary tumor growth in rats by adrenalectomy. *Cancer Res.,* 36:1414–1417.
16. Chen, H. J., Bradley, C. J., and Meites, J. (1977): Stimulation of growth of carcinogen-induced mammary cancers in rats by thyrotropin-releasing hormone. *Cancer Res.,* 37:64–66.
17. Chomczynski, P., and Topper, Y. J. (1974): A direct effect of prolactin and placental lactogen on mammary epithelial nuclei. *Biochem. Biophys. Res. Commun.,* 60:56–63.
18. Clemens, J. A., Welsch, C. W., and Meites, J. (1968): Effects of hypothalamic lesions on incidence and growth of mammary tumors in carcinogen-treated rats. *Proc. Soc. Exp. Biol. Med.,* 127:969–972.
19. Cohen, N., and Hilf, R. (1975): Effect of estrogen treatment on DMBA-induced mammary tumor growth and biochemistry in intact and diabetic rats (38535). *Proc. Soc. Exp. Biol. Med.,* 148:339–343.
20. Cohen, N., and Hilf, R. (1974): Influence of insulin on growth and metabolism of 7,12-dimethylbenz*(a)*anthracene-induced mammary tumors. *Cancer Res.,* 34:3245–3252.
21. Costlow, M. E., Buschow, R. A., and McGuire, W. L. (1976): Prolactin receptors and androgen-induced regression of 7,12-dimethylbenz*(a)*anthracene-induced mammary carcinoma. *Cancer Res.,* 36:3324–3329.
22. Costlow, M. E., Buschow, R. A., and McGuire, W. L. (1974): Prolactin receptors in an estrogen receptor-deficient mammary carcinoma. *Science,* 184:85–86.
23. Costlow, M. E., Buschow, R. A., and McGuire, W. L. (1976): Prolactin receptors in 7,12-dimethylbenz*(a)*anthracene-induced mammary tumors following endocrine ablation. *Cancer Res.,* 36:3941–3943.
24. Costlow, M. E., Buschow, R. A., and McGuire, W. L. (1975): Prolactin stimulation of prolactin receptors in rat liver. *Life Sci.,* 17:1457–1466.
25. Costlow, M. E., Buschow, R. A., Richert, N. J., and McGuire, W. L. (1975): Prolactin and estrogen binding in transplantable hormone-dependent and autonomous rat mammary carcinoma. *Cancer Res.,* 35:970–974.

26. Costlow, M. E., and Gallagher, P. E. (1977): Prolactin receptors in primary cultures of 7,12-dimethylbenz*(a)*anthracene-induced rat mammary carcinoma. *(submitted).*
27. Costlow, M. E., and McGuire, W. L. (1977): Autoradiographic localization of prolactin receptors in 7,12-dimethylbenz*(a)*anthracene-induced rat mammary carcinoma. *J. Natl. Cancer Inst.,* 58:1173–1175.
28. Costlow, M. E., and McGuire, W. L. (1977): Autoradiograhic localization of the binding of ^{125}I-labeled prolactin to rat tissues *in vitro. J. Endocrinol.,* 75:221–226.
29. Costlow, M. E., Sluyser, M., and Gallagher, P. E. (1977): Prolactin receptors in mammary tumors of GR mice. *Endocrine Res. Commun.,* 4:285–294.
30. Cowie, A. T., and Tindall, J. S. (1971): *The Physiology of Lactation.* Edward Arnold, London.
31. Dao, T. L., Sinha, D., Christakos, S., and Varela, R. (1975): Biochemical characterization of carcinogen-induced mammary hyperplastic alveolar nodules and tumors in the rat. *Cancer Res.,* 35:1128–1134.
32. DeSombre, E. R., Kledzik, G., Marshall, S., and Meites, J. (1976): Estrogen and prolactin receptor concentrations in rat mammary tumors and response to endocrine ablation. *Cancer Res.,* 36:354–358.
33. Diamond, E. J., Giladi, M., Khon, S., and Hollander, V. P. (1977): Estradiol binding in ovariectomy responsive and nonresponsive rat mammary carcinoma. *Cancer Res.,* 37:1852–1856.
34. Diamond, E. J., Koprak, S., Shen, S. K., and Hollander, V. P. (1976): The conversion of an ovariectomy-nonresponsive to an ovariectomy-responsive mammary tumor strain. *Cancer Res.,* 36:77–80.
35. Dickey, R. P., and Minton, J. P. (1972): L-dopa effect on prolactin, follicle-stimulating hormone, and luteinizing hormone in women with advanced breast cancer: A preliminary report. *Am. J. Obstet. Gynecol.,* 114:267–269.
36. Dilley, W. G., and Kister, S. J. (1975): *In vitro* stimulation of human breast tissue by human prolactin. *J. Natl. Cancer Inst.,* 55:35–36.
37. Djiane, J., and Durand, P. (1977): Prolactin-progesterone antagonism in self regulation of prolactin receptors in the mammary gland. *Nature,* 266:641–643.
38. Ehni, G., and Eckles, N. E. (1959): Interruption of pituitary stalk in the patient with mammary cancer. *J. Neurosurg.,* 16:628–652.
39. Elias, J. L. (1959): Effect of insulin and hydrocortisone on organ cultures of adult mouse mammary gland. *Proc. Soc. Exp. Biol. Med.,* 101:500–502.
40. Englesman, E., Heuson, J. C., Blonk-van de Wijst, J., Drochmons, A., Maas, H., Cheix, F., Sobrinho, L. G., and Nowakouski, H. (1975): Controlled clinical trial of L-dopa and nafoxidine in advanced breast cancer: An E.O.R.T.C. study. *Br. J. Med.,* 2:714–715.
41. Fidler, T. J., and Falconer, I. R. (1969): The effect of intraductal prolactin on protein and nucleic acid biosynthesis in the rabbit mammary gland. *Biochem. J.,* 115:58–59.
42. Finkelstein, M., Geier, A., Horn, H., Levij, I. S., and Ever-Hadani, P. (1975): Effect of testosterone and estradiol-17β on synthesis of DNA, RNA and protein in human breast in organ cultures. *Int. J. Cancer,* 15:78–90.
43. Forsyth, I. A. (1971): Reviews of the progress of dairy science. Section A. Physiology. Organ culture techniques and the study of hormone effects on the mammary gland. *J. Dairy Res.,* 3:419–444.
44. Frantz, A. G., Habif, D. V., Hyman, G. A., and Suh, H. K. (1972): Remission of metastatic breast cancer after reduction of circulating prolactin in patients treated with L-dopa. *Clin. Res.,* 20:864.
45. Frantz, A. G., Habif, D. V., Hyman, G. A., Suh, H. K., Sassin, J. F., Zimmerman, E. A., Noel, G. L., and Kleinberg, D. L. (1973): Physiological and pharmacological factors affecting prolactin secretion, including suppression by L-dopa in the treatment of breast cancer. In: *Human Prolactin,* edited by J. L. Pasteels and C. Robyn, pp. 273–290. Excerpta Medica, Amsterdam.
46. Frantz, W. L., MacIndoe, J. H., and Turkington, R. W. (1974): Prolactin receptors: Characteristics of the particulate fraction binding activity. *J. Endocrinol.,* 60:485–497.
47. Frantz, W. L., Payne, P., and Dombroske, O. (1975): Binding of ovine ^{125}I-prolactin to cultured anterior pituitary tumour cells and normal cells. *Nature,* 255:636–638.
48. Frantz, W. L., and Turkington, R. W. (1972): Formation of biologically active ^{125}I-prolactin by enzymatic radioiodination. *Endocrinology,* 91:1545–1548.
49. Gibson, S. L., and Hilf, R. (1976): Influence of hormonal alterations of host on estrogen-

binding capacity in 7,12-dimethylbenz*(a)*anthracene-induced mammary tumors. *Cancer Res.,* 36:3736–3741.

50. Goldenberg, I. S., Waters, M. N., Ravdin, R. S., Ansfield, F. J., and Segoloff, A. (1973): Androgenic therapy for advanced breast cancer in women. *J.A.M.A.,* 223:1267–1268.
51. Goldenberg, I. (1964): Testosterone propionate therapy in breast cancer. *J.A.M.A.,* 188:1069–1077.
52. Grahame, R. E., and Bertalanffy, F. D. (1972): Cell division in normal and neoplastic mammary gland tissue in the rat. *Anat. Rec.,* 174:1–8.
53. Guerzon, P. G., and Pearson, O. H. (1974): Lergotrile mesylate, a new prolactin inhibitor drug. *Clin. Res.,* 22:632a.
54. Harada, Y. (1976): Pituitary role in the growth of metastasizing MRMT-1 mammary carcinoma in rats. *Cancer Res.,* 36:18–22.
55. Hawkins, R. A., Hill, A., Freedman, B., Killen, E., Buchan, P., Miller, W. R., and Forrest, A. P. M. (1977): Oestrogen receptor activity and endocrine status in DMBA-induced rat mammary tumours. *Eur. J. Cancer,* 13:223–228.
56. Heuson, J. C., Coume, A., and Heimann, R. (1967): Cell proliferation induced by insulin in organ culture of rat mammary carcinoma. *Exp. Cell Res.,* 45:351–360.
57. Heuson, J. C., Coume, A., and Staquet, M. (1972): Clinical trial of 2-Br-α-ergocryptine (CB-154) in advanced breast cancer. *Eur. J. Cancer,* 8:155–156.
58. Heuson, J. C., and Legros, N. (1970): Effect of insulin and of alloxan diabetes on growth of the rat mammary carcinoma *in vivo. Eur. J. Cancer,* 6:349–351.
59. Heuson, J. C., and Legros, N. (1971): Effect of insulin on DNA synthesis and DNA polymerase activity in organ culture of rat mammary carcinoma, and the influence of insulin pretreatment and of alloxan diabetes. *Cancer Res.,* 31:59–65.
60. Heuson, J. C., Legros, N., and Heimann, R. (1972): Influence of insulin administration on growth of the 7,12-dimethylbenz*(a)*anthracene-induced mammary carcinoma in intact, oophorectomized and hypophysectomized rats. *Cancer Res.,* 32:233–238.
61. Heuson, J. C., Legros, H., Heuson-Stiennon, J. A., Leclercq, G., and Pasteels, J. L. (1976): Hormone dependency of rat mammary tumors. In: *Breast Cancer: Trends in Research and Treatment,* edited by J. C. Heuson, W. H. Mattheiem, and M. Rozencweig, pp. 81–93. Raven Press, New York.
62. Heuson, J. C., and Legros, N. (1972): Influence of insulin deprivation on growth of the 7,12-dimethylbenz*(a)*anthracene-induced mammary carcinoma in rats subjected to alloxan diabetes and food restriction. *Cancer Res.,* 32:226–232.
63. Heuson, J. C., Waelbroeck-Van Gaver, C., and Legros, N. (1970): Growth inhibition of rat mammary carcinoma and endocrine changes produced by 2-Br-α-ergocryptine, a suppressor of lactation and nidalion. *Eur. J. Cancer,* 6:353–356.
64. Hilf, R., Michel, I., and Bell, C. (1967): Biochemical and morphological response of normal and neoplastic mammary tissue to hormonal treatment. *Recent Prog. Horm. Res.,* 23:229–295.
65. Holcomb, H., Costlow, M. E., Buschow, R. A., and McGuire, W. L. (1976): Prolactin binding in rat mammary gland during pregnancy and lactation. *Biochim. Biophys. Acta.,* 428:104–112.
66. Holdaway, I. M., and Friesen, H. G. (1976): Correlation between hormone binding and growth response of rat mammary tumor. *Cancer Res.,* 36:1562-1567.
67. Holdaway, I. M., and Friesen, H. G. (1977): Hormone binding by human mammary carcinoma. *Cancer Res.,* 37:1946–1952.
68. Horwitz, K. B., and McGuire, W. L. (1977): Progesterone and progesterone receptors in experimental breast cancer. *Cancer Res.,* 37:1733–1738.
69. Huggins, C., Briziarelli, G., and Sutton, H., Jr. (1959): Rapid induction of mammary carcinoma in the rat and the influence of hormones on the tumors. *J. Exp. Med.,* 109:25–41.
70. Huggins, C., and Yang, N.C. (1962): Induction and extinction of mammary cancer. *Science,* 137:257–262.
71. Jabara, A. G. (1967): Effects of progesterone on 9,10-dimethyl-1,2-benzanthracene-induced mammary tumours in Sprague-Dawley rats. *Br. J. Cancer,* 21:418-429.
72. Jacobs, S., and Cuatrecasas, P. (1976): The mobile receptor hypothesis and "cooperativity" of hormone binding. Application to insulin. *Biochim. Biophys. Acta,* 433:482–495.
73. Keenan, E. J., Kemp, E. D., Pauley, R. J., and Leung, B. S. (1977): Subcellular distribution of specific prolactin binding sites in the lactating mammary gland. *Endocrinology,* 100:88.

74. Kelly, P. A., Bradley, C., Shiu, R. P. C., Meites, J., and Friesen, H. G. (1974): Prolactin binding to rat mammary tumor tissue. *Proc. Soc. Exp. Biol. Med.*, 146:816–819.
75. Kelly, P. A., LeBlanc, G., Ferlond, L., Labrie, F., and Delean, A. (1977): Androgen inhibition of basal and estrogen-stimulated prolactin binding in rat river. *Mol. Cell Endocrinol.*, 9:195–204.
76. Kim, U., and Furth, J. (1976): The Role of prolactin in carcinogenesis *Vitam. Horm.*, 34:107–136.
77. Klaiber, M. S., Gruenstein, M., Meranze, D. R., and Shimkin, M. B. (1969): Influence of hypothalmic lesions on the induction and growth of mammary cancers in Sprague-Dawley rats receiving 7,12-dimethylbenz(*a*)anthracene. *Cancer Res.*, 29:999–1001.
78. Kledzik, G. S., Bradley, C. J., Marshall, S., Campbell, G. A., and Meites, J. (1976): Effects of high doses of estrogen on prolactin-binding activity and growth of carcinogen-induced mammary cancers in rats. *Cancer Res.*, 36:3265–3268.
79. Kledzik, G., Marshall, S., Gelato, M., Campbell, G., and Meites, J. (1975): Prolactin binding activity in the crop sacs of juvenile, mature, parent and prolactin-injected pigeons. *Endocrine Res. Commun.*, 2:345–355.
80. Koyama, H., Sinha, D., and Dao, T. L. (1972): Effect of hormones and 7,12-dimethylbenz(*a*)anthracene on rat mammary tissue grown in organ culture. *J. Natl. Cancer Inst.*, 48:1671–1680.
81. Lasfargues, E. Y. (1957): Cultivation and behavior *in vitro* of the normal mammary epithelium of the adult mouse. *Anat. Rec.*, 127:117–125.
82. Lesniak, M. A., and Roth, J. (1976): Regulation of receptor concentration by homologous hormone. *J. Biol. Chem.*, 251:3720–3729.
83. Leung, B. S., and Sasaki, G. H. (1975): On the mechanism of prolactin and estrogen action in 7,12-dimethylbenz(*a*)anthracene-induced mammary carcinoma in the rat. II. *In vivo* tumor responses and estrogen receptor. *Endocrinology,* 97:564–572.
84. Leung, B. S., and Sasaki, G. H. (1973): Prolactin and progesterone effect on specific estradiol binding in uterine and mammary tissues *in vitro. Biochem. Biophys. Res. Commun.*, 55:1180–1187.
85. Lewis, D., and Hallowes, R. C. (1974): Correlation between the effects of hormones on the synthesis of DNA in explants from induced rat mammary tumours and the growth of the tumours. *J. Endocrinol.*, 62:225–240.
86. Lippman, M. E., and Bolan, G. (1975): Oestrogen-responsive human breast cancer in long-term tissue culture. *Nature,* 256:592–593.
87. Lippman, M., Bolan, G., and Huff, K. (1976): The effects of estrogens and antiestrogens on hormone-responsive human breast cancer in long-term tissue culture. *Cancer Res.*, 36:4595–4601.
88. Lipsett, M. B., and Gergenstall, D. M. (1960): Lack of effect of human growth hormone and ovine prolactin on cancer in man. *Cancer Res.*, 20:1172–1178.
89. Luft, R., Olivecrona, H., and Sjögren, B. (1952): Hypofysektomi pa Människa. *Nord. Med.*, 47:351–354.
90. MacLeod, R. M., Allan, M. S., and Hollander, V. P. (1964): Hormonal requirements for the growth of mammary adenocarcinoma (MTW-9) in rats. *Endocrinology,* 75:249–258.
91. Matsuzawa, A., and Yamamoto, T. (1974): A transplantable pregnancy-dependent mammary tumor line (TPD MT-4) in strain DDD mice. *Gann,* 65:307–315.
92. Matsuzawa, A., and Yamamoto, T. (1977): No growth of a pregnancy-dependent mouse mammary tumor (TPD MT-4) without pituitary hormones. *J. Natl. Cancer Inst.*, 58:1087–1091.
93. Matsuzawa, A., and Yamamoto, T. (1975): Response of a pregnancy-dependent mouse mammary tumor to hormones. *J. Natl. Cancer Inst.*, 55:447–453.
94. McCormick, G. M., and Moon, R. C. (1967): Hormones influencing postpartum growth of 7,12-dimethylbenz(a)anthracene (DMBA)-induced rat mammary tumors. *Cancer Res.*, 27:626–631.
95. McGuire, W. L., Carbone, P. P., and Vollmer, E. P. (editors) (1975): *Estrogen Receptors in Human Breast Cancer.* Raven Press, New York.
96. McGuire, W. L., Julian, J. A., and Chamness, G. C. (1971): A dissociation between ovarian dependent growth and estrogen sensitivity in mammary carcinoma. *Endocrinology,* 89:969–973.
97. McGuire, W. L., Horwitz, K. B., Pearson, O. H., and Segaloff, A. (1977): Current status of estrogen and progesterone receptors in breast cancer. *Cancer,* 39:2934–2947.

98. McGuire, W. L., Raynaud, J.-P., and Baulieu, E. E. (editors) (1977): *Progress in Cancer Research and Therapy, Vol. 4, Progesterone Receptors in Normal and Neoplastic Tissues.* Raven Press, New York.
99. Meites, J. (1972): Relation of prolactin to mammary tumorigenesis and growth in rats. In: *Prolactin and Carcinogenesis,* edited by A. D. Boyns and K. Griffiths, pp. 56–57. Alpha Omega Alpha Publishers, Cardiff, Wales.
100. Meites, J., Cassell, E., and Clark, J. (1971): Estrogen inhibition of mammary tumor growth in rats; counteraction of prolactin. *Proc. Soc. Exp. Biol. Med.,* 137:1225–1227.
101. Meites, J., Lu, K. H., Wuttke, W., Welsch, C. W., Nagasawa, H., and Quadri, S. K. (1972): Recent studies on functions and control of prolactin secretions in rats. *Recent Prog. Horm. Res.,* 28:471–526.
102. Meites, J., Nicoll, C. S., and Talwalker, P. K. (1963): The central nervous system and the secretion and release of prolactin. In: *Advances in Neuroendrocrinology,* edited by A. V. Nalbandov, p.238. University of Illinois Press, Urbana.
103. Minton, J. P. (1974): The response of breast cancer patients with bone pain to L-dopa. *Cancer,* 33:358–363.
104. Minton, J. P., Bronn, D. G., and Kibbey, W. E. (1976): L-dopa effect in painful bony metastases. *N. Engl. J. Med.,* 294:340.
105. Miyachi, Y., Vaitukaitis, J. L., Nieschlag, E., and Lipsett, M. B. (1972): Enzymatic radioiodination of gonadotropins. *J. Clin. Endocrinol.,* 34:23–28.
106. Mobbs, B. G. (1966): The uptake of tritiated oestradiol by dimethylbenzanthracene-induced mammary tumors of the rat. *J. Endocrinol.,* 36:409–414.
107. Mukherjee, A. S., Washburn, L. L., and Banerjee, M. R. (1973): Role of insulin as a "permissive" hormone in mammary gland development. *Nature,* 246:159–160.
108. Murray, R. M. L., Mozaffarian, G., and Pearson, O. H. (1972): Prolactin levels with L-dopa treatment in metastatic breast carcinoma. In: *Prolactin and Carcinogenesis,* edited by A. R. Boyns and K. Griffiths, pp. 158–161. Alpha Omega Alpha Publishers, Cardiff, Wales.
109. Nagasawa, H., and Meites, J. (1970): Effects of hypothalmic estrogen implant on growth of carcinogen-induced mammary tumors in rats. *Cancer Res.,* 30:1327–1329.
110. Nagasawa, H., and Yanai, R. (1970): Effects of prolactin or growth hormone on growth of carcinogen-induced mammary tumors of adreno-ovariectomized rats. *Int. J. Cancer,* 6:488–495.
111. Nolin, J. M., Campbell, G. T., Nansel, D. D., and Bogdanove, E. M. (1977): Does androgen influence prolactin secretion? *Endocrine Res. Commun.,* 4:61–70.
112. Nolin, J. M., and Witorsch, J. (1976): Detection of endogenous immunoreactive prolactin in rat mammary epithelial cells during lactation. *Endocrinology,* 99:949–958.
113. Oka, T., and Topper, Y. J. (1972): Hormone-dependent accumulation of rough endoplasmic reticulum in mouse mammary epithelial cells *in vitro. J. Natl. Cancer Inst.,* 48:1225–1230.
114. Oka, T., and Topper, Y. J. (1972): Is prolactin mitogenic for mammary epithelium? *Proc. Natl. Acad. Sci. U.S.A.,* 69:1693–1696.
115. Osborne, C. K., Bolan, G., Monaco, M. E., and Lippman, M. E. (1976): Hormone responsive human breast cancer in long-term tissue culture: Effect of insulin. *Proc. Natl. Acad. Sci. U.S.A.,* 33:4536–4540.
116. Parke, L., and Forsyth, I. A. (1975): Assay of lactogenic hormones using receptors isolated from rabbit liver. *Endocrine Res. Commun.,* 2:137–149.
117. Pasteels, J.-L., Heuson, J.-C., Heuson-Stiennon, J., and Legros, N. (1976): Effects of insulin, progesterone and estradiol on DNA synthesis in organ cultures of 7,12-dimethylbenz(*a*)anthracene-induced rat mammary tissues. *Cancer Res.,* 36:2162–2170.
118. Pearson, O. H., and Ray, B. S. (1959): Results of hypophysectomy in the treatment of a metastatic mammary carcinoma. *Cancer,* 12:85–92.
119. Pearson, O. H., Llerena, O., Llerena, L., Molina, A., and Butler, T. (1969): Prolactin-dependent rat mammary cancer: A model for man? *Trans. Assoc. Am. Physicians,* 82:225–237.
120. Pearson, O. H., Ray, B. S., Harrold, C. C., West, C. D., Li, M.C., MacLean, J. P., and Lipsett, M. B. (1955): Hypophysectomy in the treatment of advanced cancer. *Trans. Assoc. Am. Physicians,* 68:101–111.
121. Pearson, O. H., West, C. D., Holland, V. P., and Treves, N. E. (1954): Evaluation of endocrine therapy for advanced breast cancer. *J.A.M.A.,* 154:234–239.
122. Posner, B. I., and Bergeron, J. J. M. (1976): Intracellular polypeptide hormone receptors. *Endocrinology,* 98:165.

123. Posner, B. I., Kelly, P. A., and Friesen, H. G. (1974): Induction of a lactogenic receptor in rat liver: Influence of estrogen and the pituitary. *Proc. Natl. Acad. Sci. U.S.A.,* 71:2407–2410.
124. Posner, B. I., Kelly, P. A., and Friesen, H. G. (1975): Prolactin receptors in rat liver: Possible induction by prolactin. *Science,* 188:57–59.
125. Posner, B. I., Kelly, P. A., Shiu, R. P. C., and Friesen, H. G. (1974): Studies of insulin, growth hormone and prolactin binding. Tissue distribution, species variation and characterization. *Endocrinology,* 95:521–531.
126. Powell, B. L., Diamond, E. J., Koprak, S., and Holland, V. P. (1977): Prolactin binding in ovariectomy-responsive and ovariectomy-nonresponsive rat mammary carcinoma. *Cancer Res.,* 37:1328–1332.
127. Prop, F. J. A., and Hendrix, S. E. A. M. (1965): Effect of insulin on mitotic rate in organ cultures of total mammary gland of the mouse. *Exp. Cell Res.,* 40:277–281.
128. Quadri, S. K., Clark, J. L., and Meites, J. (1973): Effects of LSD, pargyline and haloperidol on mammary tumor growth in rats. *Proc. Soc. Exp. Biol. Med.,* 142:22–26.
129. Quadri, S. K., Kledzik, G. S., and Meites, J. (1974): Counteraction by prolactin of androgen-induced inhibition of mammary tumor growth in rats. *J. Natl. Cancer Inst.,* 52:875–878.
130. Rajaniemi, H., Okasanen, A., and Vanha-Perttula, T. (1974): Distribution of ^{125}I-prolactin in mice and rats. Studies with whole-body and microautoradiography. *Horm. Res.,* 5:6–20.
131. Riley, P. A., Latter, T., and Sutton, P. M. (1973): Hormone assays on breast tumor cultures. *Lancet,* 2:818.
132. Rillema, J. A., and Linebaugh, B. E. (1977): Characteristics of the insulin stimulation of DNA, RNA and protein metabolism in cultured human mammary carcinoma cells. *Biochim. Biophys. Acta,* 475:74–80.
133. Rivera, E. M., Elias, J. J., Bern, H. A., Napalkov, N. P., and Pitelka, D. R. (1963): Toxic effects of steroid hormones on organ cultures of mouse mammary tumor, with a comment on the occurrence of viral inclusion bodies. *J. Natl. Cancer Inst., 31:671–687.*
134. Rolland, R., Gunsalus, G. L., and Hammond, J. M. (1976): Demonstration of specific binding of prolactin by porcine corpora lutea. *Endocrinology,* 98:1083–1091.
135. Rolland, R., and Hammond, J. M. (1975): Demonstration of a specific receptor for prolactin in porcine granulosa cells. *Endocrine Res. Commun.,* 2:281–298.
136. Roth, J. (1973): Peptide hormone binding to receptors: A review of direct studies *in vitro. Metabolism,* 22:1059–1073.
137. Rudland, P. D., Hallowes, R. C., Durbin, H., and Lewis, D. (1977): Mitogenic activity of pituitary hormones on cell cultures of normal and carcinogen-induced tumor epithelium from rat mammary glands. *J. Cell Biol.,* 73:561–577.
138. Sakai, S., Kohmoto, K., and Johke, T. (1975): A receptor site for prolactin in lactating mouse mammary tissues. *Endocrinol. Jpn.,* 22:379–387.
139. Sanders, S., and Attramodal, A. (1968): The *in vivo* uptake of oestradiol-17β by hormone responsive and unresponsive tumors of the rat. *Acta Pathol. Microbiol. Scand.,* 74:169–178.
140. Sasaki, G. H., and Leung, B. J. (1975): On the mechanism of hormone action in 7,12-dimethylbenz*(a)*anthracene-induced mammary tumor. I. Prolactin and progesterone effects on estrogen receptor *in vitro. Cancer,* 35:645–651.
141. Sasaki, G. H., and Leung, B. S. (1974): Prolactin stimulation of estrogen receptor *in vitro* in 7,12-dimethylbenz(*a*)anthracene-induced mammary tumor. *Res. Commun. Chem. Pathol. Pharmacol.,* 8:409–412.
142. Scatchard, G. (1949): The attraction of proteins for small molecules and ions. *Ann. N.Y. Acad. Sci.,* 51:600–672.
143. Schulein, M., Daehnfeldt, J. L., and Briand, P. (1976): Biochemical changes during regression and regrowth of hormone dependent GR mouse mammary tumors. *Int. J. Cancer,* 17:120–128.
144. Schultz, K. D., Czygan, P. J., del Pozo, E., and Friesen, H. G. (1973): Varying response of human metastasizing breast cancer to the treatment with 2-Br-α-ergocryptine (CB-154) (case report). In: *Human Prolactin,* edited by C. Robyn and J. L. Pasteels, pp. 268–271. Excerpta Medica, Amsterdam.
145. Shafie, S., and Brooks, S. C. (1977): Effect of prolactin on growth and the estrogen receptor level of human breast cancer cells (MCF-7). *Cancer Res.,* 37:792–799.
146. Sherman, B. N., Stagner, J. I., and Jochimsen, P. R. (1978): Lactogenic hormone binding to human breast cancer: Correlation with estrogen receptor. *(submitted for publication).*

147. Shiu, R. P. C., and Friesen, H. G. (1976): Blockade of prolactin action by antiserum to its receptors. *Science,* 192:259–261.
148. Shiu, R. P. C., and Friesen, H. G. (1974): Properties of a prolactin receptor from the rabbit mammary gland. *Biochem. J.,* 140:301–311.
149. Shiu, R. P. C., Kelly, P. A., and Friesen, H. G. (1973): Radioreceptor assay for prolactin and other lactogenic hormones. *Science,* 180:968–971.
150. Sinha, D., Cooper, D., and Dao, T. L. (1973): The nature of estrogen and prolactin effect on mammary tumorigenesis. *Cancer Res.,* 33:411–414.
151. Smith, R. D., Hilf, R., and Senior, A. E. (1977): Prolactin binding to DMBA-induced mammary tumors in diabetic rats. *Cancer Res.,* 37:4070–4074.
152. Smith R. D., Hilf, R., and Senior, A. E. (1976): Prolactin binding to mammary gland, 7,12-dimethylbenz*(a)*anthracene-induced mammary tumors, and liver in rats. *Cancer Res.,* 36:3726–3731.
153. Smith, R. D., Hilf, R., and Senior, A. E. (1977): Prolactin binding to R3230AC mammary carcinoma and liver in hormone-treated and diabetic rats. *Cancer Res.,* 37:595–598.
154. Sterenthal, A., Dominguez, J. M., Weisman, C., and Pearson, O. H. (1963): Pituitary role in the estrogen dependency of experimental mammary cancer. *Cancer Res.,* 23:481–484.
155. Stoll, B. A. (1972): Brain catecholamines and breast cancer: A hypothesis. *Lancet,* 1:431.
156. Takizawa, S., Furth, J. J., and Furth, J. (1970): Biological and technical aspects of nucleic acid synthesis in cultures of mammary tumors. *Cancer Res.,* 30:211–220.
157. Takizawa, S., Furth, J. J., and Furth, J. (1970): DNA synthesis in autonomous and hormone-responsive mammary tumors. *Cancer Res.,* 30:206–210.
158. Talwalker, P. K., and Meites, J. (1961): Mammary lobulo-alveolar growth induced by anterior pituitary hormones in adreno-ovariectomized and adreno-ovariectomized-hypophysectomized rats (26783). *Proc. Soc. Exp. Biol. Med.,* 107:880–883.
159. Terenius, L. (1968): Selective retention of estrogen isomers in estrogen-dependent breast tumors of the rat demonstrated by *in vitro* methods. *Cancer Res.,* 28:328–337.
160. Thorell, J. I., and Johansson, B. G. (1971): Enzymatic iodination of polypeptides with ^{125}I to high specific activity. *Biochim. Biophys. Acta,* 251:363–369.
161. Turkington, R. W. (1974): Prolactin receptors in mammary carcinoma cells. *Cancer Res.,* 34:758–763.
162. Turkington, R. W. (1968): Hormone-induced synthesis of DNA by mammary gland *in vitro. Endocrinology,* 82:540–546.
163. Turkington, R. W. (1970): Stimulation of RNA synthesis in isolated mammary cells by insulin and prolactin bound to sepharose. *Biochem. Biophys. Res. Commun.,* 41:1362–1367.
164. Turkington, R. W., and Hilf, R. (1968): Hormonal dependence of DNA synthesis in mammary carcinoma cells *in vitro. Science,* 160:1457–1458.
165. Turkington, R. W., and Riddle, M. (1970): Expression of differentiated function by mammary cancer cells *in vitro. Cancer Res.,* 30:127–132.
166. Turkington, R. W., Underwood, L. E., and VanWyk, J. J. (1971): Elevated serum prolatcin levels after pituitary-stalk section in man. *N. Engl. J. Med.,* 285:707–710.
167. Vignon, F., and Rochefort, H. (1976): Regulation of estrogen receptors in ovarian-dependent rat mammary tumors. I. Effects of castration and prolactin. *Endocrinology,* 98:722–729.
168. Vignon, F., and Rochefort, H. (1974): Regulation des "recepteurs" des oestrogines dans les tumeurs mammaires: Effect de la prolactine *in vivo. C.R. Acad. Sci.* [*D*] *(Paris),* 278:103–106.
169. Volk, H., Deupree, R. H., Goldenberg, I. S., Wilde, R. C., Carabasi, R. A., and Escher, G. C. (1974): A dose response evaluation of delta-1-testolactone in advanced breast cancer. *Cancer,* 33:9–13.
170. Welsch, C. W., Clemens, J. A., and Meites, J. (1968): Effects of multiple pituitary homographs on progesterone on 7,12-dimethylbenz*(a)*anthracene-induced mammary tumors in rats. *J. Natl. Cancer Inst.,* 41:465–471.
171. Welsch, C. W., DeIturri, G. C., and Brennan, M. J. (1976): DNA synthesis of human, mouse and rat mammary carcinoma *in vitro. Cancer,* 38;1272–1281.
172. Welsch, C. W., DeIturri, G. C., and Meites, J. (1973): Comparative effects of hypophysectomy, ergocornine and ergocornine-reserpine treatments on rat mammary carcinoma. *Int. J. Cancer,* 12:206–212.
173. Welsch, C. W., and McManus, M. J. (1977): Stimulation of DNA synthesis by placental

lactogen or insulin or organ cultures of benign human breast tumors. *Cancer Res.*, 37:2257–2261.

174. Welsch. C. W., and Nagasawa, H. (1977): Prolactin and murine tumorigenesis: A review. *Cancer Res.*, 37:951–963.
175. Welsch, C. W., and Rivera, E. M. (1972): Differential effects of estrogen and prolactin on DNA synthesis in organ cultures of DMBA-induced rat mammary carcinoma (36201). *Proc. Soc. Exp. Biol. Med.*, 139:623–626.
176. Witorsch, R. J., Smith, J. P., and Nolin, J. M. (1976): Evidence for androgen-dependent intracellular binding of prolactin in rat ventral prostate gland. *Endocrinology*, 101:929–938.
177. Witorsch, R. J. (1977): Immunohistochemical demonstration of prolactin binding in some sex accessory organs of the male rat. *Endocrinology*, 100:281.
178. Yani, R., and Hagasawa, H. (1976): Importance of progesterone in DNA synthesis of pregnancy-dependent mammary tumors in mice. *Int. J. Cancer*, 18:317–321.
179. Young, S., Baker, R. A., and Helfenstein, J. E. (1965): The effect of androgens on induced mammary tumors in rats. *Br. J. Cancer*, 19:155–159.
180. Zava, D. T., and McGuire, W. L. (1977): Estrogen receptors in androgen-induced breast tumor regression. *Cancer Res.*, 37:1608–1610.

NONPITUITARY PROTEIN HORMONES

Endocrine Control in Neoplasia, edited by
R. K. Sharma and W. E. Criss.
Raven Press, New York © 1978.

Insulin and Insulin Receptors in Mammary Cancer

*Russell Hilf, **Joan T. Harmon, and *Samir M. Shafie

** Biochemistry Department and University of Rochester Cancer Center, University of Rochester School of Medicine and Dentistry, Rochester, New York 14642; and ** Diabetes Branch, National Institute of Arthritis, Metabolic and Digestive Diseases, National Institutes of Health, Bethesda, Maryland 20014*

Growth of certain rodent mammary adenocarcinomas can be affected by alteration of the insulin status of the host. In an attempt to explore these effects at the cellular level, we initiated studies on insulin binding and its regulation. For these studies, we used isolated enzymatically dissociated tumor cells that were obtained from intact or hormonally modified tumor-bearing hosts. Conditions for optimum binding of labeled insulin were established *in vitro.* Under these conditions, we demonstrated the existence of specific receptors for insulin based on data defining the saturability, reversibility, affinity, and specificity of binding of the labeled ligand. An important observation was the finding that estrogens play a role in regulation of insulin binding. Removal of endogenous estrogens resulted in enhanced insulin binding, and administration of estrogens resulted in a reduction of insulin binding; these effects were observed in the absence of alterations in circulating insulin levels. The insulin-estrogen relationship also extends to a permissive role of insulin in maintenance of estrogen and prolactin receptors in these experimental tumors. Further exploration of the insulin-estrogen axis *in vivo* and in short-term culture *in vitro,* as shown by our preliminary data, should yield additional information pertinent to regulation of hormone receptors and their relationship to tumor growth, results that could have widespread therapeutic implications for the human disease.

INTRODUCTION

Development and differentiation of the normal mammary gland are controlled by concerted actions of several hormones acting in a temporal relationship. The best known elucidation of this complex process was set forth by Lyons et al. (32), whose studies in triply operated (ovariectomized-adrenalectomized-hypophysectomized) rats demonstrated that there are requirements for estrogens, progesterone, glucocorticoids, prolactin, and growth hormone in fulfilling the morphological criteria of lobuloalveolar development. A role for insulin was not considered in these studies, which dealt mainly with pituitary hormones and their target tissue products. However, a role for insulin in lactogenesis *in vivo* was suggested by the data of Kumareson and Turner (31), who found that injection of insulin to postpartum rats increased total milk yield, and by the data of Martin and Baldwin (33), who demonstrated that induction of diabetes by alloxan caused a rapid decrease in lactational performance, which was assessed by measurement of lactose, casein, and lipids. The most extensive evidence supporting a role for insulin in lactogenesis came from the studies of Topper and his colleagues (51), who used the mouse mammary gland explanted *in vitro,* a system originally developed by Elias (14) and Rivera and Bern (41). It became clear that insulin was required for maintenance, cellular proliferation, and production of differentiated products, the latter being produced in concert with prolactin and glucocorticoids. It was shown that insulin significantly increases DNA synthesis in the rat mammary gland *in vitro* (20). Thus, if insulin acts as a mitogen toward the normal mammary gland, it would be of interest to determine if insulin also acts as a mitogen toward mammary tumors.

In a continuing series of experiments both *in vitro* and *in vivo,* Heuson and his colleagues convincingly demonstrated that insulin stimulated DNA synthesis in DMBA-induced tumors and that tumor growth *in vivo* was dependent on insulin (24–27)[1]. We have confirmed their findings *in vivo,* although the number of tumors classified as insulin-dependent may be influenced by the severity of the alloxan-induced diabetes and the attendant weight loss (4). In addition, we observed that the transplantable R3230AC tumor was also affected by the insulin status of the host; the tumor grew faster in the diabetic host, and its growth was retarded by treatment with insulin (6). In other experiments we observed that simultaneous injections of insulin and estrogen were additive in causing increased inhibition of growth of the R3230AC tumor (6), whereas estrogen treatment of diabetic animals bearing DMBA-induced tumors resulted in regression of all lesions, an event that did not occur with either treatment alone (5). Thus, although the roles of insulin may be different in these two model tumor systems, we certainly concur with the conclusions reached by Heuson et al. (25,27) that insulin should be considered as another hormonal factor important in the growth of breast cancer. Other earlier reports also implicated insulin as a factor that could alter neoplastic growth (23).

RESULTS AND DISCUSSION

Insulin Binding to Mammary Tumor Cells

It is now well accepted that if a tissue responds to a hormone, a receptor for that hormone should be identifiable in the tissue. The concept of a receptor is not new, as it was proposed by pharmacologists to aid in explaining responses to drugs (at the end of the nineteenth century Ehrlich proposed the presence

---

[1] See also chapter by Legros and Heuson, *this volume.*

of receptors to explain the affinity of certain ligands for certain organs). The modern advances in this area were achieved by techniques that enabled investigators to obtain hormonal ligands with high radiospecific activities and thereby begin to examine the interactions of ligands with receptors at physiological levels of hormones. To examine the role of insulin on mammary tumor growth, studies were initiated in our laboratory to identify and characterize the interaction of insulin with dissociated cells prepared from the R3230AC adenocarcinoma and, in later experiments, from DMBA-induced tumors. In these experiments we were guided by the studies of many investigators, as summarized in several recent reviews (7,8,10,42). Our purpose was to establish an experimental system that would enable us to study binding of the hormone and measure hormone-induced responses; for insulin we chose to use enzymatically dissociated cells for binding assays and substrate transport measurements. Cells were prepared by digesting tumor tissue with collagenase and hyaluronidase; the final cell preparations used exhibited viability greater than 85%, as estimated by trypan blue exclusion (21). Insulin was labeled stoichiometrically with either ^{131}I-Na or ^{125}I-Na by chloramine T, following the method of Freychet et al. (16,18). The separated monoiodoinsulin had radiospecific activity of 140 to 180 μCi/μg; it was 99% precipitable with trichloroacetic acid and was indistinguishable from unlabeled insulin by radioimmunoassay, yielding one radioactive peak after polyacrylamide gel electrophoresis. At the outset of our investigations, conditions that yielded optimum levels of specific insulin binding were established. We examined the relationships between binding and various factors: number of cells used; time course; effects of temperature and pH; shaking of the incubation mixture; methods for separating bound ligand from free ligand; reduction of nonspecific binding relative to total binding; addition of reagents to the incubation medium to reduce the extent of ligand degradation during the binding assay. Details of the results have been published (22,45,46). The data reported here are expressed as specific insulin binding, which is calculated as the difference between total binding (labeled insulin alone) and the binding in the presence of 1,000-fold excess unlabeled insulin (nonspecific binding). Most binding assays were performed with 10^{-10} M to 10^{-9} M labeled insulin, with or without 10^{-7} M to 10^{-6} M unlabeled insulin. In our experience with cells from intact rats, the nonspecific binding was usually approximately 25% of the total binding, and the total binding represented 3 to 6% of the labeled ligand added to the incubation system. It is also worth noting that the alteration in binding resulting from hormonal perturbations was due entirely to differences in total binding, the nonspecific binding remaining quite constant.

Specificity of Insulin Binding

One approach to defining the specificity of a ligand-receptor interaction is to examine the amount of insulin bound in the presence of structurally related or unrelated polypeptides. We measured the effects, over a wide concentration

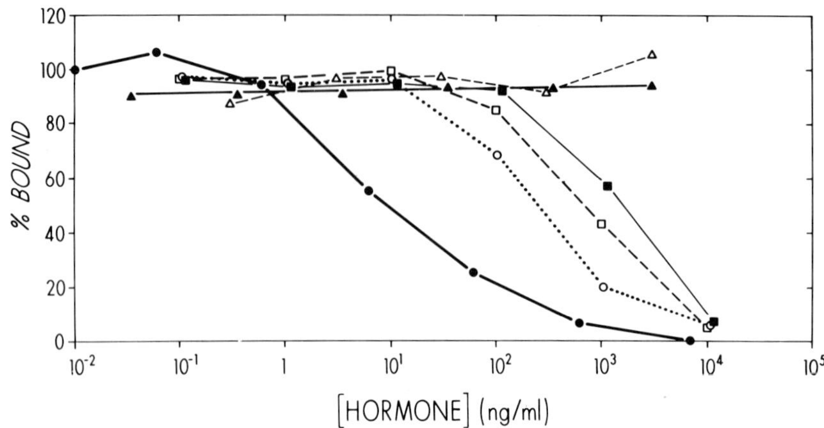

FIG. 1. Competition for ^{125}I-insulin binding to R3230AC tumor cells by insulin, insulin analogs, and other polypeptide hormones. Inhibition of labeled hormone binding, expressed as percentage of maximum bound, is plotted as a function of concentration (ng/ml) of unlabeled hormone. Specific binding in absence of unlabeled insulin is 100%; in the presence of 1,000-fold excess of unlabeled insulin, it is 0%. Each point is the average of triplicate samples: porcine insulin *(filled circles);* porcine proinsulin *(open circles);* guinea pig insulin *(open squares);* porcine desoctapeptide insulin *(filled squares);* ovine prolactin *(open triangles);* porcine and bovine glucagon *(filled triangles).*

range, of unlabeled insulin, proinsulin, guinea pig insulin, desoctapeptide insulin, glucagon, and prolactin on the binding of ^{131}I-insulin (10^{-10} M) to dissociated tumor cells (22). The data (Fig. 1) show that glucagon and prolactin did not compete for binding of labeled insulin, whereas the other polypeptides demonstrated their ability to inhibit binding of the labeled ligand in the following order: insulin > proinsulin > guinea pig insulin > desoctapeptide insulin. From the competition curves (Fig. 1) it was possible to estimate the relative potency (molar concentration of unlabeled insulin needed to inhibit binding by 50% divided by molar concentration of analog required to achieve 50% labeled insulin bound): insulin, 1.00; proinsulin, 0.053; guinea pig insulin, 0.011; desoctapeptide insulin, 0.005. Although we have not examined the biological potency of each of these analogs on the tumor cells, it is certainly of interest that the data obtained here on their estimated potency are in good agreement with their bioactivity reported for fat cells and rat liver membranes (16,17). These results also imply that the structural features of the membrane in the mammary tumor cell required for insulin binding are probably similar to those found in normal cells.

Kinetic Characterization of Insulin Binding

The approach most commonly employed in estimating the affinity of a hormone ligand for its receptor is to measure the amount of hormone bound at steady-state conditions over a wide range of different concentrations of labeled ligand, preferably (in our opinion) over a range that is also physiologically relevant. The data thus obtained could be analyzed according to the method of Scatchard (43); when graphically depicted, they would yield a straight line for one class of receptors but would present other than a straight line for two or more classes of independent sites. Since Scatchard analysis for specific insulin binding invariably yields a curvilinear plot, the latter interpretation was initially invoked by several investigators (7). An alternative explanation for the curvilinear behavior of the Scatchard analysis was proposed by DeMeyts et al. (9–13) in which site-site interactions (negative cooperativity) could account for the diversion from linearity. If the latter is true for insulin receptors, it is necessary to employ other methods to estimate the affinity of insulin for its receptor; such an approach has been proposed by DeMeyts and Roth (12).

As shown in Fig. 2, Scatchard analysis of insulin binding to dissociated cells from the R3230AC tumor gave a curvilinear plot, a result similar to those reported for other tissues. If two or more classes of sites are assumed, the slope of the low-capacity, high-affinity portion of the curve (initial linear portion) can be estimated, yielding a value of 1.2×10^{10} M^{-1}. Also shown in Fig. 2 are the results obtained for insulin binding to tumor cells from diabetic and ovariectomized animals. All three plots demonstrate roughly parallel behavior, and analysis of the initial linear portions of the curves gave similar slopes: 1.03×10^{10} M^{-1} and 1.00×10^{10} M^{-1} for diabetic and ovariectomized rats, respectively (no difference in parallelism by analysis of covariance). We interpret this finding to indicate similar affinities of tumor cells for insulin over this concentration range of insulin, and the results suggest that there may be differences in the numbers of sites, since the capacity for insulin binding was higher in cells from diabetic rats and highest in those from ovariectomized rats (45). The number of sites is usually estimated from the Scatchard analysis by linear

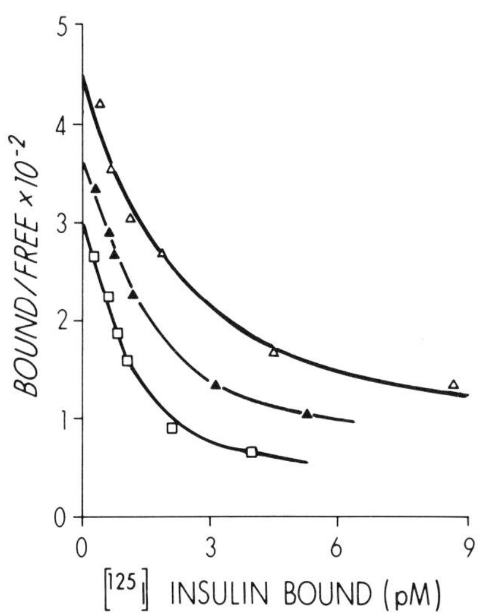

FIG. 2. Scatchard analysis for insulin binding to R3230AC tumor cells from intact *(squares)*, diabetic *(filled triangles)*, and ovariectomized *(open triangles)* rats. Cells (2×10^6) were incubated at 20°C for 45 min with ^{125}I-insulin (10^{-11} M to 10^{-9} M) in 1 ml medium 199 plus 1% bovine serum albumin. Bound/free ratio of ^{125}I-insulin is plotted versus amount of insulin bound; nonspecific binding (measured in presence of 1,000-fold excess unlabeled insulin) has been subtracted.

projection to the X-axis intercept, which in the case of curvilinear plots is subject to uncertainty. However, we have made such estimates and found that there were 1173, 1884, and 2791 sites/cell for intact, diabetic, and ovariectomized rats, respectively.

One approach to estimating the existence of negative cooperativity is to examine the kinetics of dissociation of bound ligand. Under the proper conditions, a difference in dissociation of labeled ligand will arise when comparing dissociations in the presence and absence (infinite dilution) of added unlabeled ligand. The presence of a saturating level of insulin should enhance dissociation, since the affinity will be reduced as the occupancy of sites reaches a maximum. This is the result obtained for R3230AC tumor cells from intact, diabetic, and ovariectomized rats (Fig. 3); it is similar to the results reported by DeMeyts et al. (10) for cultured lymphocytes. A dose-related increase in the amount of ligand dissociated (10^{-10} M labeled insulin was used for binding) was also observed, with a peak at 10^{-7} M unlabeled insulin, with less dissociation observed above and below the 10^{-7} M concentration of insulin (22). Thus the degree of dissociation was influenced by the amount of unlabeled insulin added to the incubation medium.

Since this behavior was compatible with the hypothesis of negative cooperative interactions, we analyzed the binding data according to the suggestion of DeMeyts and Roth (12) to obtain an estimate of the average affinity. Comparison of the average affinity profiles ($\bar{K}$) for tumors from intact, diabetic, and ovariectomized rats revealed similar values, ranging from 2 to 3×10^9 M^{-1} for the three groups, estimated over a range of insulin concentrations that reached approximately 40% occupancy. It is of interest that the three graphic representa-

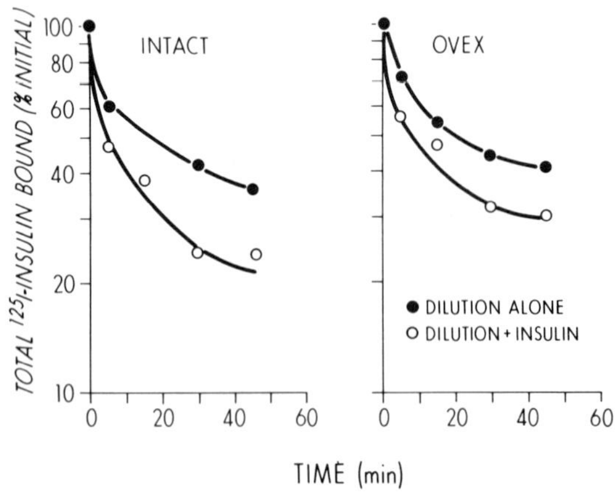

FIG. 3. Time course of dissociation of bound ^{125}I-insulin from R3230AC tumor cells of intact and ovariectomized rats. Cells were initially incubated (45 min at 20° C with 10^{-10} M ^{125}I-insulin), pelleted, and resuspended in 8 ml of medium 199 above (dilution only) *(filled circles)* or in the presence of *(open circles)* 10^{-7} M unlabeled insulin. Triplicate samples were obtained at each time point; data are presented as percentage of total bound at zero time (100%).

tions of the affinity profiles were also roughly parallel and resembled those recently published by Bar et al. (1). However, it must be pointed out that the hypothesis of negative cooperativity based on enhanced dissociation of bound ligand by excess unlabeled insulin has recently been challenged. Pollet et al. (38) reported that the dissociation rate of bound insulin was largely independent of binding site occupancy over a physiological range of insulin and that conditions could be found in which enhanced dissociation was demonstrated when binding site occupancy was actually decreased. Such behavior would not be compatible with the proposed negative cooperativity. Regardless of which hypothesis one favors for insulin binding, our data simply indicate that the characteristics of the interaction of insulin with its receptors in these tumor cells are similar to those seen in other tissues and are similar in tumor cells from intact, diabetic, and ovariectomized rats. The difference in binding observed between tumors from intact rats and those from hormonally modified hosts is most likely due to an increase in the number of binding sites.

Effect of Estrogen on Insulin Binding

Our interest in exploring a possible relationship between insulin and estrogen actions was prompted by earlier reports. Heuson and Legros (26) reported that estrogen treatment failed to reverse the regression of DMBA-induced tumors resulting from removal of insulin. In our laboratory we observed that growth of the R3230AC adenocarcinoma, which was inhibited by either estrogen treatment or insulin treatment alone, was significantly reduced by simultaneous administration of estrogen plus insulin; the two hormone therapies appeared to be additive in causing inhibition of neoplastic growth (6). We also reported that estrogen treatment of diabetic rats bearing DMBA-induced tumors resulted in regression of all tumors, which is suggestive of a role for both hormones in control of neoplastic growth (5). As a first approach to examining the relationship between these two hormones, we studied insulin binding in R3230AC tumors from ovariectomized rats. Cells prepared from tumors implanted into ovariectomized rats demonstrated insulin binding two to three times higher than that seen in tumor cells from intact animals. This is shown in Fig. 2, in which the Scatchard analysis yielded a curvilinear plot. As was indicated previously, analysis of this binding isotherm from ovariectomized rats indicated that the slopes of the linear components were similar to those for intact or diabetic rats; the same was found for the average affinity profile ($\bar{K}$). No differences in degradation of labeled ligand were observed among these experimental groups. Examination of the time course of binding clearly showed that the binding capacity of cells from ovariectomized rats was elevated at each time point examined. We therefore concluded that removal of ovarian hormones resulted in enhanced binding capacity for insulin, probably attributable to an increased number of receptors.

We initiated experiments designed to examine the temporal relationship between ovariectomy and enhanced insulin binding (45). Tumors were obtained

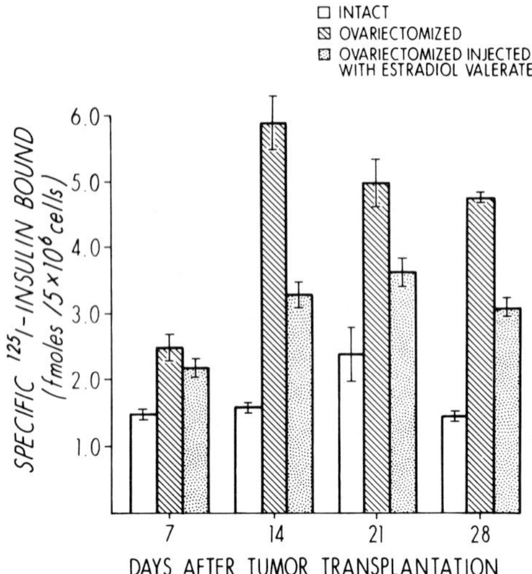

FIG. 4. Effect of ovariectomy and estrogen treatment on insulin binding capacity of R3230AC mammary tumor cells. Dissociated cells were incubated at 20°C with 10^{-10} M ^{125}I-insulin for 45 min. Specific ^{125}I-insulin binding (fmoles/5 $\times$ 10^6 cells) was measured in relation to days after tumor implantation in untreated intact female rats *(open bars),* ovariectomized rats *(hatched bars),* and ovariectomized rats sacrificed 4 days after a single subcutaneous injection of 1 mg estradiol valerate *(stippled bars).* Each value is the mean of at least four measurements; vertical lines are SEM.

at 1, 2, 3, and 4 weeks after implantation into ovariectomized rats, and ^{125}I-insulin binding to dissociated cells prepared from these tumors was measured. As shown in Fig. 4, specific insulin binding was significantly higher in neoplastic cells from ovariectomized rats, with the greatest increase in binding occurring between 1 and 2 weeks after implantation. Tumor cells from ovariectomized rats bound approximately 2.5 times more insulin than cells from intact rats. To assess the effects of estrogen (since ovariectomy would also remove the major source of progesterone), tumor-bearing rats were administered a single injection of estradiol valerate, a long-acting estrogen; tumor cells were prepared from animals sacrificed 4 days after injection of this estrogen. These results are also shown in Fig. 4; they demonstrate that estrogen treatment was effective in reducing insulin binding capacity in tumors obtained at 2, 3, and 4 weeks after implantation into ovariectomized rats. It should be noted that estrogen therapy did not completely return insulin binding to the levels seen in cells from intact animals, which implies that either the dose or time employed was not ideal or that other factors, i.e., progesterone, may also play a role in regulation of insulin binding.

It is now clear that insulin binding is subject to regulation by a variety of factors, one of which is the hormone itself. Data from a variety of human and animal models indicate that there is an inverse relationship between the number of receptors and the serum concentration of insulin (1,42). Since we observed an apparent increase in insulin binding in tumors from ovariectomized rats, it was essential that we determine if such an increase could be attributed to a decrease in serum insulin levels. We measured insulin levels by a radioimmunoassay procedure and found that the levels of insulin in serum from ovariectomized rats were indistinguishable from those in intact rats sacrificed at comparable times after tumor implantation. It is also of interest that serum insulin levels from animals that had been injected with estradiol valerate were not different from those in intact or ovariectomized animals. Therefore the alteration in insulin binding that resulted from removal of ovarian hormones or administration of estrogens was not due simply to changes in circulating insulin levels. It would appear then, that a simple self-modulating model for regulation of insulin receptors is not adequate to explain hormonal regulation of insulin binding. Indeed, it has been proposed that numerous other factors may contribute to fluctuations in binding capacity (1). Further, some recent studies have provided evidence for alterations in receptor levels that are not compatible with simple "down regulation" (2,50).

Since we observed an apparent decrease in insulin binding in response to estrogen treatment *in vivo,* we wished to examine this more carefully under experimental conditions that would lend themselves to more direct control. For this we chose short-term tissue culture of dissociated tumor cells, since this offered us an opportunity to investigate the effects of hormones directly *in vitro.* We also wished to determine if the amount of insulin bound to freshly dissociated cells was an accurate estimation, since the use of enzymes to dissociate the cells can cause some loss of membrane protein. Examination of cells grown in culture for 3, 4, and 6 days (in the presence of 10% fetal calf serum) showed that twice as much ^{125}I-insulin was bound in these cells as in freshly dissociated cells. Since nonspecific bindings were similar in all cases, it appeared that the increase in binding after cell culture was due to increased specific hormone binding, probably as a result of membrane regeneration and/or cell cycle stage. It is of interest that the addition of 10^{-8} M estradiol-17β on day 1 and 3 hr prior to harvesting cells on day 6 caused a decrease in insulin binding per cell (Table 1). These data, although preliminary, suggest that the effects of estrogen *in vivo* in reducing insulin binding were also demonstrated *in vitro.* This finding will require confirmation and extension.

We have also initiated studies of insulin-estrogen relationships in DMBA-induced tumors (46). In this experimental system all lesions do not behave in the same manner. Each lesion must be followed after hormonal alteration of the host in order to categorize the tumor as regressing ($>$ 20% reduction in size), static, or growing ($>$ 20% increase in size). We have analyzed binding of ^{125}I-insulin to dissociated tumor cells from intact rats and have found approximately 2 fmoles of specific insulin binding per 2×10^6 cells, a value two to three times higher than that observed for the R3230AC tumor from intact rats. Insulin binding to biopsy samples of tumors obtained prior to induction of diabetes was measured, and these data were compared to binding data obtained

TABLE 1. *Insulin binding to cultured R3230AC tumor cells*[a]

Days in culture	Hormone addition	Specific insulin binding (fmoles/10^6 cells)
0 (freshly dissociated cells)	—	0.46 ± 0.024[b]
3	—	1.00 ± 0.019
4	—	1.04 ± 0.015
6	—	0.98 ± 0.017
6	10^{-8} M estradiol-17β	0.80 ± 0.021

[a]Tumors were obtained from intact rats, and cells were prepared by enzymatic dissociation. Cells were plated in T_{75} Falcon flasks and fed on alternate days with medium 199 supplemented with 10% fetal calf serum. Estradiol-17β was added 1 day after placing cells in culture, with each additional feeding, and 3 hr prior to harvesting cells on day 6.

[b]Mean ± SEM.

on the same lesions after hormonal perturbation of the host. This experimental approach enabled us to characterize the biological behavior of each lesion and its response to removal of insulin or ovarian hormones. The traumatic effects of biopsy on tumor growth and insulin binding were first assessed in growing tumors of intact animals. Specific insulin bindings were similar in both biopsy and postbiopsy samples (obtained 2 weeks later) from the same neoplasm. The results of removal of insulin on specific ^{125}I-insulin binding in DMBA-induced tumors that regressed, those that remained static, and those that continued to grow are presented in Table 2. An increase (approximately 155%) in insulin binding capacity was observed in insulin-dependent regressing tumors, whereas a decrease of 64% of the prediabetic level was seen in insulin-independent growing tumors. Tumors that remained static showed no significant change in insulin binding capacity (< 6% change). These results indicate that neoplastic cells classified as insulin-dependent demonstrate an inverse relationship between insu-

TABLE 2. *Effect of diabetes or ovariectomy on insulin binding to DMBA-induced tumors*[a]

Tumor response	Specific ^{125}I-insulin bound (fmoles/5 × 10^6 cells)	
	At biopsy	After treatment
To diabetes		
Growing	6.9 ± 0.60[b]	4.4 ± 0.70
Static	6.6 ± 0.80	6.3 ± 0.60
Regressing	6.1 ± 0.60	9.4 ± 0.70
To ovariectomy		
Growing	6.2 ± 0.20	7.9 ± 0.37
Static	6.7 ± 0.25	6.3 ± 0.48
Regressing	6.2 ± 0.33	4.4 ± 0.34

[a]Biopsy samples of tumors were obtained 2 days prior to induction of diabetes or surgical ovariectomy and again at 8 to 15 days after hormonal perturbation of the host. Tumor response was estimated by caliper measurements, and each lesion was classified as stated.

[b]Mean ± SEM (4 to 19 measurements).

lin binding capacity and endogenous levels of insulin, which suggests that this spectrum of cells has maintained a regulatory response similar to those reported for other cells (42). However, the lesions that were insulin-independent demonstrated the opposite behavior regarding the relationship between insulin binding and endogenous insulin levels. These results may be a reflection of two or more families of cells in any one carcinogen-induced lesion, with insulin-independent cells having lower levels of insulin receptors. Diabetes would be likely to select for insulin-independent cells, as is seen by their continued growth in the absence of insulin, and that would eventuate in lesions containing more cells with reduced insulin binding capacity.

The effect of ovariectomy on insulin binding to DMBA-induced tumors was examined using the approach indicated above with biopsy samples obtained prior to and after ovariectomy (Table 2). The results obtained indicated that there was a direct relationship between the change in insulin binding and growth response to ovariectomy. Ovariectomy-induced tumor regression was accompanied by a significant decrease in specific insulin binding, whereas ovarian-independent tumors, those that continued to grow after ovariectomy, demonstrated a modest but significant increase in insulin binding. As before, tumors that remained static after the hormone ablative procedure showed no change in insulin binding. Since ovariectomy had no effect on serum insulin levels, regardless of the biological behavior of the individual lesion, the change in insulin binding cannot be attributed to a simple "down regulation" model for regulation of insulin receptor. It is pertinent that our proposal of negative regulation of insulin receptor by estrogens, based on the data presented for the R3230AC tumor, was supported, at least in part, by the data obtained with the ovarian-independent DMBA-induced tumors, which more closely resemble the ovarian-independent R3230AC tumor. However, it is also likely that DMBA-induced tumors are comprised of more than one cell population and that the results obtained are influenced by the relative distribution of cell types present after hormonal perturbation of the host. Experiments to examine this proposal, using tissue culture techniques *in vitro* after hormonal perturbation *in vivo*, are currently in progress.

Insulin and Regulation of Hormonal Control in Mammary Cancer

In the data that have been presented we have been concerned primarily with the actions of insulin on mammary tumor growth and response and the ability of estrogen to play a role in the regulation of insulin receptors. However, it is apparent that insulin may play a facilitative or permissive role in the actions of other hormones, and it is appropriate to review briefly some of the data that are pertinent to a discussion of breast cancer. Since hormone receptors are protein in nature, it is entirely possible that insulin may effect the response of a target cell by influencing the levels of receptors, based on the generally accepted protein anabolic effects of insulin (15). In experiments in our laboratory the effects of removal of insulin on estrogen binding capacity of DMBA-induced tumors were examined (19). In those lesions classified as static or regressing after the host was made diabetic, the estrogen binding capacity was significantly decreased (approximately 70% reduction) as compared to that measured in growing tumors from intact or diabetic rats. These data can be interpreted as indicating a role for insulin in maintaining estrogen receptors, or they could mean that there exist at least two neoplastic cell populations in which the cells that are independent of insulin have low estrogen receptor content. Although we have no direct evidence at this time to rule out the latter explanation, we favor the former proposal on the basis of the following evidence: (a) there was a reduction in estrogen binding in R3230AC tumors from diabetic hosts, and the R3230AC tumor is a uniformly epithelial transplantable tumor that has been maintained for 15 years; (b) in MCF-7 cells in culture, estrogen receptor levels were significantly reduced in the absence of insulin, and they returned to normal levels in the presence of added insulin (44); (c) we have preliminary data indicating that the estrogen binding capacity of DMBA-induced tumors from diabetic rats given replacement insulin therapy is comparable to the estrogen binding capacity of tumors from intact rats. Additional studies will be required to determine if the effects of insulin on estrogen receptors are specific or if they result from a general effect of insulin on protein synthesis.

A clear-cut role for prolactin in mammary tumorigenesis and growth has been demonstrated in rodents (52). As with the estrogen receptor approach to ascertain hormone dependence, attention has turned recently to measurement of specific prolactin binding to normal and neoplastic breast tumors to identify dependence on prolactin. It has also become apparent that regulation of prolactin binding may arise from prolactin itself (29). In a series of experiments Smith and colleagues (48,49) demonstrated that prolactin binding was significantly reduced in membrane particles prepared from R3230AC mammary adenocarcinomas, DMBA-induced mammary tumors, and livers obtained from diabetic rats, as compared to tissues obtained from intact rats. Additional data showed that the apparent degrees of affinity (Scatchard analysis of the binding data) of prolactin for liver and DMBA-tumor membranes were similar and were not affected by diabetes. These data, and the fact that there were no differences in the distributions of protein, prolactin binding, and 5′-nucleotidase (an enzyme localized in plasma membranes) between tissues prepared from normal and diabetic rats, led to the conclusion that the removal of insulin produced a decrease in the number of prolactin binding sites (49). Thus it would appear that insulin may also influence the sensitivity of certain mammary tumors to prolactin.

Insulin and Human Breast Cancer

Since data obtained by study of animal mammary tumors should have ultimate application to the human disease, it is advisable to cite briefly those data in the clinical literature that suggest or imply a role for insulin in breast cancer. There are data, which can be classified as epidemiologic, that suggest either an enhanced or a decreased incidence of breast cancer in diabetics. More recent and perhaps better controlled studies have shown that glucose tolerance was abnormal in a high percentage of women with breast cancer (3,37). Muck et al. (34,35) examined a large number of women with breast cancer and compared them to women with benign breast diseases, correcting for age and body weight. They concluded that the incidence of diabetes was about two times higher in women with breast cancer, approaching 21 to 22% of the patients studied, compared to an incidence ranging from 1 to 3% for women with fibroadenoma or fibrocystic disease and up to 14% for patients with papillomas. It would appear that women with breast cancer have a higher incidence of diabetes than the general population, but the question still to be answered is whether this observation indicates that diabetes bears a cause relationship, an effect relationship, or no relationship to cancer of the breast.

Insulin has also been studied as a therapeutic agent, and there are a few reports, somewhat anecdotal, on its usefulness in advanced carcinoma. Insulin was claimed to induce tumor regression in some cases and improvement of the patient in almost all cases (23,30,36). These types of reports need confirmation under the same rigorous experimental protocols used in current studies of cancer chemotherapeutic agents, but a most intriguing report has recently appeared that should renew interest in exploring the role of insulin in breast cancer growth. Rhomberg (40) studied 130 women with progressive metastatic breast cancer who were treated with hormones and/or cytostatic drugs. Thirty of these women had either subclinical or manifest diabetes. He concluded that the course of the disease in the 30 diabetic patients was protracted and that their survival times were significantly longer than those of the nondiabetic patients with comparable disease. It was also concluded that the diabetic patients had more favorable responses to hormone therapy, since 18 of 24 showed remission with hormonal therapy, compared to less than one-third of the other patients. Diabetic patients were controlled primarily by oral hypoglycemic agents or by diet alone, and in general the type of diabetes was classified as having "mild clinical characteristics." This report raises several intriguing possibilities, particularly in light of experimental data that have been obtained with animal models. Cohen and Hilf (5) reported that estrogen therapy was more effective in causing regression of DMBA-induced tumors in diabetic rats than in intact rats. In another study, Cohen and Hilf (6) reported that combined therapy with insulin and estrogen was additive in decreasing growth of the R3230AC mammary adenocarcinoma. Although these results may seem at odds with one another regarding the role of insulin, we have recently observed that insulin may play a role in maintaining estrogen receptors in mammary tumors (see the preceding section on regulation), and this may be a mechanism whereby enhanced sensitivity to estrogen therapy would be manifest. Regardless of the mechanism, this report by Rhomberg (40) surely demands further investigation.

ACKNOWLEDGMENTS

The research reported here was supported by U.S. Public Health Service grants CA-16660 and CA-11180, National Cancer Institute, NIH. Dr. S. M. Shafie is the recipient of National Institutes of Health fellowship IF32 CA-05941, and Dr. J. T. Harmon is the recipient of fellowship IF32 AM-05571. The authors wish to thank the following individuals for their contributions: Dr. M. Root, Eli Lilly Company, for the gift of porcine insulin; Dr. W. Dulin, Upjohn Company, for the supply of streptozotocin; Mr. A. Kharroubi, Corning Medical Diagnostics, for the gift of the Immophase insulin RIA bit; W. Swanson and H. Ochej, Animal Tumor Research Facility, University of Rochester Cancer Center (CA-11198), for their continuing cooperation and help in tumor biopsy and transplantation.

REFERENCES

1. Bar, R. S., Gorden, P., Roth, J., Kahn, C. R., and DeMeyts, P. (1976): Fluctuations in the affinity and concentration of insulin receptors on circulating monocytes of obese patients. *J. Clin. Invest.*, 58:1123–1135.
2. Broer, Y., Freychet, P., and Rosselin, G. (1977): Insulin and glucagon-receptor interactions in the genetically obese Zucker rat: Studies of hormone binding and glucagon-stimulated cyclic AMP levels in isolated hepatocytes. *Endocrinology,* 101:236–249.
3. Carter, A. C., Lefkon, B. W., Farlin, M., and Feldman, E. B. (1975): Metabolic parameters in women with metastatic breast cancer. *J. Clin. Endocrinol. Metab.*, 40:260–264.
4. Cohen, N. D., and Hilf, R. (1974): Influence of insulin on growth and metabolism of 7,12-dimethylbenz(a)anthracene-induced mammary tumors. *Cancer Res.*, 34:3245–3252.
5. Cohen, N. D., and Hilf, R. (1975): Effect of estrogen treatment on DMBA-induced mammary tumor growth and biochemistry in intact and diabetic rats. *Proc. Soc. Exp. Biol. Med.*, 148:339–343.
6. Cohen, N. D., and Hilf, R. (1975): Influence of insulin on estrogen-induced responses in the R3230AC mammary carcinoma. *Cancer Res.*, 35:560–567.
7. Cuatracasas, P. (1974): Membrane receptors. *Annu. Rev. Biochem.*, 43:169–214.
8. Cuatracasas, P., Hollenberg, M. D., Chang, K. J., and Bennett, V. (1975): Hormone receptor complexes and their modulation of membrane function. *Recent Prog. Horm. Res.*, 31:37–94.
9. DeMeyts, P. (1976): Cooperative properties of hormone receptors in cell membranes. *J. Supramol. Struct.*, 4:241–258.
10. DeMeyts, P. (1976): Insulin and growth hormone receptors in human cultured lymphocytes and peripheral blood monocytes. In: *Methods in Receptor Research,* edited by M. Blecher, pp. 301–383. Marcel Dekker, New York.
11. DeMeyts, P., Bianco, A. R., and Roth, J. (1976): Site-site interactions among insulin receptors. Characterization of the negative cooperativity. *J. Biol. Chem.*, 251:1877–1888.
12. DeMeyts, P., and Roth, J. (1975): Cooperativity in ligand binding: A new graphic analysis. *Biochem. Biophys. Res. Commun.*, 43:400–408.
13. DeMeyts, P., Roth, J., Neville, D. M., Jr., Gavin, J. R., III, and Lesniak, M. A. (1973): Insulin interactions with its receptors: Experimental evidence for negative cooperativity. *Biochem. Biophys. Res. Commun.*, 55:154–161.
14. Elias, J. J. (1959): Effect of insulin and cortisol on organ cultures of adult mouse mammary gland. *Proc. Soc. Exp. Biol. Med.*, 101:500–502.
15. Fain, J. N. (1974): Mode of action of insulin. In: *MTP International review of Science, Vol. 8, Biochemistry of Hormones,* edited by H. V. Rickenberg, pp. 1–23. Butterworth, London.
16. Freychet, P., Roth, J., and Neville, D. M., Jr. (1971): Monoiodoinsulin: Demonstration of its biological activity and binding of fat cells and liver membranes. *Biochem. Biophys. Res. Commun.*, 43:400–408.

17. Freychet, P., Roth, J., and Neville, D. M., Jr. (1971): Insulin receptors in the liver: Specific binding of ^{125}I-insulin to the plasma membrane and its relation to insulin bioactivity. *Proc. Natl. Acad. Sci. U.S.A.,* 68:1833–1837.
18. Freychet, P., Roth, J., and Neville, D. M., Jr. (1972): Insulin interactions with liver plasma membranes: Independence of binding of the hormone and its degradation. *J. Biol. Chem.,* 247:3953–3961.
19. Gibson, S. L., and Hilf, R. (1976): Influence of hormonal alteration of host on estrogen-binding capacity in 7,12-dimethylbenzanthracene-induced mammary tumors. *Cancer Res.,* 36:3736–3741.
20. Hallowes, R. C., Wang, D. Y., and Lewis, D. J. (1973): The lactogenic effects of prolactin and growth hormone on mammary gland explants from virgin and pregnant Sprague-Dawley rats. *J. Endocrinol.,* 57:253–264.
21. Harmon, J. T., and Hilf, R. (1976): Insulin binding and glucose transport in the R3230AC mammary adenocarcinoma. *J. Supramol. Struct.,* 4:233–240.
22. Harmon, J. T., and Hilf, R. (1976): Identification and characterization of the insulin receptors in the R3230AC mammary adenocarcinoma of the rat. *Cancer Res.,* 36:3993–4000.
23. Harmon, J. T., and Hilf, R. (1978): Insulin and mammary cancer. In: *Influences of Hormones in Tumor Development,* edited by J. A. Kellen and R. Hilf. CRC Press, Cleveland *(in press).*
24. Heuson, J. C., Coune, A., and Heimann, R. (1967): Cell proliferation induced by insulin in organ culture of rat mammary carcinoma. *Exp. Cell Res.,* 45:351–360.
25. Heuson, J. C., and Legros, N. (1970): Effect of insulin and of alloxan diabetes on growth of the rat mammary carcinoma *in vivo. Eur. J. Cancer,* 6:349–351.
26. Heuson, J. C., and Legros, N. (1972): Influence of insulin deprivation on growth of the DMBA-induced mammary carcinoma in rats subjected to alloxan diabetes and food restriction. *Cancer Res.,* 32:226–232.
27. Heuson, J. C., Legros, N., and Heimann, R. (1972): Influence of insulin administration on growth of 7,12-dimethylbenz*(a)*anthracene-induced mammary carcinoma in intact, oophorectomized and hypophysectomized rats. *Cancer Res.,* 32:233–238.
28. Hilf, R., Harmon, J. T., Matusik, R. J., and Ringler, M. B. (1976): Hormonal control of mammary cancer. In: *Control Mechanisms in Cancer,* edited by W. E. Criss, T. Ono, and J. R. Sabine, pp. 1–24. Raven Press, New York.
29. Kelly, P. A., Posner, B. I., and Friesen, H. G. (1975): Effects of hypophysectomy, ovariectomy, and cycloheximide on specific binding sites for lactogenic hormones in rat liver. *Endocrinology,* 97:1408–1415.
30. Koroljow, S. (1962): Two cases of malignant tumors with metastases apparently treated successfully with hypoglycemic coma. *Psychiatr. Q.,* 36:262–270.
31. Kumareson, P., and Turner, C. W. (1965): Effect of graded levels of insulin on lactation in the rat. *Proc. Soc. Exp. Biol. Med.,* 119:415–416.
32. Lyons, W. R., Li, C. H., and Johnson, R. E. (1958): The hormonal control of mammary growth and lactation. *Recent Prog. Horm. Res.,* 14:219–254.
33. Martin, R. J., and Baldwin, R. L. (1971): Effects of alloxan diabetes on lactational performance and mammary tissue metabolism in the rat. *Endocrinology,* 88:863–867.
34. Muck, B. R., Trotnow, S., Eggar, H., and Hommel, G. (1976): Altered carbohydrate metabolism in breast cancer and benign breast affections. *Arch. Gynaekol.,* 221:83–91.
35. Muck, B. R., Trotnow, S., and Hommel, G. (1975): Cancer of the breast, diabetes and pathological glucose tolerance. *Arch. Gynaekol.,* 220:73–81.
36. Neufeld, O. (1962): Insulin therapy in terminal cancer: A preliminary report. *J. Am. Geriatr. Soc.,* 10:274–276.
37. Pearson, O. H., Llerana, O., Samaan, N., and Gonzalez, D. (1968): Serum growth hormone and insulin levels in patients with breast cancer. In: *Prognostic Factors in Breast Cancer,* edited by A. P. M. Forrest and P. B. Kunkler, pp. 421–430. Williams & Wilkins, Baltimore.
38. Pollet, R. J., Standaert, M. L., and Haase, B. A. (1977): Insulin binding to the human lymphocyte receptor. Evaluation of the negative cooperativity model. *J. Biol. Chem.,* 252:5828–5834.
39. Posner, B. I., Kelly, P. A., and Friesen, H. G. (1974): Induction of a lactogenic receptor in rat liver: Influence of estrogen and the pituitary. *Proc. Natl. Acad. Sci. U.S.A.,* 71:2407–2410.
40. Rhomberg, W. (1975): Metastasierendes Mammakarzinom und Diabetes mellitus—eine prognostisch günstige Kranksheitskombination. *Dtsch. Med. Wochenschr.,* 100:2422–2427.
41. Rivera, E. M., and Bern, H. A. (1961): Influence of insulin on maintenance and secretory stimulation of mouse mammary tissues by hormones in organ-culture. *Endocrinology,* 69:340–353.

42. Roth, J., Kahn, C. R., Lesniak, M. G., Gorden, P., DeMeyts, P., Megyesi, K., Neville, D. M., Jr., Gavin, J. R., III, Soll, A. H., Freychet, P., Goldfine, I. D., Bar, R. S., and Archer, J. A. (1975): Receptors for insulin, NSILA-S, and growth hormone: Applications to disease states in man. *Recent Prog. Horm. Res.,* 31:95–139.
43. Scatchard, G. (1974): The attractions of proteins for small molecules and ions. *Ann. N.Y. Acad. Sci.,* 51:660–672.
44. Shafie, S. M., and Brooks, S. C. (1976): The relationship of insulin to regulations of breast tumor cells by 17β-estradiol. *Fed. Proc.,* 35:1628.
45. Shafie, S. M., Gibson, S. L., and Hilf, R. (1977): Effect of insulin and estrogen on hormone binding in the R3230AC mammary adenocarcinoma. *Cancer Res.,* 37:4655–4663.
46. Shafie, S. M., and Hilf, R. (1978): Relationship between insulin and estrogen binding to growth response in 7,12-dimethylbenz*(a)*anthracene-induced rat mammary tumors. *Cancer Res.,* 38:759–764.
47. Smith, R. D., Hilf, R., and Senior, A. E. (1976): Prolactin binding to mammary gland, 7,12-dimethylbenz*(a)*anthracene-induced mammary tumors, and liver in rat. *Cancer Res.,* 36:3726–3731.
48. Smith, R. D., Hilf, R., and Senior, A. E. (1977): Prolactin binding to R3230AC mammary carcinoma and liver in hormone-treated and diabetic rats. *Cancer Res.,* 37:595–598.
49. Smith, R. D., Hilf, R., and Senior, A. E. (1977): Prolactin binding to 7,12-dimethylbenz*(a)*anthracene-induced mammary tumors and liver in diabetic rats. *Cancer Res.,* 37:4070–4074.
50. Sun, J. V., Tepperman, H. M., and Tepperman, J. (1977): A comparison of insulin binding by liver plasma membranes of rats fed high glucose diet or a high fat diet. *J. Lipid Res.,* 18:533–539.
51. Topper, Y. J., and Oka, T. (1974): Some aspects of mammary gland development in the mature mouse. In: *Lactation. A Comprehensive Treatise, Vol. I,* edited by B. L. Larson and V. R. Smith, pp. 327–348. Academic Press, New York.
52. Welsch, C. W., and Nagasawa, H. (1977): Prolactin and murine mammary tumorigenesis: A review. *Cancer Res.,* 37:951–963.

Endocrine Control in Neoplasia, edited by
R. K. Sharma and W. E. Criss.
Raven Press, New York © 1978.

Hormone Action in Breast Cancer Explants

N. Legros and J. C. Heuson

Service de Médecine et Laboratoire d'Investigation Clinique H. J. Tagnon, Institut Jules Bordet, Bruxelles, Belgique*

Organ culture was successfully used for the study of hormone dependence in experimental mammary tumors. In mice, hyperplastic alveolar nodules survive only in the presence of certain hormones. On the other hand, mammary tumors survive in the absence of hormones in the medium. Nevertheless, they respond to certain hormonal stimuli such as insulin, which enhances DNA synthesis, and 17β-estradiol, which inhibits this effect. In rats, the transplantable mammary tumor R3230AC reacts to the combination of insulin, hydrocortisone, and prolactin by an augmentation of the synthesis of milk proteins, but these hormones do not affect cell proliferation. Also in rats, the dimethylbenz*(a)*anthracene-induced mammary tumors belong to either of two categories. Some are insulin-independent *in vitro* and also fail to react to other hormones. Others are insulin-dependent and also react to prolactin, progesterone, or 17β-estradiol, the first two hormones being stimulating and the last inhibiting. These hormone effects are quite variable from tumor to tumor. With regard to human breast cancer, organ culture proves a difficult technique to handle. Short-term cultures (24–48 hr) are inadequate to demonstrate or assess hormone dependence of the tissue. With long-term cultures (>2 days), difficulties are met because of the scirrhous nature of many breast cancers. In rare "soft tumors" with a loose stroma, survival does not require hormone addition. In the scirrhous ones, survival is possible only if collagen is dissolved around the epithelial tumor cells under the effect of either added estradiol-17β or added exogenous collagenase. Estradiol-17β is able to induce production of collagenolytic activity around tumor cells that is probably enzymatic in nature. Survival is then ensured by proper diffusion of nutrients and oxygen into these cells. There is evidence from previously reported data that this estrogen-dependent collagenolytic system may play a role in the survival and spread of breast cancer *in vivo.* Aside from this observation, long-term organ culture of human breast cancer with today's techniques proves (as does short-term culture) unsuitable for demonstrating or assessing hormone dependence in individual patients for the purpose, for example, of providing a guide to therapy.

* This service is a member of the European Organization for Research on Treatment of Cancer (E. O. R. T. C.).

INTRODUCTION

Between 30 and 40% of patients with breast cancer in the advanced phase or at the time of dissemination respond favorably to endocrine surgical procedures (ovariectomy, adrenalectomy, hypophysectomy) or to administration of various hormones. The hormone-dependent mechanisms underlying these therapeutic responses are far from being known. Therefore it is impossible at present to forecast which patients will benefit from such treatments. Various methods have been developed for the purpose of defining the hormone dependence of a given tumor by *in vitro* studies. Of these, organ culture would seem appropriate, since it saves tissue architecture and especially the relationships between tumor epithelial cells and neighboring connective tissue. This method has the further advantage in that it permits assessment of the direct effects of hormones on tissue cell proliferation without interference of the multiple endocrine interactions that prevail within the whole organism. It enables the cultured tissue to be kept alive for several days and allows the long-term effects of the various hormones tested to be observed.

Organ culture has successfully been applied to experimental mammary tumors. The animal models most frequently studied have been spontaneous tumors of the mouse, the transplantable tumor R3230AC of the rat, and the 7,12-dimethylbenz*(a)*anthracene-induced mammary tumor of the rat.

On the other hand, with regard to human breast cancer, long-term organ culture proves quite difficult, especially in cases of the scirrhous type. This is the reason why various authors have proposed, as an alternative, very short-term organ culture for the purpose of studying these tumors *in vitro.*

This chapter will analyze the effects of various hormones either alone or in combination on experimental mammary tumors, as well as on human breast cancer, maintained in organ culture for varying durations of time.

SPONTANEOUS MOUSE TUMORS

Mammary carcinogenesis in the C3H mouse and related strains results from the action of carcinogenic viruses such as Bittner's milk factor. Tumor induction involves two consecutive steps: on the one hand, formation of preneoplastic lesions, the so-called hyperplastic alveolar nodules, and on the other hand, their transformation into cancer. Although preneoplastic lesions are hormone-dependent (5,42,43), the mammary tumors from which they derive usually have become autonomous (6). These various tissues have been studied in culture by Elias and Rivera (11). They cultured normal mammary tissue, preneoplastic nodules, and tumor tissue from C3H/HeCrgl mice in the presence of various hormones and hormone combinations. The results of the different treatments were assessed by histological criteria. Explants from spontaneous mammary tumors display very good survival in synthetic medium that is uninfluenced by hormone addition, whereas hyperplastic nodules and prelactating mammary gland degenerate in nonenriched medium. Addition of cortisol and ovine prolactin maintains the alveoli of the nodules and the prelactating gland and stimulates their secretory activity. In contrast, addition of estrone, progesterone, and growth hormone, either singly or in combination, does not modify the appearance of tissues *in vitro.* It is worthy of note that the prelactating gland requires higher hormone concentrations for full maintenance than do the hyperplastic nodules. This observation may mean that, in terms of hormone dependence *in vitro,* the requirements are decreasing with neoplasia, being less in preneoplastic tissue than in the normal gland, and still less in full-grown cancer. These observations are in agreement with *in vivo* findings, namely that hyperplastic nodules survive in a hormonal milieu that is inadequate for mammary tissue (43) and that hypophysectomy in C3H/HeCrgl mice results in regression of alveolar nodules (43) but is ineffective on mammary tumors (8).

One fundamental characteristic of neoplastic tissue is its unrestrained proliferation. Yet in mammary carcinomas the rate of cell proliferation can be altered by various endocrine factors. In order to assess the precise role of the hormonal environment on growth of mammary tumor cells, Turkington and Hilf (53) studied the effects of hormones on DNA synthesis in cultures of mammary tumors from C3H/HeJ mice. They found that insulin markedly stimulates DNA synthesis. This effect becomes manifest after 12 hr of incubation and progressively increases for at least 96 hr of culture. This enhancement of DNA synthesis does not result from insulin-induced augmentation of glucose transfer across the cell membrane, since it is also observed when fructose instead of glucose is added to the culture medium. This stimulating effect of insulin can be modified by the addition of steroids. 17β-Estradiol at 10^{-11}M (levels provided by adrenal steroidogenesis) strongly inhibits the stimulating effect of insulin; at a concentration of 10^{-10} M (levels corresponding approximately to those in the adult female) it allows maximal effect of insulin; at a concentration of 10^{-8} M (pharmacological levels) it again inhibits the insulin stimulating effect. Similar inhibitions have been observed with other estrogens in the following order of relative potencies: 17β-estradiol 1.0; estriol 1.0; diethylstilbestrol 0.5; estrone 0.4. Autoradiographic investigations indicate that the responses to insulin and to estrogens reflect a change in the number of cells engaged in DNA synthesis rather than a change in the rate of replication per cell. Turkington and Ward (56) further analyzed the mechanism of hormone action; they looked for an effect of insulin on processes directly related to DNA synthesis. They studied the activity of DNA polymerase in cultures of these same mammary tumors of C3H/HeJ mice. They observed parallel increases in DNA synthesis and DNA polymerase activity under the influence of insulin, which is consistent with the view of insulin acting directly on the enzymatic machinery of DNA synthesis.

Another aspect of the hormone dependence of C3H/HeJ mammary tumors is that of cell differentiation. It is well known that *in vitro,* under the influence of prolactin and in the presence of insulin and hydrocortisone, the normal mammary epithelium differentiates into secretory alveolar cells that synthesize casein, α-lactalbumin, and lactose synthetase protein A. Under the same culture conditions, no increased production of casein or α-lactalbumin could be observed in mouse mammary carcinoma (55). The neoplastic mammary cells dividing *in vitro* at the same rate as normal mammary cells, the absence of stimulation of differentiation, is therefore unrelated to the proliferative state. When the mammary precursor cells are stimulated by hormonal inducers of cell differentiation, they react by producing differentiated and secretory daughter cells that very seldom divide. On the other hand, since the C3H tumor cells fail to differentiate in response to the appropriate hormonal stimuli, the daughter cells retain the characteristics of precursor cells; they continue to divide and form masses of undifferentiated neoplastic cells. According to Turkington and Riddle (55), these results provide support for the concept that C3H mouse tumor cells are unable to limit their number through a normal sequence of cell differentiation. Welsch and associates also studied the C3H/HeJ mouse mammary tumor with regard to its *in vitro* response to insulin and prolactin. They confirmed Turkington's results insofar as insulin was found to increase DNA synthesis. Prolactin in the presence of insulin did not significantly alter ^{3}H-thymidine incorporation into explants. These results are consistent with *in vivo* observations showing that administration of prolactin (40) or antiprolactin drugs (58) to tumor-bearing mice does not modify tumor growth.

In summary, normal mammary glands of mouse, as well as hyperplastic alveolar nodules, survive in organ culture only if hormones are added to the medium; in contrast, tumors do not need supplementation for survival. Tumors are nevertheless responsive to certain hormonal stimuli. Thus insulin added to the culture medium increases DNA synthesis and DNA polymerase activity. Prolactin is ineffective, but 17β-estradiol, only at very precise concentrations, inhibits the stimulating effect of insulin. Prolactin in the presence of insulin and hydrocortisone *in vitro* induces secretory differentiation of the normal mammary epithelium, but it fails to display this effect in tumors. This observation is consistent with the theory that C3H mouse mammary tumors are made up of cells that are unable to limit their number through a normal sequence of cell differentiation.

TRANSPLANTABLE RAT MAMMARY TUMOR R3230AC

The transplantable tumor R3230AC is derived from a spontaneous mammary tumor of the Fisher rat. This tumor was discovered and its properties described by Hilf (27,28). It is autonomous and grows at identical rates in male and female rats whether or not they are castrated. However, it is hormone-responsive, its growth and differentiation being influenced by hormone administration. Thus administration of 17β-estradiol and/or prolactin inhibits tumor growth and induces an intense secretory response characterized by extensive vacuolization of the cells and distension of the acini, with accumulation of liquid containing casein, α-lactalbumin, and galactosyl transferase, each of these proteins being specifically synthesized by the alveolar cells of the normal mammary gland.

This tumor has been studied in organ culture. Explants show a fast rate of DNA synthesis that is independent of the presence of insulin (53). DNA polymerase activity behaves in a parallel way (56). 17β-Estradiol in the presence or absence of insulin fails to influence DNA synthesis significantly over a wide range of concentrations (10^{-6} to 10^{-13} M) (53). On the other hand, this hormone affects cell differentiation. Thus 17β-estradiol added *in vitro* increases casein synthesis and lactose synthetase activity (54). However, it should be stressed that in absolute values these metabolic activities represent hardly 10% of those recorded in cultures of normal lactating mammary glands. Addition of insulin, hydrocortisone, and prolactin to the culture medium also enhances casein synthsis (55).

It appears, therefore, that various hormones stimulate cell differentiation in the R3230AC tumor both *in vitro* and *in vivo,* with increased synthesis of milk proteins. Under these conditions tumor regression occurs *in vivo,* whereas DNA synthesis is unaffected *in vitro. In vivo* tumor regression will then merely be the consequence of the production of differentiated cells that will subsequently stop dividing.

CARCINOGEN-INDUCED RAT MAMMARY TUMORS

In 1959 Huggins et al. (29) showed that oral administration of a carcinogenic hydrocarbon readily induced multiple mammary carcinomas in the Sprague-Dawley rat. The carcinogen most commonly used at present for mammary carcinogenesis in this strain is 7,12-dimethylbenz*(a)*anthracene (DMBA). DMBA-induced rat mammary tumors are hormone-dependent; they regress as a consequence of various endocrine manipulations: ovariectomy or hypophysectomy (29); induction of alloxan diabetes (22); administration of hormones (29, 30,51) or hormone antagonists (9,26,52). On the other hand, their growth is accelerated by administration of insulin (23), prolactin (45), or progesterone (31,32). Thus they represent an interesting model for *in vitro* studies.

Heuson et al. (19) described the effects of insulin on explants of DMBA-induced rat mammary tumors *in vitro.* They defined two types of tumors in regard to their responses to insulin. These are designated insulin-dependent, in which active proliferation occurs only in the presence of this hormone, and insulin-independent, in which active proliferation occurs in unsupplemented medium and is unaltered by the addition of insulin. These tumor types have the same histological appearance, and both develop in rats irrespective of age and physiological status (18). The difference seems to be inherent in the tumor tissue itself. The stimulating effect of insulin on growth of the dependent type of tumor is not mediated through an increase in glucose transfer across the cell membrane. Thus increased concentrations of glucose in the culture medium do not mimic the insulin effect, nor does replacement of glucose by fructose, of which entry into cells is not dependent on insulin. Likewise, when glucose concentration in the culture medium is lowered to rate-limiting levels for cell proliferation, addition of pyruvate (which like fructose does not require the presence of insulin) restores cell proliferation toward normal only if insulin is present (20). This led Heuson and Legros (21) to search for an effect of insulin on enzymatic processes more directly linked with cell proliferation. They selected DNA polymerase and found that its activity paralleled the rate of DNA synthesis as influenced by insulin in dependent tumors, whereas it remained unaffected by insulin in independent tumors. This bundle of observations suggests that insulin-dependent growth of rat tumors is unrelated to an effect of insulin on carbohydrate metabolism; rather, it is related to processes more directly connected with the DNA synthesis machinery (21). The lack of insulin dependence of some tumors is unexplained. It is conceivable that the mature mammary gland may be composed of two cell types giving rise to either insulin-dependent or -independent tumors. Insulin dependence of rat mammary tumors, as revealed by organ culture experiments, seems to have its counterpart *in vivo.* Thus induction of alloxan diabetes in tumor-bearing animals results in rapid regression of the tumors that show insulin dependence *in vitro.* In contrast, the tumors that continue to grow in diabetic rats prove insulin-independent *in vitro* (21). Lewis and Hallowes (34) and Welsch et al. (59) confirmed this insulin dependence in organ culture of DMBA-induced mammary tumors of the rat.

Prolactin plays a major part in regulating growth of the DMBA rat tumor *in vivo.* Therefore prolactin has been studied in organ culture of this tumor. Welsch and Rivera (60) showed that explants cultured in the presence of insulin *and* prolactin have significantly higher rates of DNA synthesis than those cultured with insulin alone. These results were confirmed in more recent work by Welsch et al. (59), who showed that growth stimulation by prolactin was inhibited by 17β-estradiol added to the culture medium at a concentration of 10^{-2} μg/ml. Lewis and Hallowes (34) studied the effect of prolactin on tumors in relation to their insulin dependence. Insulin-independent tumors were uninfluenced by prolactin or prolactin plus 17β-estradiol (10^{-6} to 10^{-2} μg/ml). Insulin-dependent tumors displayed different behaviors toward prolactin: about half were uninfluenced by prolactin and 17β-estradiol, but the other half were further stimulated by prolactin, this effect being inhibited by 17β-estradiol (10^{-4} or 10^{-3} μg/ml). These observations were confirmed by Pasteels et al. (44): insulin-independent tumors were uninfluenced by other hormones in organ culture, but DNA synthesis in the presence of insulin was enhanced by prolactin in about 25% of the dependent tumors. In the latter, 17β-estradiol often abolished the stimulating effect of prolactin. Several authors have shown that "pharmacological" doses of estrogen inhibit growth of mammary tumors *in vivo* in castrated and noncastrated rats (38,41,51). Meites (37) suggested that estrogens might derive this action from inhibition of the stimulating effect of prolactin, which is in keeping with the foregoing results of organ culture experiments.

Progesterone, under certain circumstances, is known to exert *in vivo* a stimulating effect on growth of the DMBA rat mammary tumor. Pasteels et al. (44) who studied this hormone in organ culture showed that in 75% of insulin-dependent tumors DNA synthesis was augmented by a combination of prolactin and progesterone, whereas this effect was significant in only 25% of tumors with either hormone alone. Thus *in vitro*, prolactin and progesterone act synergistically. The *in vitro* effect of progesterone seems to have its counterpart *in vivo:* administration of progesterone accelerates tumor growth in tumor-bearing rats (31,32) and maintains tumors in about half the rats that are lactating after oophorectomy (36). These experiments were carried out in animals with intact pituitary; on the basis of the *in vitro* results demonstrating synergism between prolactin and progesterone, one may speculate that progesterone would fail to activate tumor growth after hypophysectomy. As far as we know, such experiments have not been done.

The histological features of hormonal effects were also studied in organ cultures of rat mammary tumors (44). Insulin-independent tumors, after 4 days of culture, displayed the same aspect as at initiation of culture, and the cultures were uninfluenced by any hormone supplementation (Figs. 1 and 2). Insulin-dependent

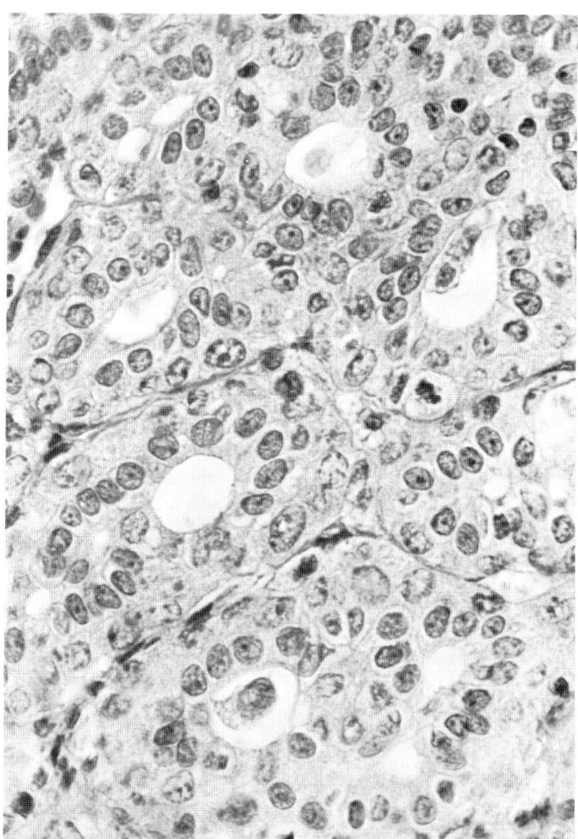

FIG. 1. Four-day organ culture of insulin-independent DMBA-induced rat mammary tumor in hormone-free medium. Tumor cells were well maintained. H&E, ×750. (Courtesy of J. A. Heuson-Stiennon and J. L. Pasteels.)

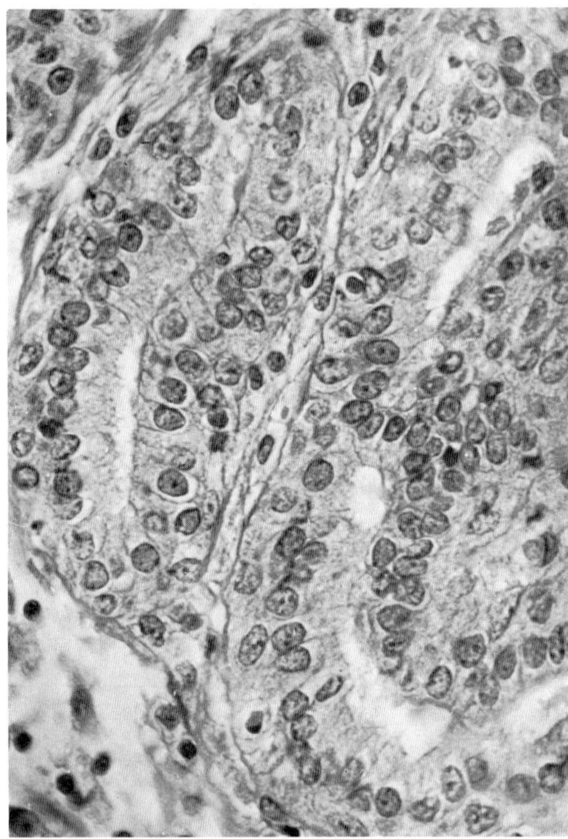

FIG. 2. Four-day organ culture of insulin-independent DMBA-induced rat mammary tumor in the presence of insulin. Supplementation of the medium with insulin did not induce any change in the histological appearance of the culture. H&E, ×750. (Courtesy of J. A. Heuson-Stiennon and J. L. Pasteels.)

tumors required the presence of insulin in the medium to maintain their initial histological characters; insulin-free cultures displayed regressive changes, with shrunken cytoplasm and nuclei and no glandular pattern (Fig. 3). In about half the tumors, prolactin in association with insulin induced an apocrine lipidic secretion without a recognizable concomitant increase in mitotic activity (Fig. 4); this prolactin-induced secretory activity was inhibited by addition of progesterone. To our knowledge, the latter property of progesterone has not been studied in the normal mammary gland.

It is concluded that organ culture of the DMBA-induced rat mammary tumor proved suitable to demonstrate the effects of various hormones on cell proliferation or differentiation and to study the underlying mechanisms. Some effects were known to occur *in vivo,* but others, such as those of insulin or progesterone,

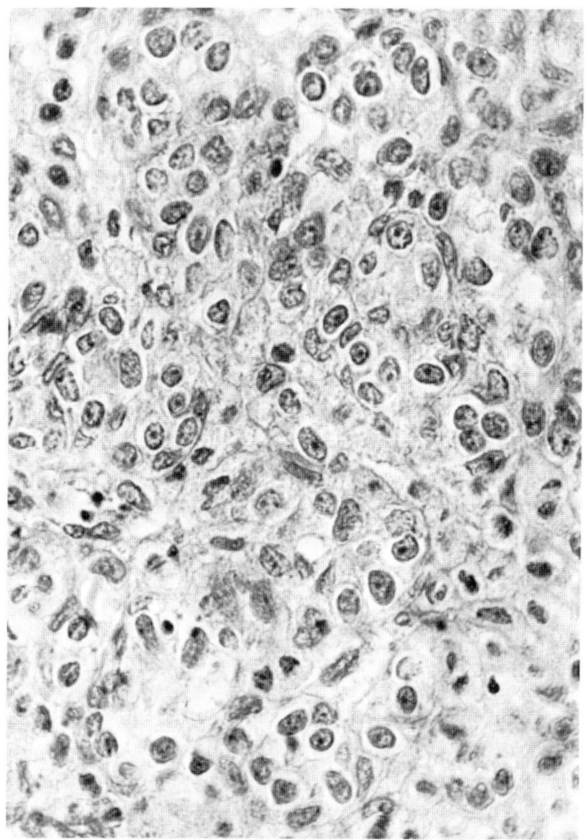

FIG. 3. Four-day organ culture of insulin-dependent DMBA-induced rat mammary tumor in hormone-free medium. Cytoplasm and nuclei are shrunken, and no glandular pattern is observed. H&E, ×750. (Courtesy of J. A. Heuson-Stiennon and J. L. Pasteels.)

were not. There seems to be good concordance between the hormonal properties under *in vitro* and *in vivo* conditions, but more work is needed before general conclusions can be drawn.

HUMAN MAMMARY TUMORS

Long-term organ cultures of human breast cancer proved very difficult to maintain, and this difficulty was probably related to the scirrhous character of these tumors. In contrast, normal mammary tissues or benign dysplasia are easily maintained in organ culture for several days without major morphological alterations (1,3,10,57). Likewise, benign fibroadenomas show good survival (10,57,61), as do malignant nonscirrhous carcinomas such as the colloid, intraductal, and medullary types that can be maintained in culture for several days

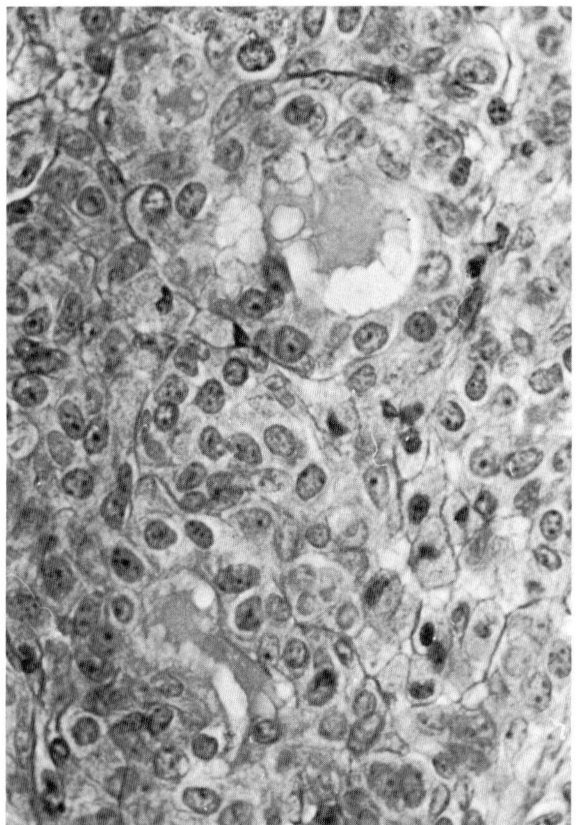

FIG. 4. Four-day organ culture of insulin-dependent DMBA-induced rat mammary tumor in the presence of insulin plus prolactin. Cells are large and well organized around glandular cavities; signs of secretory activity are visible mainly as lipid droplets at apical parts of the cells. H&E, ×750. (Courtesy of J. A. Heuson-Stiennon and J. L. Pasteels.)

(24,57,61). Survival of these nonscirrhous cancers seems unaffected by added hormones (24).

Short-Term Cultures

The difficulty of maintaining scirrhous carcinomas in organ culture for long periods led some authors to study short-term cultures (24–48 hr). Stoll (49) measured the levels of acid phosphatase and lactic dehydrogenase in explants cultured with 17β-estradiol or progesterone. In general, survival was poor, and hormones did not affect enzyme levels. Chayen et al. (7) made cultures in the presence of 17β—estradiol or drostanolone or both. They distinguished two types of tumors: those surviving without added hormones and those requiring the presence of estradiol. In the latter, drostanolone inhibited the estradiol beneficial effect. Salih et al. (47) evaluated pentose shunt activity by histochemistry and used histological criteria to assess hormonal effects in short-term cultures of breast carcinomas. They also described estrogen-dependent and -independent tumors and reported that this property correlated with the patients' responses to endocrine treatments. Their conclusions were seriously questioned (50). The same authors (46) claimed that some tumors were prolactin-dependent, whereas Flax et al. (15), in the same laboratory, found androgen-dependent tumors; both groups correlated these properties with clinical responses of the patients to endocrine treatments. Their conclusions were also much criticized with regard to methodology in both biological and clinical aspects (25). Beebey et al. (4), Masters et al. (35), and Montessori et al. (39) reported experiments of the same kind, but they found results quite different from those of Salih and Flax. Beebey et al. failed to observe any hormone sensitivity; the other two groups found sensitivity in only a small proportion of tumors, which could not be correlated with clinical responses. Lagios (33) measured the mitotic index on histological preparations and found, after 48 hr of culture, that some tumors were dependent on estradiol, testosterone, *and* prolactin. However, it should be noted that survival seemed not to exceed 48 hr and that therefore the proliferative activity was assessed at a time when it was sharply decreasing. Finally, Welsch et al. (59) measured ^{3}H-thymidine incorporation into DNA of breast cancer explants cultured in the presence of various combinations of insulin, prolactin, and hydrocortisone. They found that insulin significantly increased DNA synthesis and that prolactin (only in the presence of insulin and hydrocortisone) enhanced DNA synthesis in 3 of 20 tumors.

Short-term organ culture does not seem, from these experiments, to have proved its value for the assessment of hormone dependence of human breast cancer or its value as a predictor of clinical responsiveness to endocrine therapies.

Long-Term Cultures

It has been a common experience that maintaining explants of human breast cancer in organ culture has been a very difficult task. Sellwood and Castro (48) carried out 4-day cultures; on histological examination they found that one-third of the cultures did not survive, and in the remaining two-thirds, only 29% of the explants were viable. Addition of testosterone, 17β-estradiol, stilbestrol, or hydrocortisone did not affect survival. Likewise, Wellings and Jentoft (57) after 5 days of culture, observed poor survival of scirrhous tumor explants that was not improved by addition of insulin, aldosterone, prolactin, or estradiol. Willcox and Thomas (61) made similar observations on 6-day organ cultures of scirrhous breast cancers. It should be stressed that under similar culture conditions, normal mammary tissues (13), mammary dysplasia (10,57), fibroadenomas (10,57,61), and nonscirrhous carcinomas (24,57,61) survived well, as judged by histological criteria, and that their survival was uninfluenced by adding hormones to the culture medium (24,57). Geier et al. (16,17) studied the metabolism of testosterone and 17β-estradiol by explants of various types of mammary tissue, whether neoplastic or not: carcinomas, cystic mastitis, fibroadenomas, and uninvaded mammary tissue obtained from mastectomy specimens. After 5 days of culture in medium 199 enriched with 20% calf serum, the explants were reported not to show signs of necrosis and to show the same histologic appearance as at initiation of culture. The metabolism of ^{14}C-testosterone (17) was studied in samples from normal mammary tissue (4 cases), samples from fibroadenomas (2 cases), and samples from carcinomas (4 cases). In all, testosterone was metabolized into androsterone, dihydrotestosterone, androstenedione, and androstanediol. The rate of conversion was higher in normal tissues than in cancer tissues. The metabolism of ^{3}H-17β-estradiol (16) was studied in samples from normal mammary tissue (3 cases), samples from fibroadenomas and cystic disease (2 and 2 cases), and samples from carcinomas (5 cases). In all, estradiol was converted into estrone; conversion was at a higher rate in normal tissues than in neoplastic tissues. The higher rates of conversion of both hormones in normal tissues could be due to greater vitality in normal tissue. This led Finkelstein et al. (14) to measure the synthesis of DNA, RNA, and protein in both cancerous and noncancerous tissue. They noted that macromolecules were synthesized at similar rates in neoplastic tissue and uninvaded tissue, even at higher rates than those seen in cultures of fibroadenomas. These observations led the authors to study the synthesis of DNA, RNA, and protein in the absence and presence of steroids in more detail. It was found that in benign tissues, testosterone inhibited the synthesis of all macromolecules, but estradiol inhibited the synthesis of DNA only; the effect of the latter hormone was variable on RNA synthesis and protein synthesis. In cancer tissue, both steroids produced variable effects, either stimulating or inhibitory, on the synthesis of macromolecules. It is our opinion that it is difficult to interpret these results, and they should be regarded with great caution. There are two major difficulties. One is that for metabolic studies, the tissues were extremely heterogeneous, containing epithelial cells, fibroblasts, inflammatory cells, etc. The other difficulty concerns the viability of these various tissue components. There was no convincing evidence presented in these reports to support the conclusion that the various tissue components were actually alive and thriving. Only one histological section was shown, and its examination suggests that cell survival was poor and that many nuclei were pyknotic.

Heuson et al. (24) developed a method for organ culture that enabled them to keep explants from human breast cancer alive for 14 days under certain conditions. This technique was applied to 94 cases of human breast carcinomas. "Soft tumors," i.e., those containing little collagen, displayed excellent survival even in the absence of any added hormone (Figs. 5 and 6). In contrast, "scirrhous tumors," i.e., those that are largely made up of dense collagen, showed poor survival of the epithelial component in the absence of any added hormone.

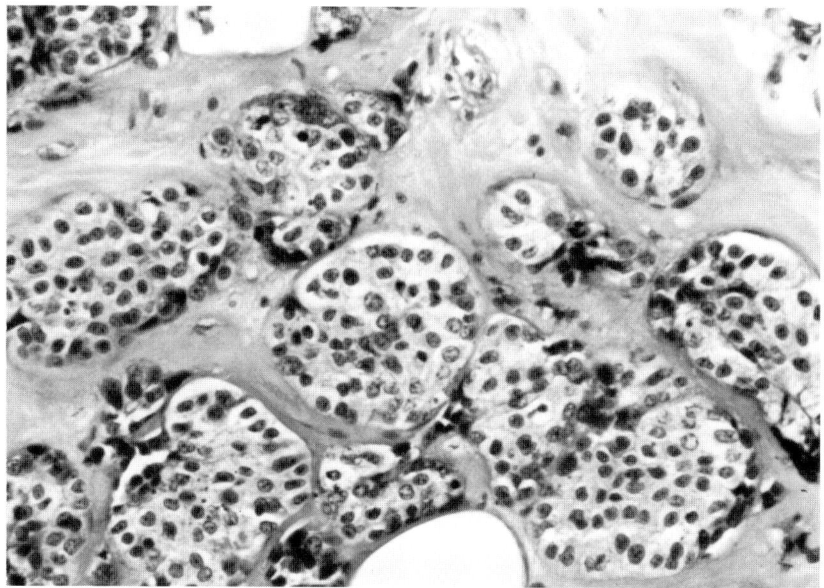

FIG. 5. Culture of soft infiltrating ductal carcinoma, initial condition. Connective tissue was sparse, with loose collagen fibrils. H&E, ×500. (Courtesy of J. A. Heuson-Stiennon and J. L. Pasteels.)

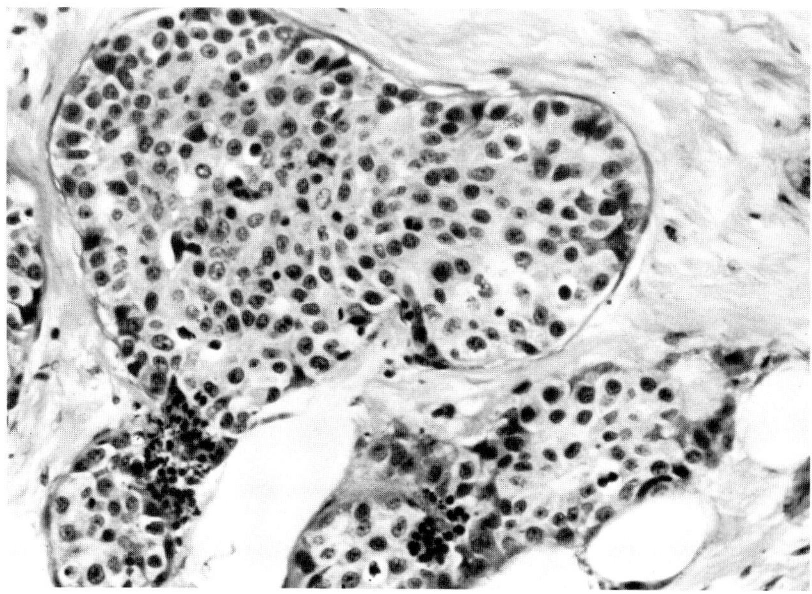

FIG. 6. Central region of a 5-day organ culture of the same tumor seen in Fig. 5 carried out in the presence of insulin and hydrocortisone. Tumor cells were well preserved, and collagen liquefaction was not necessary for maintenance of viable cells in the center of the explant. H&E, ×500. (Courtesy of J. A. Heuson-Stiennon and J. L. Pasteels.)

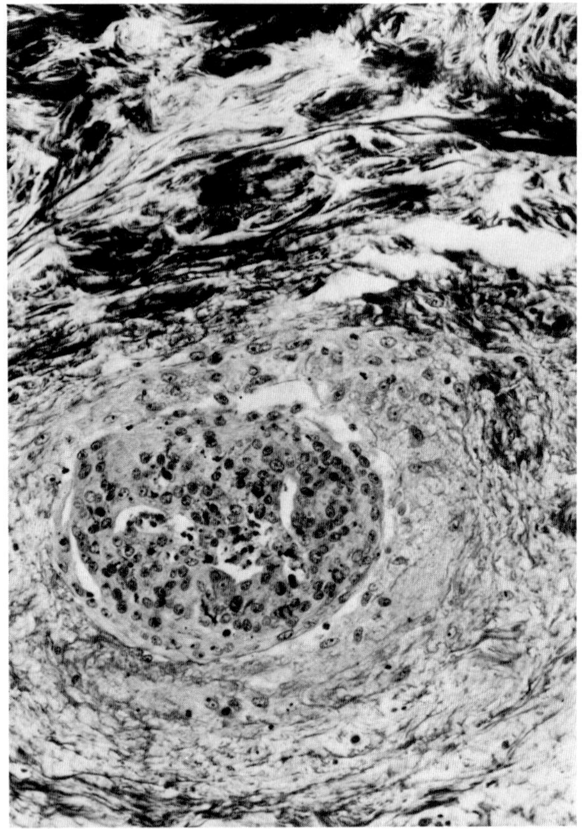

FIG. 7. Seven-day organ culture of scirrhous carcinoma carried out in the presence of insulin, prolactin, and 17β-estradiol. Cancer epithelial cells survived in the central area of the explant surrounded by a halo of dissolved collagen. Intact dense collagen fibers were present far from the cancer cells. Van Gieson, ×200. (Courtesy of J. A. Heuson-Stiennon and J. L. Pasteels.)

Only a few islets of this tissue component survived at the periphery of the explants. Addition of insulin, prolactin, or hydrocortisone in various combinations failed to induce any histologically detectable changes in the tumors, whether soft or scirrhous. However, further addition of estradiol, although ineffective on soft tumors, brought about spectacular changes in the cultures of scirrhous explants. The epithelial cells survived even in the centers of the explants, and these islets of epithelial neoplastic cells were surrounded by halos of dissolved collagen (Fig. 7). On the other hand, if purified collagenase was added at the start of culture for 1 or 2 days, the collagen of scirrhous explants was totally dissolved and excellent survival of the remaining epithelial cancer cells was obtained, no addition of any hormone being required at all. It is concluded that human breast cancer is not dependent on hormones for survival in culture, provided that the epithelial cancer cells are not choked by dense collagen. When they are, estradiol ensures their survival by inducing them to synthesize collagenolytic enzymes that dissolve collagen. Nutrients and oxygen can then freely diffuse from the medium into them. This estrogen-dependent collagenolytic enzyme system might play an important part in the mechanisms that govern hormone dependence of breast cancer.

Aspegren (2) studied ^{3}H-thymidine incorporation into explants of human breast cancer as influenced by estradiol, testosterone, or progesterone; he cultured in parallel and under identical conditions explants of human fibroblastic sarcomas. Both tumor types showed responses to these hormones, but the responses were either stimulation or inhibition. Since sarcomas are supposedly hormone-insensitive, it was concluded that the *in vitro* test used lack specificity.

From this review, it would appear that organ culture does not provide a useful and practical means for assessment of hormone dependence in human breast cancer. However, it may give valuable pieces of information of clinical interest, such as demonstration of an estrogen-dependent collagenolytic system in scirrhous carcinomas.

CONCLUSIONS

In experimental mammary tumors, hormone dependence was successfully studied by the method of organ culture. Good correlation was often found between *in vitro* effects of hormones and tumor responses to the same hormonal stimuli *in vivo.* Organ culture may therefore be considered to be a useful tool for studying enhancing or inhibiting stimuli (hormonal or cytostatic) on growth of these experimental tumors.

On the other hand, organ culture of human breast cancer has encountered numerous difficulties, and its *in vivo* behavior in relation to hormones remains to be explained. Thus breast cancer shows good survival *in vitro* without hormone supplementation, provided it is a "soft" tumor such that the epithelial neoplastic component is not choked to death by dense surrounding collagen. However, scirrhous explants can be maintained if the dense collagen is eliminated early in culture by the addition of exogenous collagenase. This survival of the breast cancer cell in a hormone-free environment does not imply that it is hormone-insensitive. Histological criteria were not found reliable to assess growth in culture of experimental tumors. More specific measurements were required, such as ^{3}H-thymidine incorporation into DNA or labeling index. These parameters were difficult to measure with any accuracy in human material, which usually contains few epithelial cells relative to stromal components; thus incorporation of labeled precursors of the synthesis of macromolecules proved to be quite low and extremely variable.

Nevertheless, one piece of information evolved from the study of human breast cancer in organ culture. It was found that 17β-estradiol in explants from scirrhous carcinomas induced production of collagenolytic activity around the epithelial tumor cells that, by loosening the stroma, improved the diffusion of nutrients and oxygen and thereby cell survival. The question now is whether this estrogen-dependent collagenolytic (enzyme?) system has any bearing on tumor growth *in vivo.* Relevant data in the literature are as follows: on one hand, in the normal mammary gland of the rodent, Elliot and Turner (12) described a "spreading factor" that had the properties of an enzyme and that would act on the collagen. According to their theory, this spreading factor would be synthesized or activated by hormones, especially estrogens, that induce both ductal and lobuloalveolar growth. The function of this enzyme would be to dissolve the collagen and allow the rapid growth of ducts and lobules. On the other hand, Emerson et al. (13) described in breast cancer patients treated with large doses of estrogens a loosening of the connective tissue surrounding the neoplastic cells. This loosening seemed to result from partial dissolution of collagen. These data are consistent with the view that the estrogen-dependent collagenolytic system described by Heuson et al. (24) might play an important part in hormonal control, growth, and spread of breast cancer. It would be of importance to be able to quantitatively assess this activity and determine if other hormones are involved in the process.

ACKNOWLEDGMENTS

This work was supported by grants from the Fonds Cancérologique de la Caisse Générale d'Epargne et de Retraite de Belgique and by NCI contract N01-CM-53,840. It was also performed under contract of the Ministère de la Politique Scientifique (Actions concertées) within the framework of the Association Euratom/University of Brussels/University of Pisa.

REFERENCES

1. Archer, F. L. (1968): Normal and neoplastic human tissue in organ culture. *Arch. Pathol.,* 85:62–71.
2. Aspegren, K. (1976): Hormone effects on human mammary cancer in organ culture. *Am. J. Surg.,* 131:575–580.
3. Barker, B. E., Fanger, H., and Farnes, P. (1964): Human mammary slices in organ culture. *Exp. Cell Res.,* 35:437–448.
4. Beeby, D. E., Easty, G. C., Gazet, J. C., Grigor, K., and Neville, A. M. (1975): An assessment of the effects of hormones on short term organ culture of human breast carcinomata. *Br. J. Cancer,* 31:317–328.
5. Bern, H. A., DeOme, K. B., Wellings, R. S., and Harkness, D. R. (1958): The effect of various hormonal treatments on the incidence of hyperplastic nodules and of "noduloids" in the mammary glands of C3H/He Crgl mice. *Cancer Res.,* 18:1324–1328.
6. Bern, H. A., and Nandi, S. (1961): Recent studies of the hormonal influence in mouse mammary tumorigenesis. *Prog. Exp. Tumor Res.,* 2:91–145.
7. Chayen, J., Altmann, F. P., Bitensky, L., and Daly, J. R. (1970): Response of human breast cancer tissue to steroid hormones in vitro. *Lancet,* 1:868–870.
8. DeOme, K. B., Bern, H. A., Elias, J. J., Nandi, S., and Faulkin, L. J. (1958): Studies on the growth potential of hyperplastic nodules of the mammary gland of the C3H/He Crgl mouse. In: *Second International Symposium on Mammary Cancer,* edited by L. Severi, pp. 595–604. Division of Cancer Research, University of Perugia, Perugia, Italy.

9. DeSombre, E. R., and Arbogast, L. Y. (1974): Effect of the antiestrogen CI 628 on the growth of rat mammary tumors. *Cancer Res.,* 34:1971–1976.
10. Elias, J. J., and Armstrong, R. C. (1973): Hyperplastic and metaplastic responses of human mammary fibroadenomas and dysplasias in organ culture. *J. Natl. Cancer Inst.,* 51:1341–1343.
11. Elias, J. J., and Rivera, E. (1959): Comparison of the responses of normal, precancerous, and neoplastic mouse mammary tissues to hormones in vitro. *Cancer Res.,* 19:505–511.
12. Elliot, J. R., and Turner, C. W. (1953): The mammary gland spreading factor. *Res. Bull. Univ. Missouri Coll. Agric.,* 537:1–52.
13. Emerson, W. J., Kennedy, B. J., Graham, J. N., and Nathanson, I. T. (1953): Pathology of primary and recurrent carcinoma of the human breast after administration of steroid hormones. *Cancer,* 6:641–670.
14. Finkelstein, M., Geier, A., Horn, H., Levij, I. S., and Ever-Hadani, P. (1975): Effect of testosterone and estradiol-17β on synthesis of DNA, RNA and protein in human breast in organ culture. *Int. J. Cancer,* 15:78–90.
15. Flax, H., Salih, H., Newton, K. A., and Hobbs, J. R. (1973): Are some women's breast cancers androgen dependent? *Lancet,* 1:1204–1207.
16. Geier, A., Horn, H., Levij, I. S., Lichtshtein, E., and Finkelstein, M. (1975): The metabolism of ^{3}H-estradiol-17β in human breast cancer in organ culture. *Eur. J. Cancer,* 11:127–130.
17. Geier, A., Horn, H., Lichtshtein, E., Levij, I. S., and Finkelstein, M. (1974): The uptake and metabolism of [4-^{14}C]testosterone in human breast cancer grown in organ culture. *Acta Endocrinol.,* 75:195–204.
18. Heuson, J. C. (1971): Contribution à l'étude de l'hormonodépendance d'une tumeur mammaire expérimentale chez le rat. Thesis, Free University of Brussels, Belgium.
19. Heuson, J. C., Coune, A., and Heimann, R. (1967): Cell proliferation induced by insulin in organ culture of rat mammary carcinoma. *Exp. Cell Res.,* 45:351–360.
20. Heuson, J. C., and Legros, N. (1968): Study of the growth-promoting effect of insulin in relation to carbohydrate metabolism in organ culture of rat mammary carcinoma. *Eur. J. Cancer,* 4:1–7.
21. Heuson, J. C., and Legros, N. (1971): Effect of insulin on DNA synthesis and DNA polymerase activity in organ culture of rat mammary carcinoma and the influence of insulin pretreatment and of alloxan diabetes. *Cancer Res.,* 31:59–65.
22. Heuson, J. C., and Legros, N. (1972): Influence of insulin deprivation on growth of the 7,12-dimethylbenz*(a)*anthracene-induced mammary carcinoma in rats subjected to alloxan diabetes and food restriction. *Cancer Res.,* 32:226–232.
23. Heuson, J. C., Legros, N., and Heimann, R. (1972): Influence of insulin administration on growth of the 7,12-dimethylbenz *(a)* anthracene-induced mammary carcinoma in intact, oophorectomized, and hypophysectomized rats. *Cancer Res.,* 32:233–238.
24. Heuson, J. C., Pasteels, J. L., Legros, N., Heuson-Stiennon, J., and Leclercq, G. (1975): Estradiol-dependent collagenolytic enzyme activity in long-term organ culture of human breast cancer. *Cancer Res.,* 35:2039–2048.
25. Heuson, J. C., and Tagnon, H. J. (1973): Androgen dependence of breast cancer. *Lancet,* 2:203–204.
26. Heuson, J. C., Waelbroeck, C., Legros, N., Gallez, G., Robyn, C., and L'Hermite, M. (1971/72): Inhibition of DMBA-induced mammary carcinogenesis in the rat by 2-Br-α-ergocryptine (CB 154), an inhibitor of prolactin, and by nafoxidine (U-11,100 A), an estrogen antagonist. *Gynecol. Invest.,* 2:130–137.
27. Hilf, R. (1968): Biochemical studies of hormone-responsive mammary tumors. *Cancer Res.,* 28:1888–1890.
28. Hilf, R., Michel, I., and Bell, C. (1967): Biochemical and morphological responses of normal and neoplastic mammary tissue to hormonal treatment. *Recent Prog. Horm. Res.,* 23:229–295.
29. Huggins, C., Briziarelli, G., and Sutton, H., Jr. (1959): Rapid induction of mammary carcinoma in the rat and the influence of hormones on the tumors. *J. Exp. Med.,* 109:25–41.
30. Huggins, C., Moon, R. C., and Morii, S. (1962): Extinction of experimental mammary cancer. I. Estradiol-17β and progesterone. *Proc. Natl. Acad. Sci. U.S.A.,* 48:379–386.
31. Huggins, C., and Yang, N. C. (1962): Induction and extinction of mammary cancer. *Science,* 137:257–262.
32. Jabara, A. G. (1967): Effects of progesterone on 9,10-dimethyl-1,2-benz*(a)*anthracene-induced marqnary tumours in Sprague-Dawley rats. *Br. J. Cancer,* 21:418–429.

33. Lagios, M. D. (1974): Hormonally enhanced proliferation of human breast cancer in organ culture. *Oncology,* 29:22–33.
34. Lewis, D., and Hallowes, R. C. (1974): Correlation between the effects of hormones on the synthesis of DNA in explants from induced rat mammary tumours and the growth of the tumours. *J. Endocrinol.,* 62:225–240.
35. Masters, J. R. W., Sangster, K., Smith, I. I., and Forrest, P. M. (1976): Human breast carcinomata in organ cultures: The effects of hormones. *Br. J. Cancer,* 33:564–566.
36. McCormick, G. M., and Moon, R. C. (1967): Hormones influencing postpartum growth of 7,12-dimethylbenz*(a)*anthracene-induced rat mammary tumors. *Cancer Res.,* 27:626–631.
37. Meites, J. (1972): Relation of prolactin and estrogen to mammary tumorigenesis in the rat. *J. Natl. Cancer Inst.,* 48:1217–1224.
38. Meites, J., Cassel, E., and Clark, J. (1971): Estrogen inhibition of mammary tumor growth in rats, counteraction by prolactin. *Proc. Soc. Exp. Biol. Med.,* 137:1225–1227.
39. Montessori, G. A., Algard, T., Van Netten, J. P., and Donald, J. C. (1977): Screening of mammary carcinoma for hormone dependency in vitro. Enzymatic activity in short-term organotypic cultures of breast biopsies from 62 patients. *Am. J. Clin. Pathol.,* 67:393–396.
40. Nagasawa, H., Kuretani, K., and Kanzawa, F. (1966): Effect of prolactin on the growth of spontaneous mammary tumor in mice. *Gann,* 57:637–640.
41. Nagasawa, H., and Yanai, R. (1974): Effects of estrogen and/or pituitary graft on nucleic acid synthesis of carcinogen-induced mammary tumors in rats. *J. Natl. Cancer Inst.,* 52:1219–1222.
42. Nandi, S., Bern, H. A., and DeOme, K. B. (1960): Effect of hormones on growth and neoplastic development of transplanted hyperplastic alveolar nodules of the mammary gland of C3H/Crgl mice. *J. Natl. Cancer Inst.,* 24:883–905.
43. Nandi, S., Bern, H. A., and DeOme, K. B. (1960): Hormonal induction and maintenance of precancerous hyperplastic alveolar nodules in the mammary glands of hypophysectomized female C3H/He Crgl mice. *Acta Unio Internationalis contra Cancrum,* 16:221–224.
44. Pasteels, J. L., Heuson, J. C., Heuson-Stiennon, J., and Legros, N. (1976): Effects of insulin, prolactin, progesterone and estradiol on DNA synthesis in organ culture of 7,12-dimethylbenz*(a)*anthracene-induced rat mammary tumors. *Cancer Res.,* 36:2162–2170.
45. Pearson, O. H., Llerena, O., Llerena, L., Molina, A., and Butler, T. (1969): Prolactin-dependent rat mammary cancer. A model for man? *Trans. Assoc. Am. Physicians,* 82:225–238.
46. Salih, H., Flax, H., Brander, W., and Hobbs, J. R. (1972): Prolactin dependence in human breast cancers. *Lancet,* 2:1103–1105.
47. Salih, H., Flax, H., and Hobbs, J. R. (1972): In-vitro oestrogen sensitivity of breast-cancer tissue as a possible screening method for hormonal treatment. *Lancet,* 1:1198–1202.
48. Sellwood, R. A., and Castro, J. E. (1974): The effect of hormones on organ cultures of human mammary carcinoma. *J. Pathol.,* 113:223–225.
49. Stoll, B. A. (1970): Investigation of organ culture as an aid to the hormonal management of breast cancer. *Cancer,* 25:1228–1233.
50. Stoll, B. A. (1972): In-vitro oestrogen sensitivity of breast cancer. *Lancet,* 1:1339.
51. Teller, M. N., Stock, C. C., and Bowie, M. (1966): Effects of 17α-thio-estradiol, 2 estradiol analogs, and 2 androgens on 7,12-dimethylbenz*(a)*anthracene-induced rat mammary tumors. *Cancer Res.,* 26:2329–2333.
52. Terenius, L. (1971): Anti-estrogen and breast cancer. *Eur. J. Cancer,* 7:57–64.
53. Turkington, R. W., and Hilf, R. (1968): Hormonal dependence of DNA synthesis in mammary carcinoma cells in vitro. *Science,* 160:1457–1459.
54. Turkington, R. W., and Riddle, M. (1969): Acquired hormonal dependence of milk protein synthesis in mammary carcinoma cells. *Endocrinology,* 84:1213–1217.
55. Turkington, R. W., and Riddle, M. (1970): Expression of differentiated function by mammary carcinoma cells. *Cancer Res.,* 30:127–132.
56. Turkington, R. W., and Ward, O. T. (1969): DNA polymerase and DNA synthesis in mammary carcinoma cells. *Biochim. Biophys. Acta,* 174:282–290.
57. Wellings, S. R., and Jentoft, V. L. (1972): Organ cultures of normal, dysplastic, hyperplastic, and neoplastic human mammary tissues. *J. Natl. Cancer Inst.,* 49:329–338.
58. Welsch, C. W., and Gribler, C. (1973): Prophylaxis of spontaneously developing mammary carcinoma in C3H/HeJ female mice by suppression of prolactin. *Cancer Res.,* 33:2939–2946.
59. Welsch, C. W., Iturri, G. C., and Brennan, M. J. (1976): DNA synthesis of human, mouse,

and rat mammary carcinomas in vitro. Influence of insulin and prolactin. *Cancer,* 38:1272–1281.

60. Welsch, C. W., and Rivera, E. M. (1972): Differential effects of estrogen and prolactin on DNA synthesis in organ cultures of DMBA-induced rat mammary carcinoma. *Proc. Soc. Exp. Biol. Med.,* 139:623–626.
61. Willcox, P. A., and Thomas, G. H. (1972): Oestrogen metabolism in cultured human breast tumours. *Br. J. Cancer,* 26:453–460.

STEROID HORMONES

Endocrine Control in Neoplasia, edited by
R. K. Sharma and W. E. Criss.
Raven Press, New York © 1978.

Human Breast Cancer and Hormone Receptors

*Keishi Matsumoto and **Haruo Sugano

**Institute for Cancer Research, Osaka University Medical School, Kita-ku, Osaka 530, Japan; and **Cancer Institute, Japanese Foundation for Cancer Research, Toshima-ku, Tokyo 170, Japan*

It is generally accepted that the incidence of breast cancer in Japan is remarkably lower than in Western countries and that Japanese women with breast cancer have a more favorable survival rate than American patients. We examined estrogen (ER), progesterone (PgR), and androgen (AR) receptors in 400 Japanese breast cancer specimens and compared the results with those obtained by investigators in Western countries.

In Japan, 55% (220/400) of breast cancers revealed measurable amounts of ER (> 2 fmoles/mg cytosol protein). There was no correlation between tumor histopathology and the presence of ER, and the ER values in primary and metastatic lesions from the same patients were similar in most cases. The response rates to endocrine therapy were 62% (16/26) for ER-positive breast tumors and 4% (1/25) for ER-negative tumors. These results are similar to those in Western patients. However, Japanese and Western postmenopausal patients differed in incidence of ER-positive tumors; i.e., the incidence in Japanese patients was similar for premenopausal and postmenopausal patients, whereas in Western patients, the incidence was higher in postmenopausal patients.

In Japan, measurable amounts of PgR (> 5 fmoles/mg cytosol protein) were found in 57% (86/150) of ER-positive breast cancers but in only 11% (12/109) of ER-negative cancers; AR (> 5) was found in 38% (13/34) of cancers with positive ER and in 23% (7/31) of cancers with negative ER. These results are also similar to those reported by Western investigators. Furthermore, McGuire et al. reported preliminary data showing that in cases where ER is positive and PgR is negative, successful response to endocrine therapy is very low, whereas in cases having both receptors, remissions are seen in a larger percentage of patients than would be predicted on the basis of ER alone. In cases where ER+ and PgR− tumors are present, our preliminary data on 20 patients support this finding.

These results show that assays of ER and/or PgR are useful markers for predicting response to endocrine therapy in breast cancer patients of any country, whether the incidence of breast cancer has been shown to be high or low.

INTRODUCTION

During the past several years several laboratories have clearly demonstrated that a certain proportion of breast cancers contain specific estrogen-, progesterone-, and/or androgen-binding proteins. These proteins, called estrogen (ER), progesterone (PgR), and androgen (AR) receptors were found to be similar to those present in target tissues of these steroids such as the uterus or prostate, and they have been shown to play an essential part in the mechanism of action of these steroids in the target tissues. Since only one-third of patients with metastatic breast cancer will respond to endocrine therapy such as ovariectomy, adrenalectomy, or hypophysectomy with objective tumor regression (11,14), determination of these receptors in breast cancers will provide a useful method for selecting or rejecting endocrine therapy with considerable confidence.

In Japan, incidence of breast cancer is remarkably lower than in Western countries (15). When women in Japan do develop breast cancer, they have a more favorable survival rate than American breast cancer patients, which is not evident from histopathology, tumor size, axillary node status, or type of primary therapy (34,59). Since ER, PgR, and AR have been shown to have some effect on the growth of breast cancer, the incidence of steroid receptors in Japanese breast cancer might be different from that in Western breast cancer. Those observations suggest that correlations of receptor measurements and clinical responses to endocrine therapy should be made in both Japanese and Western breast cancer patients.

It is now generally appreciated that ER are found in 50 to 80% of human breast cancers and that 55 to 60% of ER+ tumors are likely to regress following endocrine therapy, whereas those tumors lacking ER usually fail to respond (response rate 0–10%). This concept was originally proposed by Jensen et al. (21), has been supported by data from their laboratory (22), the laboratory of McGuire et al. (32), and other Western workers (24,28), as well as by data from Japan, including data from our laboratories (38). In the present review, the collective data, especially on Japanese breast cancers, are summarized.

There is no doubt that ER determinations are helpful in selecting patients with metastatic breast cancer for endocrine treatment. However, this method is not completely satisfactory, since approximately 40% of ER-positive breast cancers fail to respond to endocrine therapy. In order to identify the 40% of ER-positive but endocrine-resistant tumors, PgR and AR as well as ER in breast cancers have been measured in Western countries and in Japan. In this review, these data accumulated to date are also summarized.

ER IN HUMAN BREAST CANCER

Experimental Procedure

Specimens from Japanese patients were processed as follows: Tumors were excised, trimmed of fat and normal tissue, frozen in liquid nitrogen, and used immediately or stored at −80° C until assay. ER in breast cancers was measured by the sucrose density gradient method or the dextran-coated charcoal method and analyzed according to Scatchard (49) or Baulieu and Raynaud (8); the methods have been reported in detail (22,28,32,38). The method for collection and assay of ER for the Japanese patients is practically identical to the method used by Western investigators. A tumor is considered ER+ in a Japanese patient if it contains more than 2 fmoles of ER per milligram of cytosol protein. The principal data (38) used in this review are the results of the U.S.–Japan Cooperative Cancer Research Program.[1]

For criteria of objective remissions of breast cancers, the published criteria of the Cooperative Breast Cancer Group were used (13). Specifically, tumor responses were classified as objective remissions only when (a) at least 50% of all directly measurable lesions decreased 50% in size or (b) osseous lesions recalcified and (c) no new lesions appeared.

ER Level in Breast Cancer

Figure 1 shows the values for ER in 350 Japanese and 400 American primary breast tumor specimens (38). In both countries the values ranged from zero to more than 1,000 fmoles/mg cytosol protein. In both countries, very high values for tumor ER are found mostly in postmenopausal patients. The wide range of values may be due to a combination of factors. For one, endogenous estrogen secreted by the patient must be considered, since high levels of endogenous estrogen would occupy ER sites and make them unavailable for assay by the techniques used. Maass et al. (27) and Sakai and Saez (48) reported that most breast tumor ER values are indeed underestimated for this reason, but they pointed out that the error is probably insufficient to explain the higher values for free cytoplasmic ER in postmenopausal patients and that false negative tumors due to masking of receptor sites are infrequent. This is supported by our data, in which blood estrogen levels as well as breast tumor ER were examined in Japanese patients (38). The peripheral blood was obtained immediately before the operation. In those patients with serum estrogen levels below 50 pg/ml in whom very high values for tumor ER were mostly found, 52% of tumors (23/44) contained ER, whereas in patients with serum levels above 50 pg/ml, 54% of tumors (13/24) contained ER. It is concluded, therefore, that endogenous estrogen levels contribute to the variation of values but rarely affect the classification of a tumor as ER+ or ER−.

When tumors from Japanese patients and American patients examined by McGuire (38) are compared, it is seen that tumors from American patients more frequently contain ER than tumors from Japanese patients, although the difference is mainly confined to the postmenopausal patients (Table 1). It seems unlikely that the discrepancy is the result of differences in assay procedures,

[1] W. L. McGuire, K. Matsumoto, H. Sugano, Y. Nomura, S. Kobayashi, O. Takatani, J. Kato, and H. Takikawa.

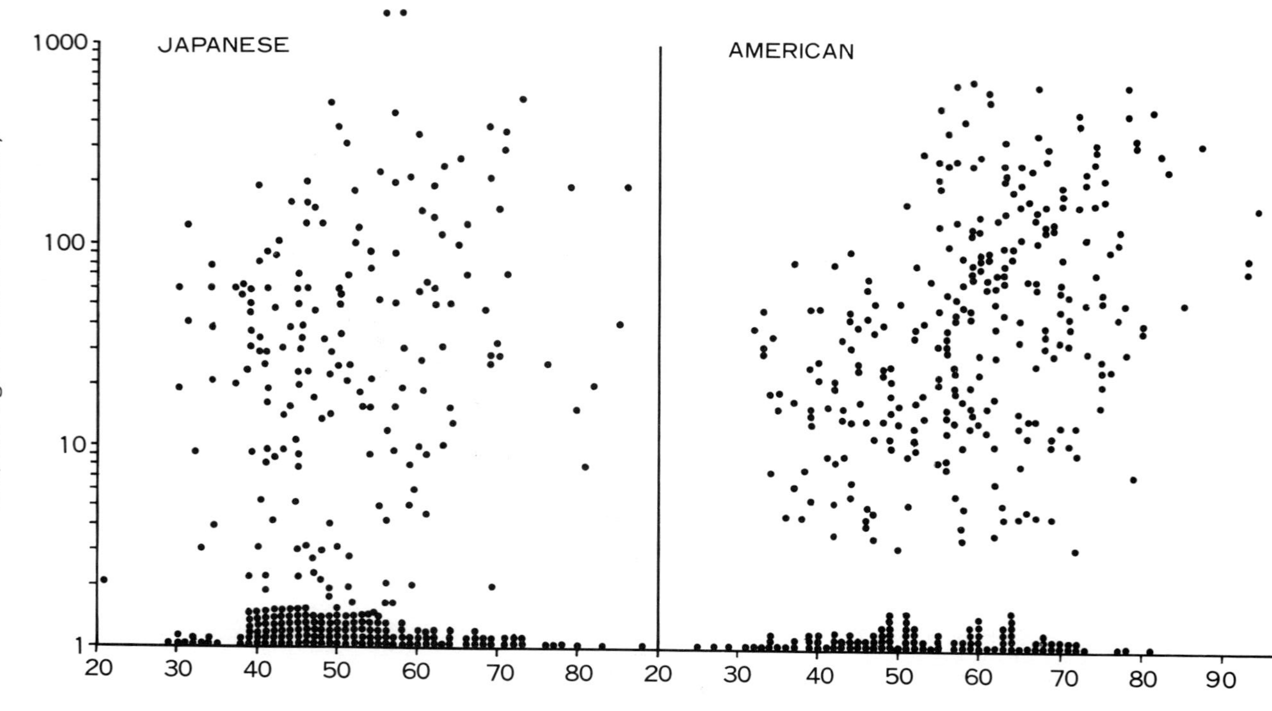

FIG. 1. ER values in primary tumor specimens listed according to patient age. Values for ER in American tumors were obtained from Nomura et al. (38).

TABLE 1. *ER in human breast cancers*

	Japanese		American[a]	
	ER+ (%)	ER− (%)	ER+ (%)	ER− (%)
Premenopausal	53	47 (194)[b]	59	41 (184)[b]
Postmenopausal	57	43 (206)	79	21 (296)
Total	55	45 (400)	71	29 (480)
Primary	56	44 (350)	73	27 (394)
Metastatic	46	54 (52)	63	37 (86)
Total	55	45 (402)	71	29 (480)

[a] Data from Nomura et al. (38). ER+ = estrogen-receptor-positive; ER− = estrogen-receptor-negative

[b] Numbers in parentheses indicate numbers of patients.

since this would have resulted in an increased frequency of tumor ER in the premenopausal American patients as well. In other Western series where the overall incidence of ER is close to the Japanese experience, the preponderance of tumor ER in postmenopausal patients still exists (50,52). This result is unexpected, since if ER in tumors is related to endocrine response and hence prolonged survival, one would have expected the frequency of ER in tumors to be higher in Japanese patients.

Table 1 also shows that in both countries the overall frequency of ER in metastatic tumors is only slightly lower than ER frequency in primary tumors. According to the collective data from Western countries (28), there was no correlation between the clinical stage, axillary lymph node status, location of the tumor in the breast, or disease-free interval and the presence of ER.

Multiple-Tumor ER Assays

We studied 32 Japanese patients in whom multiple-tumor ER determinations were made in primary and metastatic tumors. The results are shown in Fig. 2. It is apparent that an ER+ primary tumor usually gives rise to an ER+ metastasis, whereas an ER− primary tumor usually gives rise to an ER− metastasis. In only 2 of 32 patients were negative ER values found in primary tumors, but positive ER values were found in their metastatic tumors. This supports previous recommendations by Western investigators that ER values in primary tumors can be used to guide therapy choices when a patient subsequently develops metastatic disease (22,24,28,32).

Histopathology and ER in Breast Cancer

The relationship between ER of breast cancer and histopathological findings was examined in 110 Japanese patients; the results are summarized in Table 2. Early studies from Western countries showed no consistent relations between

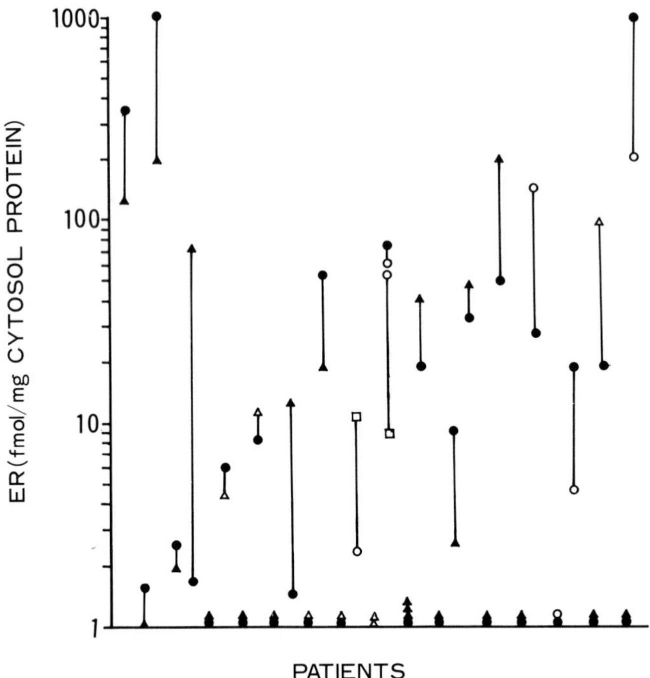

FIG. 2. Comparison of breast tumor ER values from different biopsies from the same Japanese patients. Multiple values from individual patients are presented in a single vertical column (vertical lines are to align columns): primary breast tumor *(filled circles);* metastatic lesion to breast *(open circles);* skin recurrence *(squares);* metastatic lymph node *(filled triangles);* metastatic liver *(open triangles).*

tumor ER and histological types or epithelial cell density of a cancer (24,28). These findings are supported by the present data from Japan. More recently, however, a strong association between ER and invasive lobular carcinoma has been described (45). This is also supported by the present data, but the data could be obtained from only 3 patients (Table 2). If this observation is confirmed in a larger number of patients, it could reflect a selective sensitivity of the distal segment of the duct to estrogens. The same authors (45) also reported a lower frequency of ER present in tumors with prominent local lymphocyte reactions. Furthermore, they suggested that morphologically undifferentiated tumors less often contained ER. However, these observations are not supported by the present data (Table 2). In summary, there is but little correlation between tumor ER and histopathological findings.

Tumor ER and Tumor Response to Endocrine Therapy

The usefulness of tumor ER data in predicting the response to endocrine therapy is compared in Japanese and American women (Table 3). In both coun-

TABLE 2. *ER and histopathology of breast cancers in Japanese patients*

	Number of cancers	ER+ (%)	ER− (%)
Histological type			
Papillotubular	12	50	50
Medullary tubular	29	55	45
Scirrhous	61	57	43
Mucous	2	100	0
Lobular	3	100	0
Squamous	1	0	100
Epithelial cellularity			
Few	46	58	42
Moderate	32	50	50
Abundant	34	70	30
Lymphocyte reaction			
None	79	55	45
Slight	19	58	42
Prominent	14	75	25
Histological grading (differentiation)			
Good	10	40	60
Moderate	57	55	45
Poor	35	65	35

tries the overall response rates of 62 and 60% for ER+ tumors and 4 and 0% for ER− tumors are remarkably similar. These data also compare favorably with the clinical correlation obtained from the collective data by Western investigators (28), as shown in Table 3. These results also seem to suggest that clinical correlations of tumor ER with tumor response are similar in any endocrine therapy, whether ablative or additive.

TABLE 3. *Objective breast cancer regressions according to ER assay and type of therapy*

	Number of regressions/number assayed					
	Japanese		American[a]		Western[b]	
	ER+	ER−	ER+	ER−	ER+	ER−
Ovariectomy	1/3	1/8	5/10	0/10	25/33	4/53
Adrenalectomy	—	0/3	—	0/1	32/66	4/33
Adrenalectomy and ovariectomy	11/16	0/11	—	—	—	—
Hypophysectomy	—	0/1	7/10	0/4	2/8	0/8
Androgen	1/3	—	3/5	0/4	12/26	2/24
Estrogen	2/2	—	—	0/1	37/57	5/58
Antiestrogen	1/2	0/2	—	—	8/20	5/27
Total	16/26	1/25	15/25	0/20	116/210	20/203
Percentage response	62%	4%	60%	0%	55%	10%

[a] Data from Nomura et al. (38).
[b] Collective data of McGuire et al. (28).

TABLE 4. *ER level and tumor response to endocrine therapy*

ER value (fmoles/ mg cytosol protein)	Number of regressions/number assayed	
	Japanese	American[a]
<2 or 3	1/25 (4)[b]	0/20 (0)[b]
2 or 3–10	6/9 (67)	3/6 (50)
>11	10/17 (59)	12/19 (63)

[a]Data from Nomura et al. (38).
[b]Numbers in parentheses are percentages.

In Table 4, data from all therapies are combined for Japanese and American patients. The response rates of 4 and 0% for ER− tumors, 67 and 50% for tumors with low ER values, and 59 and 63% for tumors with high ER values are similar in both countries. It is not clear why patients with low tumor ER values respond as well as those with higher ER values. On the contrary, a positive relationship between ER concentration and the probability of response to endocrine therapy has been reported by Leclercq and Heuson (24). This point should be clarified in future studies.

ER in Male Breast Cancer

ER has been studied extensively in breast cancers from women, as is shown in this review. However, there is little information available about ER in male breast cancers, mainly because this is a rare neoplasm. In this review, data on ER in male breast cancer gleaned from an extensive review of the literature are summarized in Table 5. ER was shown to be positive in 5 of 5 Japanese and 26 of 31 Western male breast cancers. Thus 31 of 36 (86%) male breast cancers contained ER. In ER+ male breast cancers, ER values ranged from 6 to 500 fmoles/mg cytosol protein (12,18,23–25,33,35,39,44,51,58). No difference

TABLE 5. *ER in male breast cancers*

Number of ER+/total cases assayed		
Japanese[a]	Western[b]	Total
5/5 (100)[c]	26/31 (84)	31/36 (86)

[a]Data from our laboratory (3/3) and from Nomura et al. (39) (2/2).
[b]Data from Hähnel and Twaddle (18) (0/2), Wittliff (58) (1/1), Korsten et al. (23) (1/1), Leung et al. (25) (2/2), Mobbs and Johnson (33) (1/1), Rosen et al. (44) (4/4), Thompson et al. (51) (1/1), Leclercq and Heuson (24) (7/10), Contesso et al. (12) (8/8), and Moseley et al. (35) (1/1).
[c]Numbers in parentheses are percentages.

was detected between the estrogen binding specificities of the cytosols from male and female cancers. This high incidence of ER in male patients is within the upper limit of that reported by Western investigators for postmenopausal patients and is higher than that for Japanese female patients. This high incidence in males is thought to be due, at least in part, to low levels of endogenous estrogens in males. However, this cannot be explained solely by the low level of endogenous estrogens, since even in postmenopausal Japanese patients an incidence of ER+ similar to that in premenopausal Japanese patients has been reported (Table 1). This high incidence may be due to special characteristics of male breast cancer itself. However, this point should be clarified by further collections of data on a large number of male breast cancers in the future.

Since the report of Farrow and Adair (16) published in 1942, not many studies have shown that response rate to endocrine ablative therapy is higher in male patients with breast cancer than in female patients; i.e., response rates of 45 to 85% in males (37) and approximately 30% in females (11,14) have been reported. This response rate in males is similar to that in female breast cancer patients with positive ER. The good response to endocrine ablation in male breast cancer appears to be related to the high incidence of ER in their tumors.

ER and α-Fetoprotein in Breast Cancer Cytosol

α-Fetoprotein is found in markedly elevated concentrations in fetal sera, in maternal sera, and in the sera of adults with hepatomas or certain germinal tumors (1–3). α-Fetoprotein is a glycoprotein with a molecular weight of 60,000 to 70,000 d (6,46). Recent studies (6,54,55) have shown that rat and mouse α-fetoproteins, as well as human α-fetoprotein, possess high estrogen-binding affinity that is similar to that of ER. However, no significant binding is observed to other steroids such as testosterone and progesterone (6). Furthermore, evidence is presented that α-fetoprotein accounts mainly, if not entirely, for the high estrogen-binding properties of uterus cytosols of immature rats, which have high levels of serum α-fetoprotein (7,53). This evidence suggests that if high concentrations of α-fetoprotein exist in the cytosol from human breast cancer, this can account for the high estrogen-binding capacity that has been considered to be due to ER.

We examined concentrations of ER and α-fetoprotein in cytosols of 72 Japanese breast cancers (36). Concentrations of α-fetoprotein were determined by radioimmunoassay (47). The concentrations of α-fetoprotein were found to be very low in all tumor cytosols examined. The values were less than 1.1 ng/mg cytosol protein (Fig. 3) and were of similar order as those in the sera of normal adults. Aussel et al. (6) reported that one molecule of 17β-estradiol is bound per molecule of α-fetoprotein. If α-fetoprotein were the major estrogen-binding protein in breast tumor cytosol having binding sites of more than 200 fmoles/mg cytosol protein, the concentration of α-fetoprotein would be more

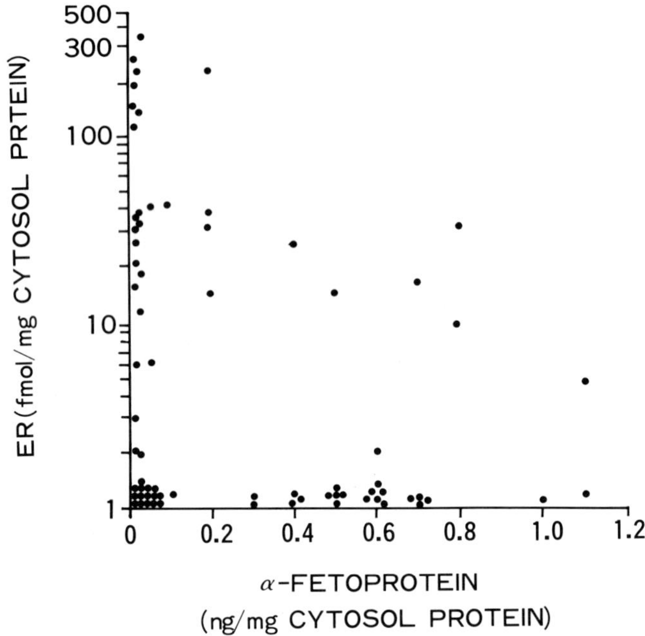

FIG. 3. Values for ER in breast cancer cytosols obtained from 72 Japanese patients listed according to α-fetoprotein values.

than 10 ng/mg cytosol protein. Furthermore, no positive relationship was found between ER and α-fetoprotein concentrations (Fig. 3). These results clearly demonstrate that ER, but not α-fetoprotein, accounts for most of the high estrogen-binding capacity in human breast cancers. However, this general conclusion may not be applicable to the breast tumors from patients having high levels of serum α-fetoprotein who are pregnant or who have complications of hepatoma, hepatitis, or liver cirrhosis. This point should be clarified in future studies.

Conclusion

A comparison of ER and clinical response between Japanese and Western breast cancer patients reveals some remarkable similarities and a few differences. In both groups of patients there is no correlation between tumor histopathology, clinical stage, axillary lymph node status, location of the tumor, or disease-free interval and the presence of ER. The ER values found in primary and metastatic lesions from the same patients are mostly similar in both groups. The overall incidence of ER+ breast cancers is slightly higher in Western patients, and this is due mainly to the higher incidence in postmenopausal Western patients than in postmenopausal Japanese patients. The survival advantage of

Japanese breast cancer patients cannot be explained by tumor ER incidence.

The correlations between tumor ER and response to endocrine therapy are remarkably similar between Japanese and Western breast cancer patients. Response to endocrine therapy is 0 to 10% in the absence of tumor ER but 55 to 60% in the presence of tumor ER. The response rate in male breast cancers, most of which contain ER, is similar to that in female breast cancers with positive ER. Our concern now should be to identify the 40 to 45% of ER+ but endocrine-resistant tumors whose growth cannot be inhibited by either ablative or additive endocrine manipulation; this should enable us to improve our ability to select endocrine therapy for appropriate patients.

PgR IN HUMAN BREAST CANCER

As described previously, about 40% of human breast cancers with positive ER fail to respond to endocrine therapy. Since binding to cytosol ER is only an early step in estrogen action, it is possible that in ER+ but endocrine-resistant tumors the lesion comes at a later step. An ideal marker of an endocrine-responsive tumor would be a measurable product of hormone action, rather than the initial step. PgR would be such an ideal marker, because in estrogen target tissues the synthesis of PgR depends on the action of estrogen (17). If so, PgR would be absent in tumors with negative ER. The presence of PgR in ER+ tumors would indicate that these tumors are capable of synthesizing at least one end product under estrogen action and that the tumors would be responsive to endocrine therapy. On the other hand, the prospect of a successful response to endocrine therapy would be very low in tumors with positive ER but no PgR. According to these theoretical bases, PgR as well as ER has been measured in breast cancer cytosols by McGuire et al. (20,29–31), other Western investigators (41–43), and Japanese investigators. Data for Japanese patients are derived from the authors (40) and from Drs. Y. Nomura, S. Kobayashi, O. Takatani, H. Okada, and H. Imura.

Experimental Procedure

For a long time a major problem in the detection of PgR in the human was the interference of progesterone binding to corticosteroid binding globulin. A simple and effective way of overriding the interference binding is to use a synthetic ^{3}H-R5020 (17,21-dimethyl-19-nor-4,9-pregnadiene-3,20-dione) not bound by corticosteroid binding globulin, which has been shown to be useful for the estimation of PgR in human breast cancers (20,29–31,42,43). Binding specificity of R5020 has been reported to be mainly restricted to PgR; it competes slightly (13%) for binding to the dexamethasone-labeled glucocorticoid receptor, but not for binding to estrogen, androgen, or mineralocorticoid receptors (5,19,42).

PgR in Japanese breast cancer was measured by the sucrose density gradient method or the dextran-coated charcoal method analyzed according to Scatchard (49), as was previously described in detail (5,19,40). The assays were carried out utilizing ^{3}H-R5020 (51 Ci/mmole) and a homogenizing medium that consisted of 25 mM Tris-HCl at pH 7.4, 1.5 mM ethylenediaminetetraacetic acid (EDTA), 10 mM thioglycerol, and 10% glycerol. The method used for the Japanese patients was practically identical to the method used for Western patients by McGuire and Raynaud. A tumor was considered PgR+ in a Japanese patient if it contained more than 5 fmoles of PgR per milligram of cytosol protein.

PgR and ER Levels in Breast Cancer

The rate of positive tumors, number of binding sites, and dissociation constant for PgR in 259 Japanese patients with breast cancers are shown in Table 6. Approximately 40% of the cancers revealed measurable amounts of PgR. This rate is within the lower range of figures reported by Western investigators, which were in the 40 to 60% range (20,29–31,41–43). This seems to be related to the finding that the rate of ER+ cancers is slightly lower in our studies than in most of the studies by Western investigators. The values for PgR ranged from 0 to 600 fmoles/mg of cytosol protein (Table 6). Scatchard plots of the binding data found the dissociation constant of R5020-PgR interaction to be 1 to 30×10^{-10} M, indicative of a high affinity of binding (Table 6).

Table 7 shows the relation between ER and PgR in breast cancers. In Japanese breast cancers, PgR were found in 57% of cancers with positive ER, but in only 11% of cancers with negative ER. These findings are fundamentally consistent with those reported by Western researchers (Table 7). As shown in Table 7, 60 to 70% of ER+ tumors in both countries had PgR. This percentage approximates the response rate to endocrine therapy based on ER+ so that this result seems to be consistent with the hypothesis that PgR is a marker of endocrine-responsive tumors. However, confirmation of this hypothesis requires

TABLE 6. *PgR and AR in Japanese breast cancers*

	PgR	AR
Positive tumors		
Rate	98/259	20/65
Percentage	38%	31%
Concentration in cytosol (fmoles/mg cytosol protein)		
Number of tumors	98	20
Mean	70	23
Range	5–581	5–137
Dissociation constant ($\times 10^{-10}$ M)		
Mean	3.7	4.0
Range	1.0–30.0	0.9–14.5

TABLE 7. *Comparison of ER and PgR in breast cancer cytosol*

	Progesterone-receptor-positive		
	Japanese	McGuire (29)	Pichon (41)
	Rate (%)	Rate (%)	Rate (%)
ER+	86/150 (57)	289/392 (73)	34/44 (77)
ER−	12/109 (11)	12/138 (9)	1/11 (9)

direct correlation of the presence of PgR with objectively defined clinical remission.

Contesso et al. (12) reported that PgR was shown to be positive in 7 of 8 male breast cancers. In our laboratory, 2 of 3 male breast cancers contained PgR. Thus 9 of 11 (82%) male breast cancers contained PgR. This point should be examined by future studies.

Tumor PgR and ER and Tumor Response to Endocrine Therapy

McGuire and Horwitz (29,30) reported preliminary data on 27 patients with breast cancers. They found that in cases where ER was positive and PgR was negative, successful response rate to endocrine therapy was very low, analogous to the response rate seen with ER− tumors. In contrast, when both receptors were present, remissions were seen in a larger percentage of patients than would be predicted on the basis of ER alone. In Japanese patients, the response rates to endocrine therapy were as follows: 3 of 5 for ER+, PgR+ tumors; 1 of 6 for ER+, PgR− tumors; 0 of 1 for ER−, PgR+ tumor; and 0 of 8 for ER−, PgR− tumors. In cases having ER+ and PgR−, our preliminary data on 20 patients support the findings obtained by McGuire and Horwitz (29,30). These data suggest that ER and PgR assays in breast cancer are better than ER alone in predicting response to endocrine therapy. However, it should be emphasized that these data are preliminary and need to be clarified by future studies.

AR IN HUMAN BREAST CANCER

There may be another reason why 40% of the breast cancer patients with positive tumor ER do not respond to endocrine therapy. The role of other hormone receptors must be considered, since ER is a part of the complex hormonal control system that influences mammary cell growth. Simultaneous analysis of these receptor proteins in addition to ER may be helpful in eliminating those patients who have positive tumor ER but who do not respond to endocrine therapy. AR as well as ER have been measured in breast cancer cytosols by Maass et al. (26,27,52), by other Western investigators (56,57), and by the authors (40).

Experimental Procedure

Since 5α-dihydrotestosterone binds to human sex steroid plasma binding protein and to its own receptor, the Western investigators used ^{3}H-5α-dihydrotestosterone and agar gel electrophoresis, which clearly differentiates between these two binding proteins (26,56,57). Since a method that involves measurement of binding sites by a dextran-coated charcoal assay meets practical requirements more satisfactorily than does agar gel electrophoresis, we used a dextran-coated charcoal assay with a synthetic androgen, ^{3}H-R1881 (17β-hydroxy-17α-methyl-estra-4,9,11-trien-3-one), 58 Ci/mmole of which does not bind to human sex steroid plasma binding protein and is not metabolized during incubation (4,9,10). According to these investigators, R1881 binding with AR is androgen-specific, but R1881 binds to PgR (4,10). However, we were able to measure AR using ^{3}H-R1881 in breast cancers with positive PgR according to the following: ^{3}H-R1881 binding with AR (e.g., obtained from rat ventral prostate) was easily displaced by unlabeled R1881, whereas unlabeled R5020 had a lower activity. ^{3}H-R1881 binding with PgR was easily displaced with unlabeled R5020. The method for assay of AR in breast cancers with negative PgR is practically the same as the method reported previously (9). Tissues were homogenized in 8 ml of buffer per gram of tissue. The buffer was 0.01 M Tris-HCl at pH 7.4, 1.5 mM EDTA, and 0.5 mM dithiothreitol. The homogenate was centrifuged at 105,000 × *g* for 60 min; 200 μl of cytosol were incubated with increasing quantities of ^{3}H-R1881 (0.05–1.5 pmoles) dissolved in 0.2 ml of the Tris buffer for 16 hr at 0 to 4° C. When the tumors contained PgR, 20 pmoles of unlabeled R5020 were included in these incubation mixtures in order to obtain the total androgen binding. Control cytosols were preincubated with 20 pmoles of nonradioactive R1881 20 min prior to adding the increasing quantities of ^{3}H-R1881 in order to obtain the nonspecific binding. The treatment with the dextran-coated charcoal was the same as used in ER and PgR assays. The results were analyzed according to Scatchard (49). A tumor was considered AR+ if it contained more than 5 fmoles of AR per milligram of cytosol protein.

AR and ER Levels in Breast Cancer

The rate of positive tumors, number of binding sites, and dissociation constant for AR in 65 Japanese breast cancer patients are shown in Table 6. Measurable amounts of AR were found in 31% of the patients. Wirtz et al. (57) and Trams and Maass (52) found AR in about 20% of breast cancers, whereas Wagner et al. (56) found AR in 55% of breast cancers. Although these investigators used ^{3}H-5α-dihydrotestosterone for detection of AR, misinterpretation of AR-positive samples caused by contamination with human sex steroid plasma binding protein can be discounted because all these researchers used agar gel electrophoresis. The rate of AR-positive cases obtained by us was at the middle of these values (Table 6). The values for AR ranged from 0 to 150 fmoles/mg of cytosol

TABLE 8. *Comparison of ER and AR in breast cancer cytosol*

	Androgen-receptor-positive		
	Japanese (40)	Trams (52)	Wagner (56)
	Rate (%)	Rate (%)	Rate (%)
ER+	13/34 (38)	34/111 (31)	9/16 (56)
ER−	7/31 (23)	9/113 (8)	4/8 (50)

protein (Table 6). Scatchard plots of the binding data found the dissociation constant of R1881-AR interaction to be 1 to 15×10^{-10} M, indicative of a high affinity of binding (Table 6).

Table 8 shows the relationship between ER and AR in breast cancers. In Japanese patients, AR were found in 38% of cancers with ER+, but in 23% of cancers with ER−. The results are not very encouraging, since as high as 23% of breast cancers with negative ER contained AR. Although Trams and Maass (52) found AR in only 8% of cancers with ER−, Wagner et al. (56) found AR in 50% of cancers with ER− (Table 8).

Tumor AR and ER and Tumor Response to Endocrine Therapy

The present available data on correlation between breast cancer AR and response to endocrine therapy reported by Engelsman and associates and Maass et al. (26,52) are not encouraging. In breast cancers examined by these investigators, 9 of 16 and 8 of 13 patients possessing ER but lacking AR responded to endocrine therapy. Therefore, it is not justified to omit endocrine treatment in ER+ and AR− patients. The situation is obviously not the same with breast cancer patients having ER but lacking PgR. Furthermore, the response rates to endocrine therapy based on AR+ and ER+ were found to be 75% (9/12) and 66% (4/6), which are only slightly higher than that based on ER+ alone. These data suggest that AR assay in breast cancer is not very useful in predicting response to endocrine therapy.

ACKNOWLEDGMENTS

These studies on Japanese patients were supported in part by grants 001040 and 101044 from the Ministry of Education. We are indebted to W. L. McGuire, Y. Nomura, S. Kobayashi, O. Takatani, H. Ochi, G. Sakamoto, J. Kato, H. Takikawa, H. Okada, and H. Imura for cooperating in these studies. We thank J. P. Raynaud of Roussel UCLAF for generously providing the R5020 and R1881.

REFERENCES

1. Abelev, G. I. (1968): Production of embryonal serum α-globulin by hepatomas. *Cancer Res.,* 28:1344–1350.
2. Abelev, G. I. (1971): α-Fetoprotein in oncogenesis and its association with malignant tumors. *Adv. Cancer Res.,* 14:295–358.
3. Abelev, G. I. (1974): α-Fetoprotein as a marker of embryo-specific differentiation in normal and tumor tissue. *Transplant. Rev.,* 20:3–37.
4. Asselin, J., Labrie, F., Gourdeau, Y., Bonne, C., and Raynaud, J. P. (1976): Binding of [^{3}H]methyltrienolone (R1881) in rat prostate and human benign prostatic hypertrophy. *Steroids,* 28:449–459.
5. Asselin, J., Labrie, F., Kelly, P. A., Philibert, D., and Raynaud, J. P. (1976): Specific progesterone receptors in dimethylbenzanthracene (DMBA)-induced mammary tumors. *Steroids,* 27:395–404.
6. Aussel, C., Uriel, J., and Mercier-Bodard, C. (1973): Rat α-fetoprotein: Isolation, characterization and estrogen-binding properties. *Biochimie,* 55:1431–1437.
7. Aussel, C., Uriel, J., Michel, G., and Baulieu, E. E. (1974): Immunological demonstration of α-fetoprotein in uterine cytosol from immature rats. *Biochimie,* 56:567–570.
8. Baulieu, E. E., and Raynaud, J. P. (1970): A 'proportion graph' method for measuring binding systems. *Eur. J. Biochem.,* 13:293–304.
9. Bonne, C., and Raynaud, J. P. (1975): Methyltrienolone, a specific ligand for cellular androgen receptors. *Steroids,* 26:227–232.
10. Bonne, C., and Raynaud, J. P. (1976): Assay of androgen binding sites by exchange with methyltrienolone (R1881). *Steroids,* 27:497–507.
11. Breast Cancer Group in Japan (1973): The effect of endocrine treatment on advanced breast cancer in Japan. *Jpn. J. Clin. Oncol.,* 3:13–18.
12. Contesso, G., Delarue, J. C., Guerinot, F., May-Levin, F., and Bohuon, C. (1977): Oestrogen and progesterone receptors in mammary pathology in man. *Nouv. Presse Med.,* 6:1951–1954.
13. Cooperative Breast Cancer Group (1961): A cooperative study to evaluate experimental steroids in the therapy of advanced breast cancer. *Cancer Chemother. Rep.,* 11:130–136.
14. Dao, T. L. (1972): Ablation therapy for hormone dependent tumors. *Annu. Rev. Med.,* 23:1–18.
15. Doll, R., Muir, C., and Waterhouse, J. (1970): Cancer incidence in five continents. *Acta Unio Internationalis contra Cancrum,* 2:341–357.
16. Farrow, J. H., and Adair, F. E. (1942): Effect of orchidectomy on skeletal metastases from cancer of the male breast. *Science,* 95:654.
17. Freifeld, M. L., Feil, P. D., and Bardin, C. W. (1974): The in vitro regulation of the progesterone receptor in guinea pig uterus. *Steroids,* 23:93–103.
18. Hähnel, R., and Twaddle, E. (1973): Estimation of the association constant of the estrogen-receptor complex in human breast cancer. *Cancer Res.,* 33:559–566.
19. Horwitz, K. B., and McGuire, W. L. (1975): Specific progesterone receptors in human breast cancer. *Steroids,* 25:497–505.
20. Horwitz, K. B., McGuire, W. L., Pearson, O. H., and Segaloff, A. (1975): Predicting response to endocrine therapy in human breast cancer: A hypothesis. *Science,* 189:726–727.
21. Jensen, E. V., DeSombre, E. R., and Jungblut, P. W. (1967): Estrogen receptors in hormone responsive tissues and tumors. In: *Endogenous Factors Influencing Host-Tumor Balance,* edited by R. W. Wessler, T. L. Dao, and S. Wood, Jr., pp. 15–30. University of Chicago Press, Chicago.
22. Jensen, E. V., Polly, T. Z., Smith, S., Block, G. E., Ferguson, D. J., and DeSombre, E. R. (1975): Prediction of hormone dependency in human breast cancer. In: *Estrogen Receptors in Human Breast Cancer,* edited by W. L. McGuire, P. P. Carbone, and E. P. Vollmer, pp. 37–54. Raven Press, New York.
23. Korsten, C. B., Engelsman, E., and Persijin, J. P. (1975): Clinical value of estrogen receptors in advanced breast cancer. In: *Estrogen Receptors in Human Breast Cancer,* edited by W. L. McGuire, P. P. Carbone, and E. P. Vollmer, pp. 93–105. Raven Press, New York.
24. Leclercq, G., and Heuson, J. C. (1976): Estrogen receptors in the spectrum of breast cancer. *Curr. Probl. Cancer,* 1:1–34.
25. Leung, B. S., Moseley, H. S., Davenport, C. E., Krippaehne, W. W., and Fletcher, W. S. (1975): Estrogen receptor in prediction of clinical responses to endocrine ablation. In: *Estrogen*

Receptors in Human Breast Cancer, edited by W. L. McGuire, P. P. Carbone, and E. P. Vollmer, pp. 107–129. Raven Press, New York.

26. Maass, H. (1977): Use of receptors as predictive tools. In: *Endocrinology, Vol. 2,* edited by V. H. T. James, pp. 410–413. Excerpta Medica, Amsterdam.
27. Maass, H., Engel, B., Trams, G., Nowakowski, H., and Stolzenback, G. (1975): Steroid hormone receptors in human breast cancer and the clinical significance. *J. Steroid. Biochem.,* 6:743–749.
28. McGuire, W. L., Carbone, P. P., and Vollmer, E. P. (editors) (1975): *Estrogen Receptors in Human Breast Cancer.* Raven Press, New York.
29. McGuire, W. L., and Horwitz, K. B. (1977): Steroid hormone receptors in breast cancer. In: *Endocrinology, Vol. 2,* edited by V. H. T. James, pp. 405–409. Excerpta Medica, Amsterdam.
30. McGuire, W. L., and Horwitz, K. B. (1977): A role for progesterone in breast cancer. *Ann. N.Y. Acad. Sci.,* 286:90–99.
31. McGuire, W. L., Horwitz, K. B., Chamness, G. C., and Zava, D. T. (1976): A physiological role for estrogen and progesterone in breast cancer. *J. Steroid. Biochem.,* 7:875–882.
32. McGuire, W. L., Pearson, O. H., and Segaloff, A. (1975): Predicting hormone responsiveness in human breast cancer. In: *Estrogen Receptors in Human Breast Cancer,* edited by W. L. McGuire, P. P. Carbone, and E. P. Vollmer, pp. 17–30. Raven Press, New York.
33. Mobbs, B. G., and Johnson, I. E. (1976): In vitro estrogen-binding by human breast carcinomas. *Can. Med. Assoc. J.,* 114:216–219.
34. Morrison, A. S., Black, M. M., Lowe, C. R., MacMahon, B., and Yuasa, S. (1973): Some international differences in histology and survival in breast cancer. *Int. J. Cancer,* 11:261–267.
35. Moseley, H. S., Fletcher, W. S., Leung, B. S., and Kippaehne, W. W. (1974): Predictive criteria for the selection of breast cancer patients for adrenalectomy. *Am. J. Surg.,* 128:143–151.
36. Nakao, K., Ochi, H., Kawashima, M., Tomino, S., Sugano, H., and Matsumoto, K. (1978): Estrogen receptor and α-fetoprotein in human breast cancer. *J. Natl. Cancer Inst.,* 60:289–290.
37. Neifeld, J. P., Meyskens, F., Tormey, D. C., and Javadpour, N. (1976): The role of orchiectomy in the management of advanced male breast cancer. *Cancer,* 37:992–995.
38. Nomura, Y., Kobayashi, S., Takatani, O., Sugano, H., Matsumoto, K., and McGuire, W. L. (1977): Estrogen receptor and endocrine responsiveness in Japanese versus American breast cancer patients. *Cancer Res.,* 37:106–110.
39. Nomura, Y., Kondo, H., Yamagata, J., and Takenaka, K. (1977): Detection of the estrogen receptor and response to endocrine therapy in male breast cancer patients. *Gann,* 68:333–336.
40. Ochi, H., Hayashi, T., Nakao, K., Yayoi, E., Kawahara, T., and Matsumoto, K. (1978): Estrogen, progesterone and androgen receptors in breast cancer in Japanese. *J. Natl. Cancer Inst.,* 60:291–293.
41. Pichon, M. F., and Milgrom, E. (1977): Characterization and assay of progesterone receptor in human mammary carcinoma. *Cancer Res.,* 37:464–471.
42. Raynaud, J. P. (1977): Receptors in breast cancer: An introduction. *Ann. N.Y. Acad. Sci.,* 286:87–89.
43. Raynaud, J. P., Bouton, M. M., Philibert, D., Delarue, J. C., Guerinot, F., and Bohuon, C. (1975): Progesterone and estradiol binding sites in human breast cancer. *J. Steroid Biochem.,* 6:xiv (abstracts).
44. Rosen, P. P., Menendez-Botet, C. J., Nisselbaum, J. S., Schwartz, M. K., and Urban, J. A. (1976): Estrogen receptor protein in lesions of the male breast. *Cancer,* 37:1866–1868.
45. Rosen, P. P., Menendez-Botet, C. J., Nisselbaum, J. S., Urban, J. A., Mike, V., Fracchia, A., and Schwartz, M. K. (1975): Pathological review of breast lesions analyzed for estrogen receptor protein. *Cancer Res.,* 35:3187–3194.
46. Ruoslahti, E., Pihko, H., and Seppälä, M. (1974): α-Fetoprotein. *Transplant. Rev.,* 20:38–60.
47. Ruoslahti, E., and Seppälä, M. (1971): Studies of carcino-fetal proteins. III. Development of a radioimmunoassay for α-fetoprotein. *Int. J. Cancer,* 8:374–383.
48. Sakai, F., and Saez, S. (1976): Existence of receptors bound to endogenous estradiol in breast cancer of premenopausal and postmenopausal women. *Steroids,* 27:99–110.
49. Scatchard, G. (1949): The attraction of proteins for small molecules and ions. *Ann. N.Y. Acad. Sci.,* 51:660–672.
50. Singhakowinta, A., Potter, H. G., Buroker, T. R., Samal, B., Brooks, S. C., and Vaitkevicius, V. K. (1976): Estrogen receptor and natural cause of breast cancer. *Ann. Surg.,* 183:34–38.

51. Thompson, E. B., Perlin, E., and Tormey, D. (1976): Steroid-binding proteins in carcinoma of the human male breast. *Am. J. Clin. Pathol.,* 65:360–363.
52. Trams, G., and Maass, H. (1977): Specific binding of estradiol and dihydrotestosterone in human mammary cancers. *Cancer Res.,* 37:258–261.
53. Uriel, J., Bouillon, D., Aussel, C., and Dupiers, M. (1976): α-Fetoprotein: The major high-affinity estrogen binder in rat uterine cytosols. *Proc. Natl. Acad. Sci. U.S.A.,* 73:1452–1456.
54. Uriel, J., Bouillon, D., and Dupiers, M. (1975): Affinity chromatography of human, rat and mouse α-fetoprotein on estradiol-sepharose adsorbents. *F.E.B.S. Lett.,* 53:305–308.
55. Uriel, J., de Nechaud, B., and Dupiers, M. (1972): Estrogen-binding properties of rat, mouse and man feto-specific serum proteins. *Biochem. Biophys. Res. Commun.,* 46:1175–1180.
56. Wagner, R. K., Görlich, L., and Jungblut, P. W. (1973): Dihydrotestosterone receptor in human mammary cancer. *Acta Endocrinol.* [*Suppl.*] *(Kbh),* 173:65.
57. Wirtz, A. Wiedemann, M., Raith, L., and Karl, H. J. (1973): Studies on the estradiol and 5α-dihydrotestosterone receptors in mammary and prostate tissues. *Acta Endocrinol.* [*Suppl.*] *(Kbh),* 177:8
58. Wittliff, J. L. (1974): Specific receptors of the steroid hormones in breast cancer. *Semin. Oncol.,* 1:109–118.
59. Wynder, E. L., Kajitani, T., Kuno, J., Lucas, J. C., Depalo, A., and Jarrow, J. (1973): A comparison of survival rates between American and Japanese patients with breast cancer. *Surg. Gynecol. Obstet.,* 117:196–200.

Endocrine Control in Neoplasia, edited by
R. K. Sharma and W. E. Criss.
Raven Press, New York © 1978.

Interaction between Hormones and Human Breast Cancer in Long-Term Tissue Culture

Marie E. Monaco and Marc E. Lippman

Medicine Branch, National Cancer Institute, National Institutes of Health, Bethesda, Maryland 20014

Human breast cancer cells in long-term culture provide a convenient model system for examining the mechanisms of action of a variety of chemotherapeutic agents, including hormones. The advantages of such a system are manifold: (a) The use of cells derived from a human neoplasm eliminates the problem of species differences. The importance of such considerations is apparent if one compares the prolactin dependence of some tumors induced by dimethylbenz*(a)*anthracene (DMBA) (38) with the lack of such dependence in human breast tumors (57). (b) The use of a cell line consisting of a single cell type allows one to distinguish between primary responses and secondary effects mediated by interaction of the agent with another cell type or organ. (c) In many tissue culture systems it is possible to do experiments under defined chemical conditions that preclude modulation of a response by unknown serum factors (18). (d) With the use of suitable selective media and subsequent cloning techniques it is often possible to isolate drug- or hormone-insensitive variant cell lines. Studies on these derivative cell lines can provide significant insights into the mechanisms of hormone and drug action. (e) Isolated cell systems are unusually advantageous for the study of significant hormone metabolism.

Tissue culture systems, like all *in vitro* models, have a major drawback: cells grown *in vitro* may differ significantly from those examined under *in vivo* conditions. There are many explanations for the discrepancies between *in vivo* and *in vitro* responses. For example, in the process of selection of cell lines, responsiveness to various trophic hormones may be lost due to the absence of the hormone itself or some "permissive" factor during the period in which the culture is established. That is, responsive cells that require the hormone for maintenance or growth will be selected against in the absence of the hormone. However, the presence of the hormone in the culture medium does not guarantee a responsive line. Since most cell cultures are inevitably selected in favor of more rapidly dividing cells, many responses may be altered by the frequently inverse relationship between "differentiated" effects and rapid growth. Viral or mycoplasma contamination may also perturb normal responses. Yet another possibility is that unique cell-cell interactions (either between homologous or heterologous cell types or stroma) may be mandatory for full expression of a given response. Finally, most cancer cell lines are heteroploid, and there is considerable variation in chromosomal makeup of cells even shortly after cloning. Thus it is best to think of tissue culture as a method for doing experiments that are difficult or impossible *in vivo.* The results must then be regarded as a structure on which to arrange testable hypotheses to be verified *in vivo.* These limitations should be kept in mind while reviewing the following data on the actions of a variety of hormones on human breast cancer cell lines. Since the interactions of steroids with these cells have recently been extensively reviewed (31,37,48), this chapter will concentrate on the interactions of peptide hormones with human breast cancer cells.

CELL LINES

Many cell lines have been derived from human breast cancers (48); however, few have met the rigid criteria of karyology, protein phenotyping, and differentiated function necessary to confirm their mammary nature. MCF-7 is one of the best characterized of these lines, but recent studies indicate that three other cell lines (ZR-75-1, ZR-75-27, and ZR-75-30) are mammary and are highly differentiated (11). MCF-7 was derived from a pleural effusion from a postmenopausal woman with metastatic breast cancer (58). Morphologically the cell line is indistinguishable from the breast cells of the original tumor, especially when grown in sponge culture (55) or on artificial capillaries (28). Evidence of its epithelial nature includes the presence of domes and desmosomes and the tendency to form acinar-like structures. These cells have a human karyotype. They also have been reported to make small amounts of the milk protein α-lactalbumin, but this function does not appear to be hormone-responsive (53); furthermore, other investigators subsequently failed to measure any α-lactalbumin (27). They do not synthesize any casein measurable by radioimmunoassay (44).

The ZR-75 cell lines were all derived from malignant effusions. They, too, have characteristic secretory epithelial morphology. They have human karyotypes in all cases virtually identical to those of the fresh malignant effusions from which they were derived. Protein phenotyping of these cell lines has revealed them to be unique and different from HeLa contamination. The ZR-75-1 line does not make casein (44).

Finally, all four lines have a number of hormone receptor proteins that are characteristic of the normal mammary gland, further supporting a mammary epithelial nature for these cells. These receptors include those for estrogens, androgens, progestins, glucocorticoids, insulin, and (in the case of MCF-7) thyroid hormone.

INTERACTION OF HORMONES AND HUMAN BREAST CANCER CELLS

Steroid Hormones

The ability of steroid hormones to alter the growth rates of some human breast tumors is well documented (41,59). Administration of estrogens, androgens, progestins, glucocorticoids, or antiestrogens provides effective therapy in at least some patients with breast cancer. Ablation of endocrine function with drugs, surgery, or radiotherapy has also been shown to be effective in modulating the growth of some breast tumors. However, the precise mechanisms involved are largely unknown.

MCF-7 cells have been shown to have receptors for all four of these steroids (4,23,32–34) and to respond to estrogens (23), androgens (32), and glucocorticoids (34). The characteristics of these receptors resemble those found in other tissues with respect to binding affinities and specificities. However, Zava et al. (70) reported that in the case of the estrogen receptor the majority of unbound receptor is found in the nucleus rather than in the cytoplasm. They suggested that this may be consistent with biologic activity of estrogen receptor without the presence of hormone.

Estrogens, androgens, and glucocorticoids are capable of modulating the growth of MCF-7 cells when tested under serum-free conditions. Physiologic concentrations of 17β-estradiol (10^{-9} M) are capable of stimulating thymidine incorporation (Fig. 1) as well as overall cell growth (23) (Fig. 2). 17α-Estradiol is inactive, and the antiestrogen tamoxifen (ICI 46,474) inhibits growth below control levels. Furthermore, the effect of tamoxifen can be reversed by addition of 100-fold less estradiol (27) (Fig. 3). Lines that lack estrogen receptor are unaffected by either estrogen or tamoxifen. In addition, the activity of a specific enzyme, thymidine kinase, which has been shown to be regulated by estrogens in other systems (29,64), is stimulated by the addition of estradiol in the same dose-dependent manner as is thymidine incorporation (35) (Fig. 3). Whether or not this enzyme plays a key role in the mechanism by which estrogen alters growth rates remains to be determined. As can be seen in Fig. 4, induction of both thymidine incorporation and thymidine kinase activity is maximal when only a fraction of the receptors are bound. Several explanations are consistent with these data. One possibility is that the cells contain spare receptors and that only a fraction need to be bound to elicit a maximal effect. A second explanation would involve the presence of residual estradiol in the cells following serum-free washes. Such estradiol present in the cells would be expected to shift the dose-response curve to the left of the binding curve while decreasing the maximal fold of observable response. Third, there may be multiple classes of receptor sites in the cytosol. A small number of sites with much higher binding affinities would be impossible to detect given the limitations of steroid-specific activities currently available.

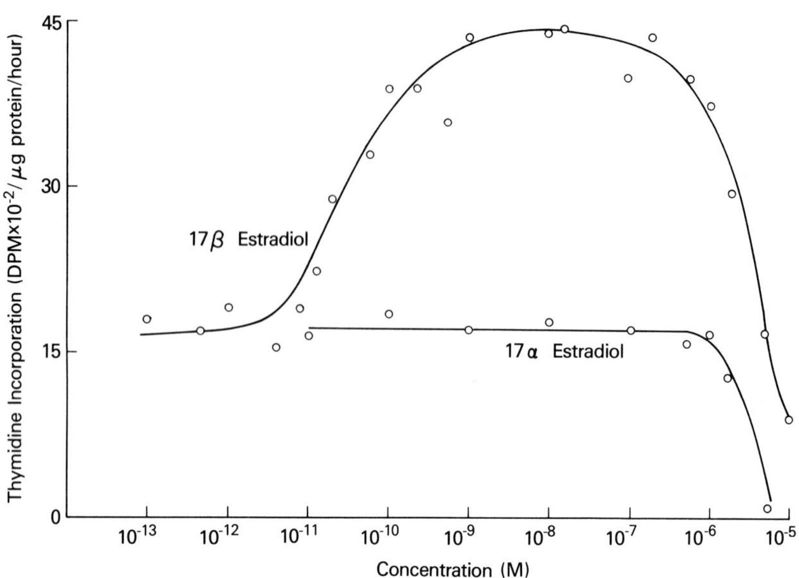

FIG. 1. Effects of 17β-estradiol and 17α-estradiol on thymidine incorporation in MCF-7 human breast cancer cells. Complete methods are described by Lippman et al. (32).

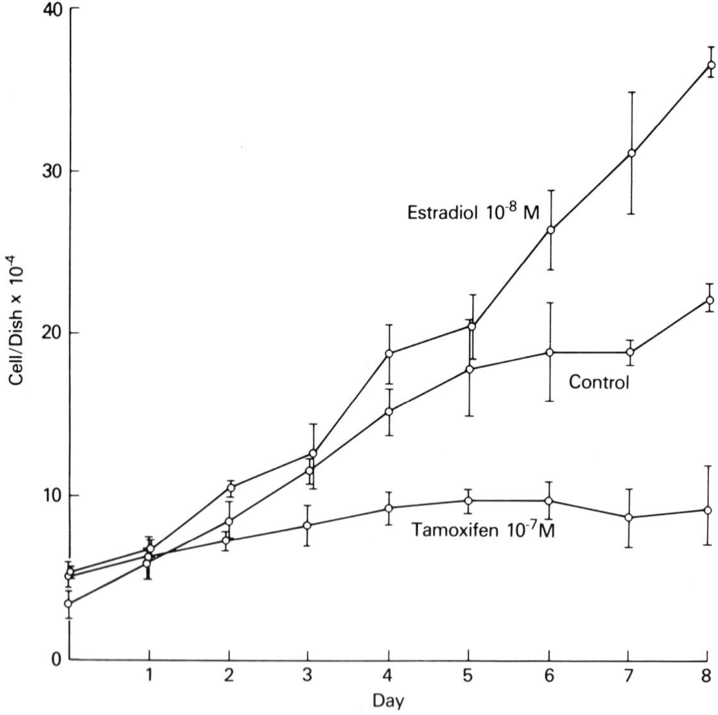

FIG. 2. Effects of estrogen and antiestrogen on cell proliferation in MCF-7 human breast cancer cells: controls, 10^{-8} M estradiol, and 10^{-7} M tamoxifen. Values represent means of triplicate determinations ± 1 SD. Complete methods are described by Lippman et al. (32).

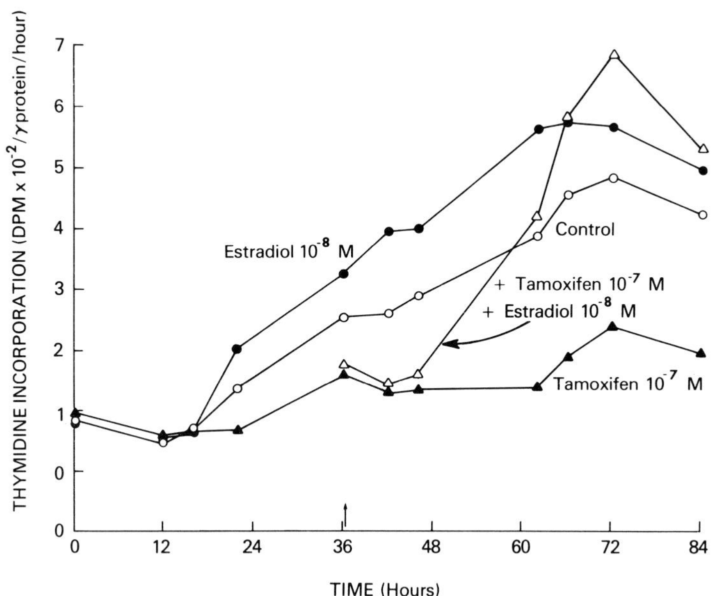

FIG. 3. Estradiol rescue of cells pretreated with tamoxifen: control *(open circles);* 10^{-8} M estradiol *(filled circles);* 10^{-7} M tamoxifen *(filled triangles);* 10^{-7} M tamoxifen added at time zero and 10^{-8} M estradiol added at 36 hr *(open triangles).* Complete methods are described by Lippman et al. (32).

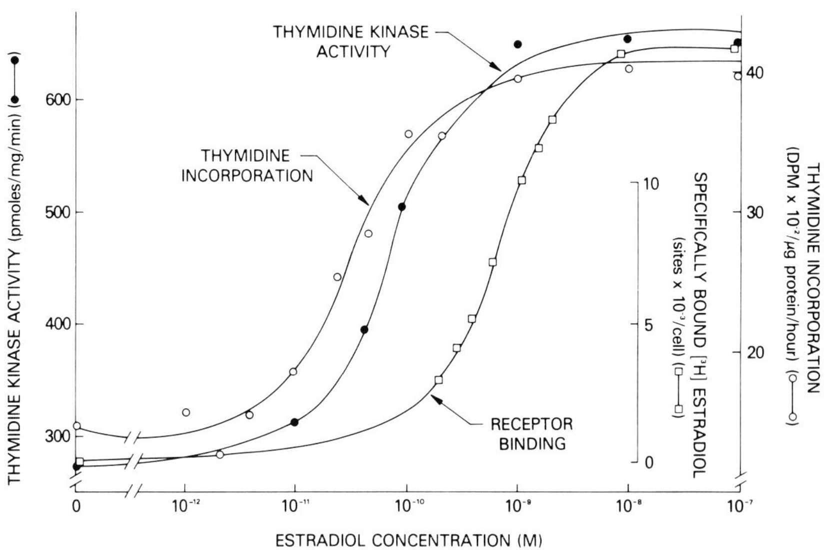

FIG. 4. Effect of 17β-estradiol on thymidine incorporation, thymidine kinase activity, and binding of 17β-estradiol to receptor in MCF-7 cells. Complete methods are described by Lippman et al. (35).

Horwitz and McGuire (24) recently reported that estrogens can modulate levels of progesterone receptor in MCF-7 cells, a situation similar to that seen in other estrogen-responsive tissues (15). However, in this instance the antiestrogen, tamoxifen, has a biphasic effect. At low concentrations (10^{-7} M), it has an estrogenic effect in that it also stimulates progesterone receptor levels. At higher concentrations (10^{-6} M), inhibition of cell growth and progesterone receptor activity is seen.

The data describing the effects of androgens on MCF-7 cell growth are somewhat controversial. Lippman et al. (32) first showed that MCF-7 cells could be stimulated by concentrations of androgen that were approximately 100 times higher than those required for binding to the androgen receptor. They suggested that this discrepancy was due to extensive metabolism of 5α-dihydrotestosterone (5α-DHT) by the cells. Figure 5 illustrates that there is indeed extensive conversion of 5α-DHT to androstanediol. Zava and McGuire (71) offered an alternative

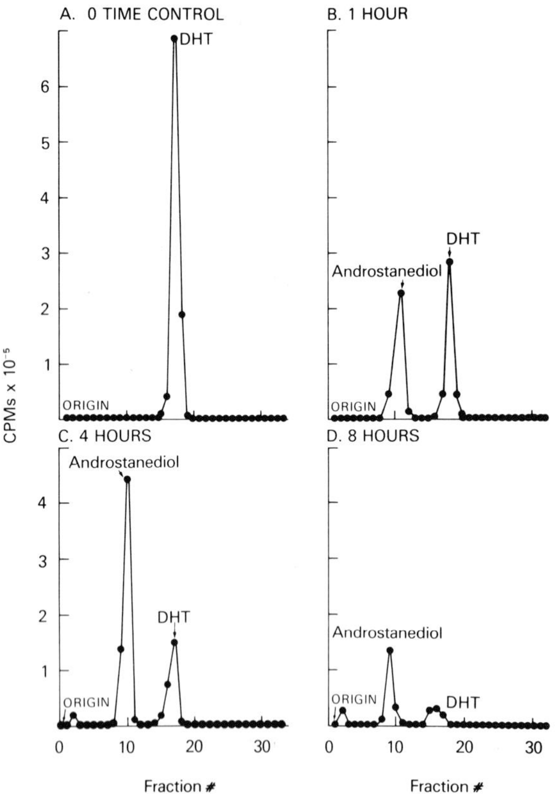

FIG. 5. Metabolism of [^{3}H]5α-DHT to [^{3}H]androstanediol by MCF-7 human breast cancer. **A** to **D:** analysis of incubation medium at 0, 1, 4, and 8 hr, respectively, following [^{3}H]5α-DHT addition. Complete methods are described by Lippman et al. (34).

explanation. They demonstrated that at concentrations required for stimulation, 5α-DHT is capable of both binding to the estrogen receptor and translocating it to the nucleus. Thus these authors maintain that androgen effects on MCF-7 cells are mediated through the estrogen receptor.

Although MCF-7 cells clearly contain a specific high-affinity progesterone receptor, no effect of progesterone on these cells has been demonstrated.

Glucocorticoids are capable of inhibiting growth of MCF-7 cells at physiologic concentrations (34). An approximately 50% inhibition is seen with dexamethasone at maximal concentrations of 10^{-7} M. That this effect is specific (i.e., mediated through the glucocorticoid receptor) is suggested by the fact that cells that lack receptor are not inhibited.

Insulin

The role of insulin, if any, in modulating the growth of human breast cancer is much less clear than the role of steroid hormones, since, at present, "insulin therapy" is not possible. However, several animal studies have suggested that insulin may be an important stimulus of the mammary gland. Normal rodent mammary gland explants require insulin for the manifestation of lactogenic responses, namely, production of casein, α-lactalbumin (61,62), and fat (16). Furthermore, it appears that an insulin-mediated wave of DNA synthesis is required before mammary cells are lactogenically competent (67). *In vivo,* alloxan-induced diabetes (39) or treatment with anti-insulin serum (40) reduces lactational performance in rats.

With respect to mammary cancer, Heuson and Legros have shown that insulin deprivation both inhibits tumor induction by DMBA and causes regression of preexistent tumors (19). Also, administration of insulin resulted in increased tumor growth (20). Harmon and Hilf demonstrated the presence of specific insulin receptors in the R3230AC rat mammary tumor (17).

There are few data on the effects of insulin on human breast cancer. Several attempts have been made to study the effects of insulin on the human mammary gland *in vitro.* Studies with normal human explants have yielded variable results. Several investigators reported an effect of insulin on maintenance, DNA synthesis, induction of hyperplasia, or mitotic activity of explants (2,6,8,10,14,65); others found no effect (13,68). Furthermore, in instances in which effects were seen on maintenance or proliferation, no concomitant effect of insulin on glucose transport was observed (65). This failure of insulin to stimulate glucose transport is in agreement with the data reported by Harmon and Hilf for the R3230AC rat mammary tumor (17). With respect to malignant human tissue, Welsch reported that thymidine incorporation was enhanced by insulin (69), whereas Heuson and Pasteels found no significant effect of insulin on survival of breast cancer explants (21,51). Invariably these explant experiments were carried out with supraphysiologic concentrations of insulin (10^{-6} M), which make interpretation of the results difficult. If no effect is seen, it is always possible that one is on the down slope of a biphasic dose-response curve. On the other hand, if an effect is documented, it is possible that one is observing an effect of insulin acting through receptors for growth peptides (42).

MCF-7 human breast cancer cells in culture provide the first acceptable model system for the study of insulin's interaction with mammary epithelium. Not only do these cells exhibit the advantages of any tissue culture system, as described in the introduction, but they also respond to insulin at physiologic concentrations. Figure 6 illustrates the dose-response curve obtained by Osborne et al. for insulin stimulation of thymidine, uridine, and leucine incorporation in MCF-7 cells (47). Stimulation is apparent with as little as 5×10^{-11} M insulin; it is maximal by 10^{-9} M. These data were later confirmed by Rillema and Linebaugh (52). That increased thymidine incorporation is a reflection of increased growth is documented in Fig. 7, which demonstrates an increase in cell number in the presence of insulin.

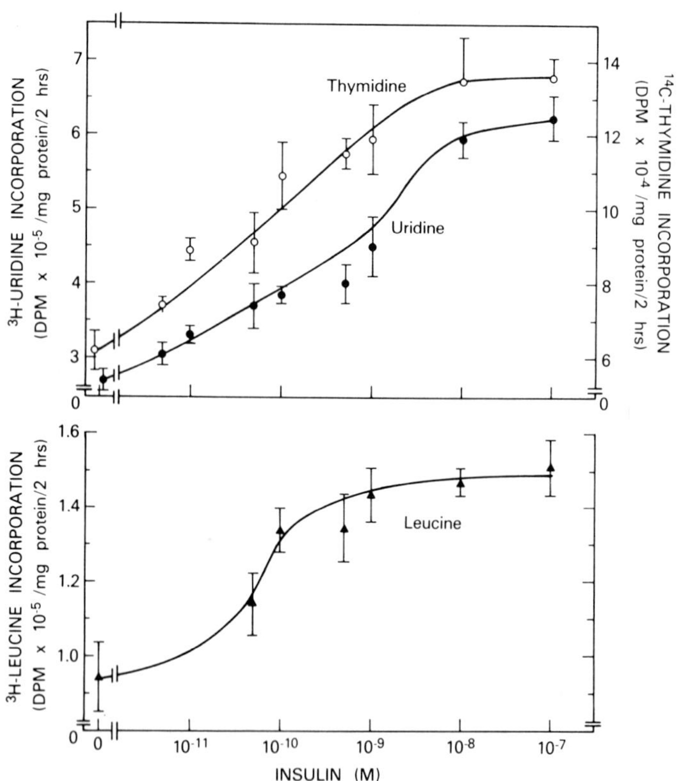

FIG. 6. Top: Effect of insulin on rates of thymidine *(open circles)* and uridine *(filled circles)* incorporation in MCF-7 human breast cancer. **Bottom:** Effect of insulin on rate of leucine incorporation. Values represent means of triplicate determinations ± 1 SD. Complete methods are described by Osborne et al. (47).

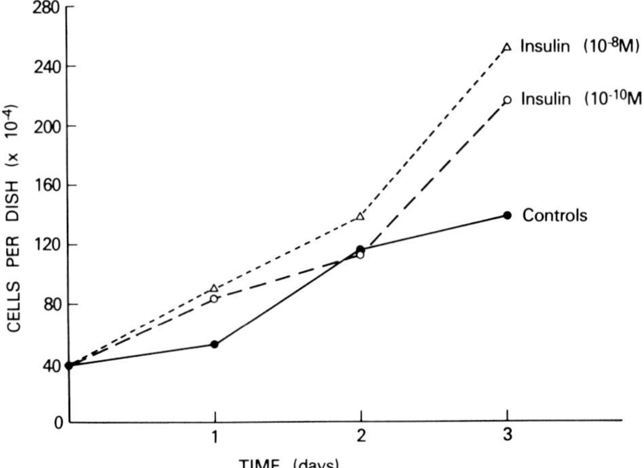

FIG. 7. Effect of insulin on growth. Insulin was added to cells in serum-free medium at time zero. Cells were harvested at times shown and counted on a hemocytometer. Complete methods are described by Osborne et al. (47).

The role of glucose transport in the mechanism of insulin's effect on growth was determined indirectly by performing experiments in glucose-free medium. Figure 8 demonstrates that the effect of insulin on incorporation of labeled thymidine and leucine is apparent even in the absence of extracellular glucose. Furthermore, when glucose transport is measured directly, there is no difference between controls and insulin-treated cells (49).

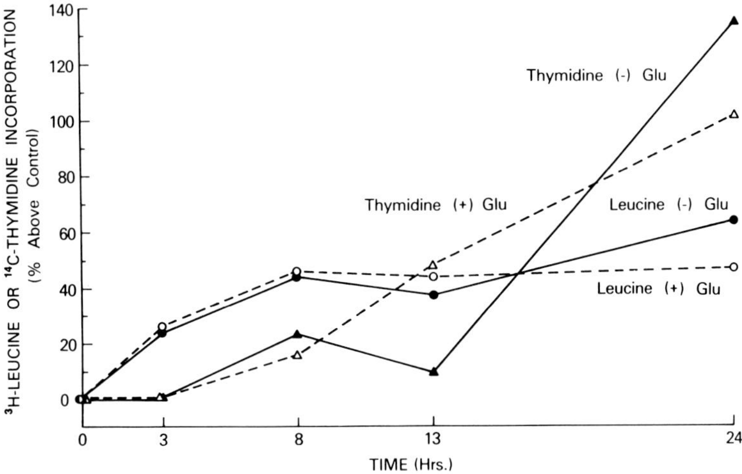

FIG. 8. Effects of insulin on rates of thymidine *(triangles)* and leucine *(circles)* incorporation in the presence *(dash lines)* and absence *(solid lines)* of glucose. Complete methods are described by Osborne et al. (47).

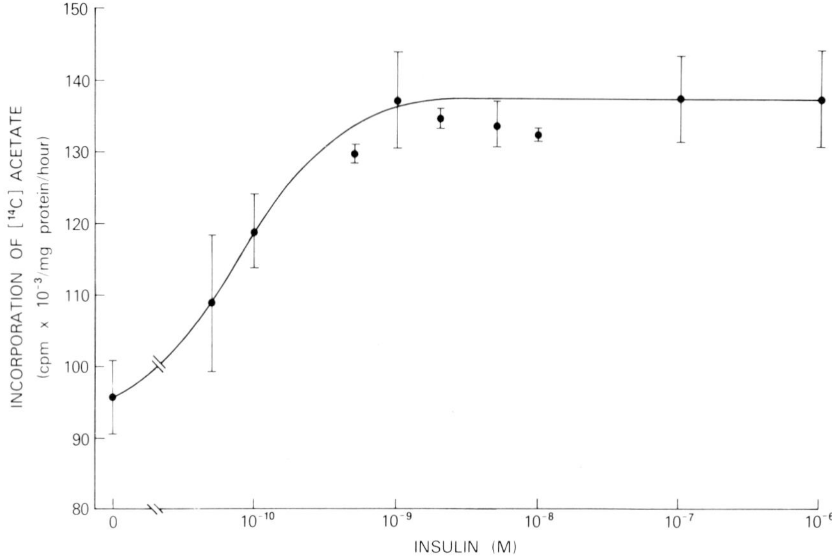

FIG. 9. Dose-response curve for insulin stimulation of acetate incorporation. Values represent means of triplicate determinations ± 1 SD. Complete methods are described by Monaco and Lippman (45).

The response of the normal mammary gland to insulin is lactogenic rather than mitogenic. Insulin is required for maintenance of lactation *in vivo* (40) and for synthesis and secretion of casein, α-lactalbumin, and fatty acids by organ explants *in vitro* (16,61,62). MCF-7 cells do not make casein, and they make little, if any, α-lactalbumin; treatment with insulin will not induce these proteins (27,44,53). However, incorporation of [^{14}C]acetate into fatty acids is stimulated by insulin in a dose-dependent manner identical to that observed for growth (Fig. 9) (45). However, whether or not this stimulation reflects an action of insulin on growth or lactogenesis is unclear, since the data do not conclusively support either interpretation. Table 1 shows the distributions of

TABLE 1. *Classes of labeled lipids synthesized by MCF-7 human breast cancer cells*

	Cells			Medium		
	PL[a]	FA	TG	PL	FA	TG
Control	60[b]	30	2	1	5	2
+ insulin	65	29	2	1	3	<1

[a]PL, polar lipids; FA, free fatty acids; TG, triglycerides. Methods are described by Monaco and Lippman (45).
[b]Percentage of total.

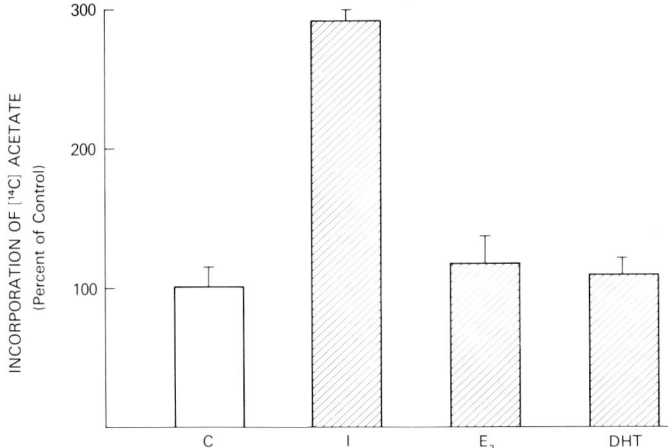

FIG. 10. Effects of mitogenic hormones on acetate incorporation into fatty acids. Abbreviations and hormone concentrations: control (C); insulin (I), 5×10^{-7} M; 17β-estradiol (E_2), 10^{-8} M; 5α-dihydrotestosterone (DHT), 10^{-6} M. Values represent means of triplicate determinations $\pm$ 1 SD. Complete methods are described by Monaco and Lippman (45).

labeled fatty acids in various lipid classes. There is very little present in the form of triglyceride, the major component of milk fat (25), and none is secreted into the medium. Under the conditions of the experiment, MCF-7 cells synthesize predominantly polar lipids, which are generally utilized in membrane synthesis. However, the synthesis of membrane-associated lipids in response to insulin does not rule out the lactogenic nature of the response. It is known that in some cultured cells the extent of triglyceride formation is a function of the environmental conditions. That is, the presence of exogenous lipid sources (serum, for example) favors triglyceride formation (54) whereas under more stringent lipid-free conditions, the cells must elaborate their own fatty acids and tend to synthesize the phospholipids required for growth. Insulin stimulation experiments are performed in lipid-free medium to preclude any possible feedback inhibition of acetate incorporation by exogenous fatty acids. Although the polar nature of the lipids synthesized by MCF-7 cells supports a growth-related role with respect to their induction by insulin, this is by no means conclusive. Furthermore, other mitogens such as 17β-estradiol and 5α-DHT do not stimulate acetate incorporation in MCF-7 cells while stimulating growth (Fig. 10). However, we cannot rule out the possibility that the mechanism of steroid induction of growth involves stimulation of fat synthesis at a time that we have not examined or that perhaps concomitant increases in the amount of protein present in the cell obliterate any increase in acetate incorporation on a per milligram of protein basis.

Table 2 compares the chain lengths of lipids isolated from milk with those synthesized by MCF-7 cells. The medium-chain fatty acids C-12 and C-14 are

TABLE 2. *Comparison of chain lengths of fatty acids made by MCF-7 and those found in human milk*[a]

Fatty acid	MCF-7	Milk
C-12	0.3	8
C-14	10	9
C-16	28	24
C-16:1	13	—
C-18	16	3.2
C-18:1	28	37
C-20	4.3	—

[a] Methods are described by Monaco et al. (43).

generally thought to be characteristic of human milk and if the human situation is similar to that observed in rodents (9), to be synthesized by the mammary epithelium rather than sequestered from serum. MCF-7 cells make C-14 but not C-12 fatty acids.

Finally, whereas insulin as well as glucocorticoid is required for induction of fat synthesis by rodent mammary glands, there is no induction in the absence of prolactin. In MCF-7 cells, addition of human placental lactogen and dexamethasone with insulin results in no further increment in acetate incorporation above that seen with insulin alone (Fig. 11). However, these cells do not contain prolactin receptors. To date, no cells in culture have been reported to contain these receptors.

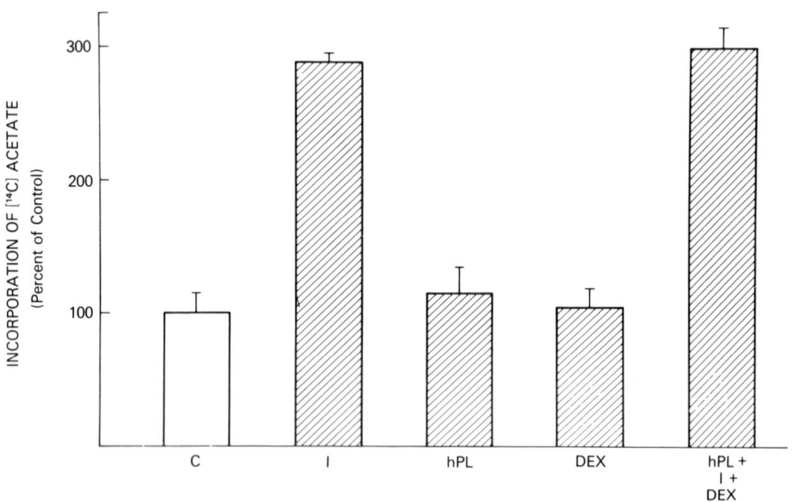

FIG. 11. Effects of lactogenic hormones on fatty acid synthesis. Abbreviations and hormone concentrations: control (C); insulin (I), 5×10^{-7} M; human placental lactogen (hPL), 1 μg/ml; dexamethasone (DEX), 10^{-7} M. Values represent means of triplicate determinations $\pm$ 1 SD. Complete methods are described by Monaco and Lippman (45).

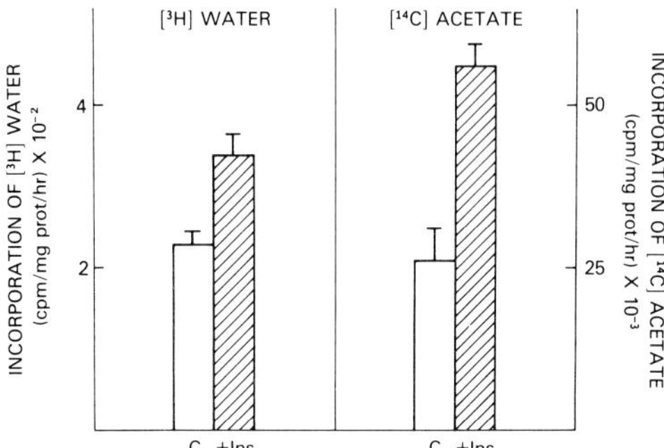

FIG. 12. Effects of insulin on incorporation of [^{3}H]water into fatty acids. Abbreviation and hormone concentrations: control (C); insulin (Ins), 5×10^{-7} M. Values represent means of triplicate determinations ± 1 SD. Complete methods are described by Monaco and Lippman (45).

Thus whether the response of MCF-7 cells to insulin reflects a lactogenic or a growth response or some aspects of both is not known.

Several aspects of the mechanism of insulin induction of fat synthesis in MCF-7 cells have been worked out. That increased acetate incorporation reflects, at least in part, increased net fat synthesis is supported by data derived from experiments with [^{3}H]water. Incorporation of [^{3}H]water is a direct measure of net fat synthesis (3). Figure 12 shows that insulin stimulates incorporation

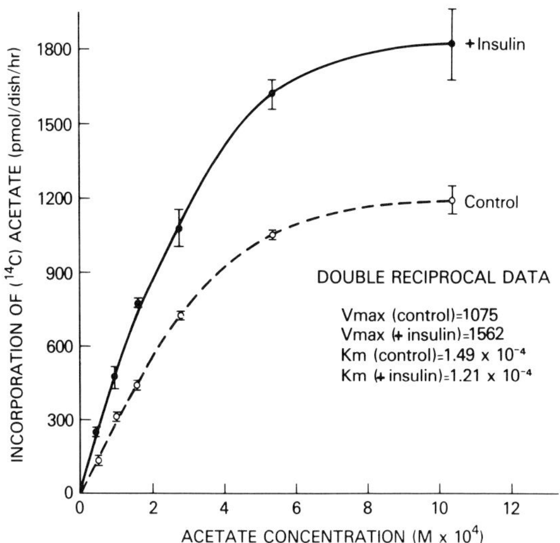

FIG. 13. Kinetics of insulin stimulation of rate of incorporation of [^{14}C]acetate into fatty acids by MCF-7 human breast cells. Values represent means of triplicate determinations ± 1 SD: control *(open circles)*; insulin *(filled circles)* (5×10^{-7} M). Complete methods are described by Monaco et al. (46).

of [^{3}H]water, although not to the same extent as it does acetate incorporation.

The overall effect of insulin on acetate incorporation involves an increase in maximal velocity rather than a decrease in K_m (Fig. 13) (46). The concentration of acetate required for half-maximal incorporation remains unchanged, but the velocity is increased at each concentration. The mechanism of insulin's action on fat synthesis does not appear to involve new RNA or protein synthesis, since antibiotics such as actinomycin D and cycloheximide do not alter the induction (45). In addition, the time course of the stimulation is relatively rapid, with an effect apparent at the earliest time studied (1 hr) and maximal effect by 4 hr of insulin treatment (Fig. 14); this supports the conclusion suggested by the antibiotic data, namely, insulin is activating a preexistent protein rather than inducing synthesis of a new one.

Figure 15 is a schematic diagram of the cytoplasmic fatty acid synthetic pathway illustrating potential points of control by insulin. Transport of substrate across the cell membrane is the first possible site of insulin activation. Increased acetate transport cannot explain all of the effect, since insulin also increases incorporation of [^{3}H]water. As in the case of growth, glucose transport does not seem to play a part, since both control and induced levels of acetate incorporation are maintained whether or not glucose is present in the medium (Fig. 16). However, supraphysiologic concentrations of glucose do seem to enhance the effect of insulin.

Another potential control point is the rate of oxidation or degradation of fatty acids. However, when cells are prelabeled with [^{14}C]acetate and disappearance of labeled fats is followed in the presence and absence of insulin, there is no difference between control and insulin-treated cells, and neither shows any degradation (43). Likewise, since the cells do not secrete fats, inhibition of secretion by insulin is ruled out.

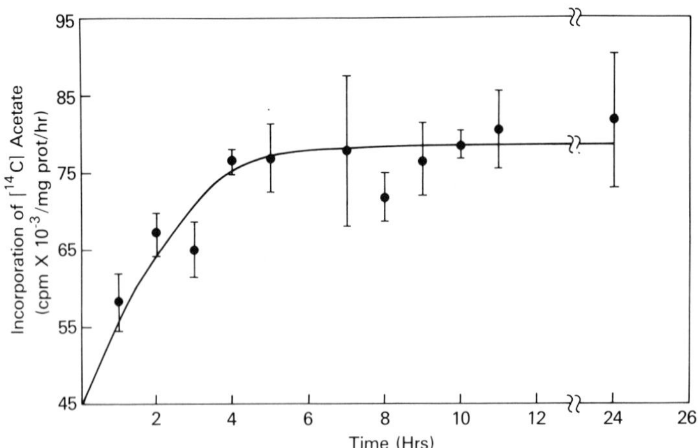

FIG. 14. Time course of insulin stimulation of acetate incorporation. Values represent means of triplicate determinations ± 1 SD. Complete methods are described by Monaco et al. (45).

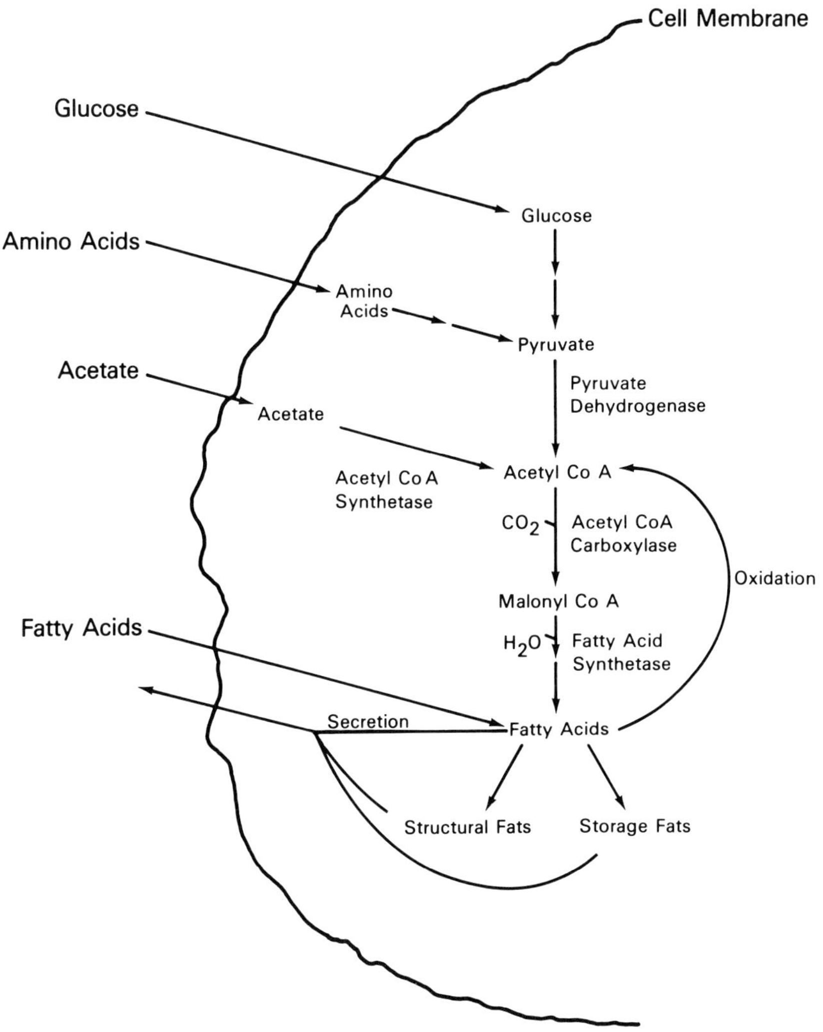

FIG. 15. Pathways of fat synthesis.

At least one locus of insulin action is probably the fatty acid synthetic enzyme acetyl coenzyme A (CoA) carboxylase. Two lines of evidence support a role for this enzyme in the mechanism of insulin action on fat synthesis. When control and insulin-treated cells are labeled with a variety of precursors, insulin enhances incorporation of all substrates that enter the pathway prior to the acetyl CoA carboxylase step, such as glucose, acetate, and acetyl CoA, whereas insulin has no effect on the incorporation of malonyl CoA into fats (43). Second, when fatty acid synthetic enzymes are assayed *in vitro,* acetyl CoA carboxylase activity is stimulated by insulin to approximately the same degree as is acetate

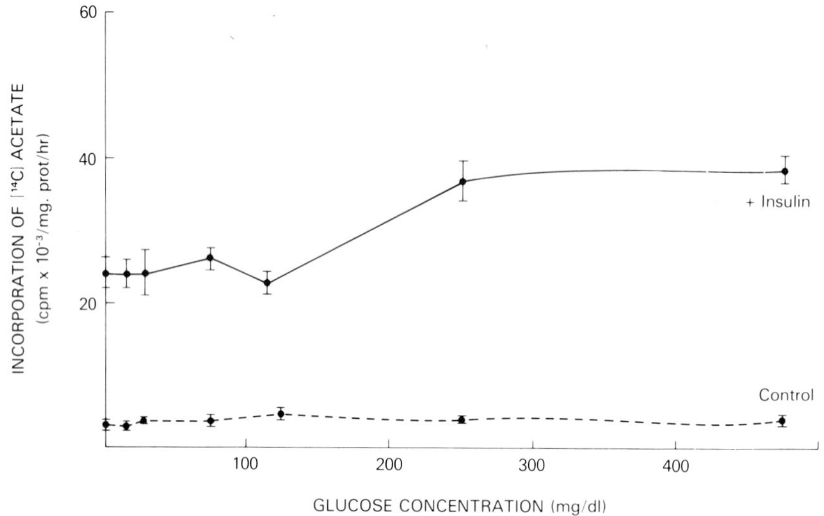

FIG. 16. Effects of glucose concentration on insulin stimulation of acetate incorporation: controls *(dash line)*; insulin *(solid line)*. Values represent means of triplicate determinations ± 1 SD. Complete methods are described by Monaco et al. (45).

incorporation. Furthermore, as predicted by labeling data (there is no stimulation by insulin of the incorporation of labeled malonyl CoA), the fatty acid synthetase activity does not change with insulin treatment. The precise mechanism of insulin stimulation of acetyl CoA carboxylase activity remains to be determined.

The first step in the interaction of insulin with a cell is believed to be binding of insulin to a specific receptor protein located on the cell membrane (79). MCF-7 cells, as well as three other human breast cancer cell lines (ZR-75-1, EVSA-T, and MDA-231), possess specific high-affinity receptors for insulin (50). Figure 17 shows the Scatchard analysis of the binding of ^{125}I-labeled insulin to these cell lines. The curvilinear Scatchard characteristic of other insulin binding reactions suggests negative cooperativity, and dilution experiments in the presence and absence of cold insulin support this interpretation.

Although all four lines have receptors, only MCF-7 and ZR-75-1 respond to insulin (Fig. 18). Furthermore, Table 3 illustrates that no correlation can be drawn between binding parameters and responsiveness. Similarly, these receptors cannot be differentiated on the basis of specificity (Fig. 19). However, when degradation is examined (Fig. 20), the two responsive cell lines degrade insulin to the largest extent, supporting the notion that degradation may be linked to subsequent activity (60). However, further experimentation will be necessary to validate this hypothesis.

Prolactin

Although prolactin is known to be required for lactogenesis in rodent mammary glands (61) and is known to play a role in the induction and growth of

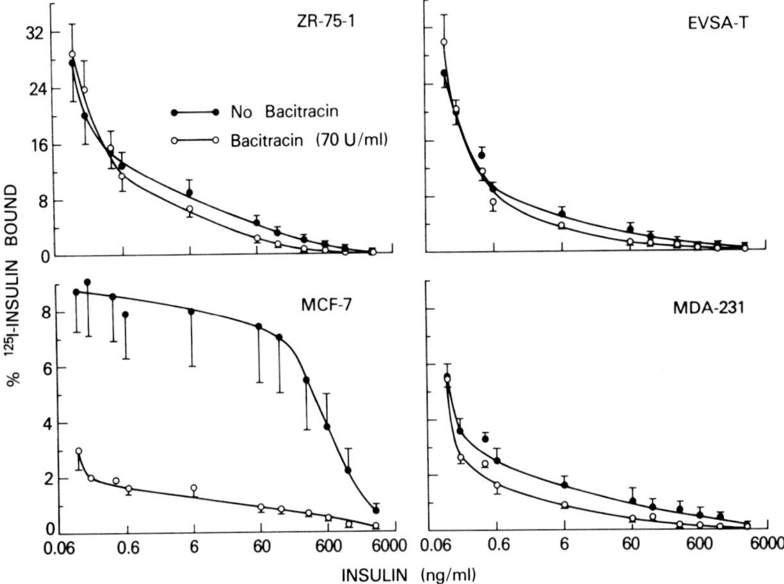

FIG. 17. Scatchard analyses of [^{125}I]insulin binding to four human breast cancer cell lines. Binding experiments were done in the presence *(open circles)* and absence *(filled circles)* of bacitracin, a protease inhibitor. Complete methods are described by Osborne et al. (50).

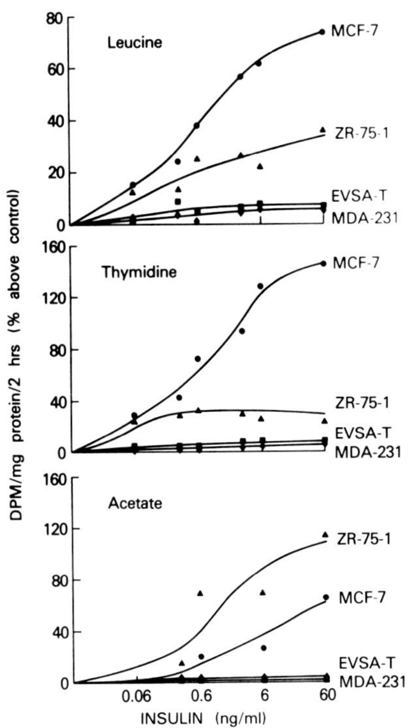

FIG. 18. Effects of insulin on rates of leucine, thymidine, and acetate incorporation. Values represent means of triplicate determinations ± 1 SD. Cell lines: MCF-7 *(circles);* ZR-75–1 *(triangles);* EVSA-T *(squares);* MDA-231 (diamonds). Complete methods are described by Osborne et al. (50).

TABLE 3. *Equilibrium binding constants*[a] *for binding of* ^{125}*I-insulin to human breast cancer cells*

Cell line	R_0[b]	K_e[c]	Biologic response
ZR-75-1	0.5 ± 0.1	8.90 ± 0.89	+
EVSA-T	0.4 ± 0.1	4.93 ± 0.77	−
MCF-7	1.3 ± 0.2	0.27 ± 0.08	+
MDA-231	0.4 ± 0.1	1.85 ± 0.20	−

[a] Values represent mean ± SE of three separate Scatchard plot analyses for each cell line.
[b] Receptor concentration (pmoles/3 × 10^6 cells).
[c] "Empty sites" affinity calculated as described by Osborne et al. (50).

rat mammary cancers (38), the importance of prolactin in human breast cancer has not been demonstrated (57). The responses of women with breast cancer to hypophysectomy do not correlate with decreased plasma prolactin levels (63). In addition, inhibition of prolactin secretion by drugs (including L-DOPA and the ergoline derivatives) does not significantly alter tumor growth (12). Several investigators demonstrated an effect of prolactin on maintenance or growth of normal and malignant human breast explants in culture (6,8,13,14,69);

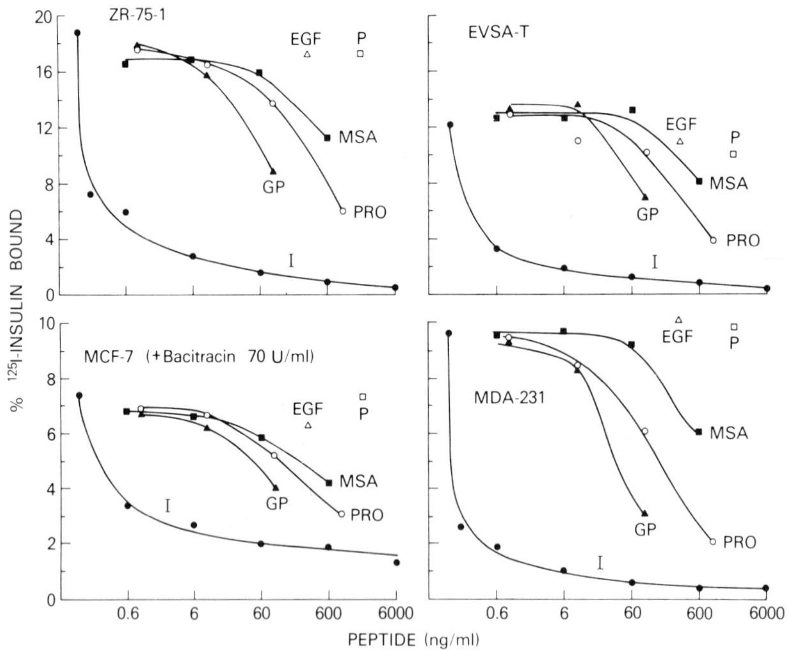

FIG. 19. Specificity of [^{125}I]insulin binding: porcine insulin (I); guinea pig insulin (GP); porcine proinsulin (PRO); multiplication-stimulating activity (MSA); epidermal growth factor (EGF); ovine prolactin (P). Bacitracin (70 units/ml) was used to inhibit degradation in the MCF-7 cells only. Complete methods are described by Osborne et al. (50).

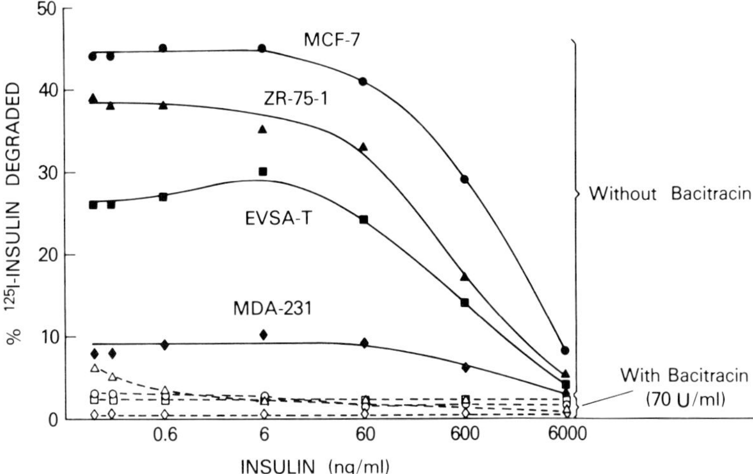

FIG. 20. Percentage of [^{125}I]insulin degraded as a function of total insulin concentration without *(solid lines)* and with *(dash line)* bacitracin: MCF-7 *(circles);* ZR-75–1 *(triangles);* EVSA-T *(squares);* MDA-231 *(diamonds).* Values represent means of three separate experiments. Complete methods are described by Osborne et al. (50).

however, pharmacologic concentrations of prolactin were required. When α-lactalbumin production by human breast cancer specimens in organ culture was quantitated by radioimmunoassay, prolactin was able to stimulate only 2 of 19 samples (26). Even in these two cases no convincing evidence was supplied that an effect on contaminating normal mammary cells was not responsible. Furthermore, Friesen and his colleagues found that only 20% of breast cancer samples contained specific prolactin binding, and this was always small quantitatively when compared with levels present in prolactin-responsive experimental mammary carcinoma (65). On the other hand, Sherman and associates reported that 60% of all human breast tumor specimens contain prolactin receptors (22).

MCF-7 cells do not have prolactin receptors, and in our hands they do not appear to respond to prolactin in terms of growth (37) or fat synthesis (45). However, Shafie and Brooks (56) reported an effect of prolactin on growth of MCF-7 cells. Observation of this activity required the simultaneous presence of cAMP. Paradoxically, theophylline had the opposite effect. The authors did not explain this discrepancy. These studies are of great potential significance regarding a role for prolactin in human breast cancer, and they are badly in need of confirmation and expansion.

Thyroid Hormone

Thyroid hormone, which is known to interact with the rodent mammary gland (66), is also able to stimulate MCF-7 cells (5). Treatment of the cells with T_3 results in increased growth as well as increased estrogen receptor levels. The nuclei of these cells contain receptor for thyroid hormones. We have recently discovered that the ZR-75-1 cell line also shows strong growth responses to T_3 (1). A role for thyroid hormones in human breast development, particularly human breast cancer, remains to be determined.

CONCLUSION

Human breast cancer cells in culture offer the first convenient model for studying the interaction of hormones with malignant mammary epithelium. An understanding of the nature of hormonal stimulation or inhibition of growth could result in more effective therapies and could preclude useless trials. For example, it has been suggested that estriol is an impeded estrogen, or antiestrogen, and as such might be useful in the treatment of breast cancer (30); however, data with MCF-7 cells indicate that estriol can stimulate growth to the same extent as estradiol (36), which forces one to rethink trials involving the administration of estriol.

REFERENCES

1. Allegra, J., and Lippman, M. E. (1978): Manuscript in preparation.
2. Barker, B. E., Fanges, H., and Farnes, P. (1964): Human mammary slices in organ culture. I. Method of culture and preliminary observations on the effect of insulin. *Exp. Cell Res.,* 35:437–448.
3. Bartley, J., and Abraham, 3. (1976): The absolute rate of fatty acid synthesis by mammary gland slices from lactating rats. *J. Lipid Res.,* 17:467–477.
4. Brooks, S. C., Locke, E. R., and Soule, H. D. (1973): Estrogen receptor in a human cell line (MCF-7) from breast carcinoma. *J. Biol. Chem.,* 248:6251–6253.
5. Burke, R. E., Zava, D. T., and McGuire, W. L. (1977): Human breast cancer cells contain thyroid hormone receptors. *Clin. Res.,* 25:461A.
6. Ceriani, R. L., Contesso, G. P., and Notaf, B. M. (1972): Hormone requirement for growth and differentiation of the human mammary gland in organ culture. *Cancer Res.,* 32:2190–2196.
7. Cuatrecasas, P. (1975): Properties of the insulin receptor of isolated fat cell membranes. *J. Biol. Chem.,* 246:7265–7274.
8. Dilley, W. G., and Kister, S. J. (1975): *In vitro* stimulation of human breast tissue by human prolactin. *J. Natl. Cancer Inst.,* 55:35–36.
9. Dils, R., Speake, B., Mayer, R., Lynch, E., Strong, C., and Forsyth, I. (1974): Hormonal control of lipogenesis: The induction of milk-fat synthesis in tissue explants of mammary glands. *Biochem. Soc. Trans.,* 2:1205–1208.
10. Elias, J. J., and Armstrong, R. C. (1973): Hyperplastic and metaplastic responses of human mammary fibroadenomas and dysplasias in organ culture. *J. Natl. Cancer Inst.,* 51:1341–1342.
11. Engel, L. W., Young, N. A., Tralka, T. S., Lippman, M. E., O'Brien, S., and Joyce, M. J. (1978): Breast carcinoma cells in continuous culture: establishment and characterization of three new cell lines *(submitted to Cancer Res.).*
12. Engelsman, E., Heuson, J. C., Blonk-Van der Wyst, J., Drochmans, A., Maass, H., Cheix, F., Sobrinho, L. G., and Nowakowski, H. (1975): Controlled clinical trial of L-dopa and nafoxidine in advanced breast cancer: An E.O.R.T.C. study. *Br. Med. J.,* 2:714–715.
13. Flaxman, B. A., Dyckman, J., and Feldman, A. (1976): Effect of prolactin on maintenance of prelactating human mammary gland *in vitro. In Vitro,* 12:467–471.
14. Flaxman, B. A., and Lasfargues, E. Y. (1973): Hormone-independent DNA synthesis by epithelial cells of adult human mammary gland in organ culture. *Proc. Soc. Exp. Biol. Med.,* 14:371–374.
15. Freifeld, M. L., Feil, P. D., and Bardin, C. W. (1974): The *in vivo* regulation of the progesterone

"receptor" in guinea pig uterus: dependence on estrogen and progesterone. *Steroids,* 23:93–103.
16. Hallowes, R., Wang, D., Lewis, D., Strong, C., and Dils, R. (1973): The stimulation by prolactin and growth hormone of fatty acid synthesis in explants from rat mammary glands. *J. Endocrinol.,* 57:265–276.
17. Harmon, J. T., and Hilf, R. (1976): Insulin binding and glucose transport in the R3230AC mammary adenocarcinoma. *J. Supramol. Struct.,* 4:233–240.
18. Hayashi, I., and Sato, G. (1976): Replacement of serum by hormones permits growth of cells in a defined medium. *Nature,* 259:132–134.
19. Heuson, J. C., and Legros, N. (1972): Influence of insulin deprivation on growth of the 7,12-dimethylbenz*(a)*anthracene-induced mammary carcinoma in rats subjected to alloxan diabetes and food restriction. *Cancer Res.,* 32:226–232.
20. Heuson, J. C., Legros, N., and Hermann, R. (1972): Influence of insulin administration on growth of the 7,12-dimethylbenz*(a)*anthracene-induced mammary carcinoma in intact, oophorectomized, and hypophysectomized rats. *Cancer Res.,* 32:233–238.
21. Heuson, J. C., Pasteels, J. L., Legros, N., Heuson-Stiennon, J. and Leclercq, G. (1975): Estradiol-dependent collagenolytic enzyme activity in long-term organ culture of human breast cancer. *Cancer Res.,* 35:2039–2048.
22. Holdaway, I. M., and Friesen, H. G. (1977): Hormone binding by human mammary carcinoma. *Cancer Res.,* 37:1946–1952.
23. Horwitz, K. B., Costlow, M. E., and McGuire, W. L. (1975): MCF-7, a human breast cancer cell line with estrogen, androgen, progesterone and glucocorticoid receptors. *Steroids,* 26:785–795.
24. Horwitz, K. B., and McGuire, W. L. (1977): Induction of progesterone receptor in a human breast cancer cell line. *Clin. Res.,* 25:295A.
25. Jenness, R. (1974): Biosynthesis and composition of milk. *J. Invest. Dermatol.,* 63:109–118.
26. Kleinberg, D. L. (1975): Human α-lactalbumin: Measurement in serum and in breast cancer organ cultures by radioimmunoassay. *Science,* 190:276–278.
27. Kleinberg, D. L., Todd, J., and Groves, M. L. (1977): Studies on human α-lactalbumin: radioimmunoassay measurements in normal human breast and breast cancer. *J. Clin. Endocrinol. Metabol.,* 45:1238–1250.
28. Knazek, R., Lippman, M. E., and Chopra, H. (1977): Formation of solid human mammary carcinoma *in vitro. J. Natl. Cancer Inst.,* 58:419–423.
29. LeGuellec, R., and Duval, J. (1976): Oestrogen induction of thymidine kinase in the pituitary of the male rat: correlation between inducer ability and oestrogenic potency. *J. Endocrinol.,* 70:149–150.
30. Lemon, H. M. (1975): Estriol prevention of mammary carcinoma induced by 7,12-dimethylbenzanthracene and procarbazine. *Cancer Res.,* 35:1341–1353.
31. Lippman, M. E. (1975): Steroid hormone receptors in human malignancy. *Life Sci.,* 18:143–152.
32. Lippman, M. E., Bolan, G., and Huff, K. (1976): The effects of estrogens and antiestrogens on hormone-responsive human breast cancer in long-term tissue culture. *Cancer Res.,* 36:4595–4601.
33. Lippman, M., Bolan, G., and Huff, K. (1976): The effects of glucocorticoids and progesterone on hormone responsive human breast cancer in long-term tissue culture. *Cancer Res.,* 36:4602–4609.
34. Lippman, M., Bolan, G., and Huff, K. (1976): The effects of androgens and antiandrogens on hormone-responsive human breast cancer in long-term tissue culture. *Cancer Res.,* 36:4610–4618.
35. Lippman, M. E., Bolan, G., Monaco, M. E., Pinkus, L., and Engel, L. (1976): Model systems for the study of estrogen action in tissue culture. *J. Steroid Biochem.,* 7:1045–1051.
36. Lippman, M., Monaco, M. E., and Bolan, G. (1977): Effects of estrone, estradiol and estriol on hormone-responsive human breast cancer in long-term tissue culture. *Cancer Res.,* 37:1901–1907.
37. Lippman, M. E., Osborne, C. K., Knazek, R., and Young, N. (1977): *In vitro* model systems for the study of hormone-dependent human breast cancer. *N. Engl. J. Med.,* 296:154–159.
38. Manni, A., Trujillo, J., and Pearson, O. (1977): Predominant role of prolactin in stimulating the growth of 7,12-dimethylbenz*(a)*anthracene-induced rat mammary tumor. *Cancer Res.,* 37:1216–1219.

39. Martin, R., and Baldwin, R. L. (1971): Effect of alloxan diabetes on lactational performance and mammary tissue metabolism in the rat. *Endocrinology,* 88:863–867.
40. Martin, R., and Baldwin, R. L. (1971): Effects of insulin and anti-insulin serum treatments on levels of metabolites in rat mammary glands. *Endocrinology,* 88:868–871.
41. McGuire, W. L., Carbone, P. P., Sears, M. E., and Escher, G. C. (1975): Estrogen receptors in human breast cancer: an overview. In: *Estrogen Receptors in Human Breast Cancer,* edited by W. L. McGuire, P. P. Carbone, and E. P. Volmer, pp. 1–7. Raven Press, New York.
42. Megyesi, K., Kahn, C. R., Roth, J., Neville, D. M., Jr., Nissley, S. P., Humbel, R. E., and Froesch, E. R. (1975): The NSILA-s receptor in liver plasma membranes. *J. Biol. Chem.,* 250:8990–8996.
43. Monaco, M. E., Bronzert, T. J., Kidwell, W. R., and Lippman, M. E. (1978): Mechanism of insulin stimulation of fatty acid synthesis in human breast cancer cells. *(in preparation).*
44. Monaco, M. E., Bronzert, D. A., Tormey, D. C., Waalkes, P., and Lippman, M. E. (1977): Casein production by human breast cancer. *Cancer Res.,* 37:749–754.
45. Monaco, M. E., and Lippman, M. E. (1977): Insulin stimulation of fatty acid synthesis in human breast cancer in long term tissue culture. *Endocrinology,* 101:1238–1246.
46. Monaco, M. E., Osborne, C. K., and Lippman, M. E. (1977): Insulin stimulation of fatty acid synthesis in human breast cancer cells. *J. Natl. Cancer Inst.,* 58:1591–1593.
47. Osborne, C. K., Bolan, G., Monaco, M. E., and Lippman, M. E. (1976): Hormone responsive human breast cancer in long-term tissue culture: effect of insulin. *Proc. Natl. Acad. Sci. U.S.A.,* 73:4536–4540.
48. Osborne, C. K., and Lippman, M. E. (1978): Human breast cancer in tissue culture: The effects of hormones. In: *Experimental Breast Cancer,* edited by W. L. McGuire. Plenum Press, New York *(in press).*
49. Osborne, C. K., and Monaco, M. E. (1977): Unpublished observation.
50. Osborne, C. K., Monaco, M. E., Lippman, M. E., and Kahn, C. R. (1978): Correlation among insulin binding degradation and biological activity in human breast cancer cells in long-term tissue culture. *Cancer Res.,* 38:94–102.
51. Pasteels, J. L., Heuson-Stiennon, J., Legros, N., Leclercq, G. and Heuson, J. C. (1976): Organ culture of human breast cancer. In: *Breast Cancer: Trends in Research and Treatment,* edited by J. C. Heuson, pp. 141–150. Raven Press, New York.
52. Rillema, J. A., and Linebaugh, B. E. (1977): Characteristics of the insulin stimulation of DNA, RNA and protein metabolism in cultured human mammary carcinoma cells. *Biochim. Biophys. Acta,* 475:74–80.
53. Rose, H. N., and McGrath, C. M. (1975): α-Lactalbumin production in human mammary carcinoma. *Science,* 190:673–675.
54. Rothblat, G. H. (1969): Lipid metabolism in tissue culture cells. *Adv. Lipid Res.,* 7:135–163.
55. Russo, J., Soule, H. D., McGrath, C., and Rich, M. A. (1976): Reexpression of the original tumor pattern by a human breast carcinoma cell line (MCF-7) in sponge culture. *J. Natl. Cancer Inst.,* 56:279–282.
56. Shafie, S., and Brooks, S. C. (1977): Effect of prolactin on growth and the estrogen receptor level of human breast cancer cells (MCF-7). *Cancer Res.,* 37:729–799.
57. Smithline, F., Sherman, L., and Kolodny, H. D. (1975): Prolactin and breast carcinoma. *N. Engl. J. Med.,* 292:784–792.
58. Soule, H. D., Vazquez, J., Long, A., Albert, S., and Brennan, M. (1973): A human cell line from a pleural effusion derived from a breast carcinoma. *J. Natl. Cancer Inst.,* 51:1409–1416.
59. Stoll, B. A. (editor) (1972): *Endocrine Therapy in Malignant Disease,* pp. 111–234. W. B. Saunders, Philadelphia.
60. Terris, S., and Steiner, D. F. (1975): Binding and degradation of ^{125}I-insulin by rat hepatocytes. *J. Biol. Chem.,* 250:8389–8398.
61. Topper, Y. (1970): Multiple hormone interactions in the development of the mammary gland *in vitro. Recent Prog. Horm. Res.,* 26:287–308.
62. Turkington, R. W., Majumber, G. C., Kadobama, N., MacIndoe, J. H., and Frantz, W. L. (1973): Hormonal regulation of gene expression in mammary cells. *Recent Prog. Horm. Res.,* 29:417–455.
63. Turkington, R. W., Underwood, L. E., and Van Wyk, J. J. (1971): Elevated serum prolactin levels after pituitary-stalk section in man. *N. Engl. J. Med.,* 285:707–710.
64. Valotaire, Y., LeGuellec, R., Kernet, H., Guellaen, G., and Duval, J. (1975): Induction of

rat pituitary thymidine kinase: another physiological response to estradiol in the male. *Mol. Cell. Endocrinol.,* 3:117–127.
65. van Bogaert, L. J. (1976): Glucose uptake by normal human breast tissue in organ culture. *Cell Tissue Res.,* 171:535–541.
66. Vonderhaar, B. K. (1977): Studies on the mechanism by which thyroid hormones enhance α-lactalbumin activity in explants from mouse mammary glands. *Endocrinology,* 100:1423–1431.
67. Vonderhaar, B. K., and Topper, Y. T. (1974): A role of the cell cycle in hormone-dependent differentiation. *J. Cell Biol.,* 63:707–712.
68. Wellings, S. R., and Jentop, V. L. (1972): Organ cultures of normal, dysplastic, hyperplastic and neoplastic human mammary tissues. *J. Natl. Cancer Inst.,* 49:329–338.
69. Welsch, C. W., De Iturri, G. C., and Brennan, M. J. (1976): DNA synthesis of human, mouse and rat mammary carcinomas *in vitro.* Influence of insulin and prolactin. *Cancer,* 38:1272–1281.
70. Zava, D. T., Chamness, G. C., Horwitz, K. B., and McGuire, W. L. (1977): Human breast cancer: biologically active estrogen receptor in the absence of estrogen. *Science,* 196:663–664.
71. Zava, D. T., and McGuire, D. L. (1977): Pharmacological effects of androgen in human breast cancer cells are mediated by estrogen receptor. In: *Proceedings 59th Annual Meeting Endocrine Society, Vol. 247,* p.180. (abstract).

Endocrine Control in Neoplasia, edited by
R. K. Sharma and W. E. Criss.
Raven Press, New York © 1978.

Steroid Hormone Action in Uterine Cancer

H. Takamizawa and S. Sekiya

Department of Obstetrics and Gynecology, Chiba University School of Medicine, Inohana, Chiba 280, Japan

Unopposed exposure of uterine endometrium to estrogen has been considered to be the causal factor in the development of adenocarcinoma. Although a carcinogenic potential for estrogen has not been proved, excess extraglandular production of estrone appears to be common in women at high risk for endometrial hyperplasia and carcinoma. Synthetic progestational agents are effective in about one-third of patients with advanced endometrial carcinoma. Direct action by hormones is suggested by *in vitro* studies, and the effect may be provoked by intracellular receptors, as is observed in normal progenitor cells.

INTRODUCTION

At present, seven kinds of carcinoma are known to be responsive to hormonal modifications: carcinomas of the breast, prostate, thyroid, endometrium, kidney, seminal vesicle, and lymphoma, as well as leukemia. These have been described by Huggins (43) and *this volume.*

Estrogen is a potent growth-stimulating agent for the uterus. Conversely, progesterone blocks the growth of endometrium and replaces its proliferative characteristics with secretory characteristics. Because of these biologically antagonistic actions of estrogen and progesterone in the endometrium (67), it has been postulated that continued estrogen stimulation unopposed by progesterone produces a gradual progression of changes from benign lesion to hyperplasia and carcinoma of the endometrium (3,31,40,59). In fact, endometrial carcinoma occurs most frequently in postmenopausal women involved with high-risk factors such as obesity, nulliparity, polycystic ovarian syndrome, functional ovarian tumors, and long-term ingestion of exogenous estrogens (72,80). Excess endogenous estrogen, particularly extraglandular production of estrone, seems to be common in these postmenopausal women (77). On the other hand, maternal ingestion of stilbestrol during early pregnancy seems to enhance the risk of vaginal adenocarcinoma developing years later in the offspring so exposed (39). However, in experimental animals treated by prolonged exposure (4,23,89) or neonatal exposure (22) to estrogen, there has been no direct evidence proving estrogen to be carcinogenic.

Synthetic progestational agents (progestagens) have produced regressive changes in the gland and stroma in endometrial hyperplasia and carcinoma *in situ* (58). Moreover, objective responses have been observed in about one-third of metastatic and recurrent adenocarcinomas after administration of large doses of progestagens (8,57,60,101). This responsiveness to hormonal therapy also appears to explain hormone dependency (30). Although direct effects of progestagens on carcinoma cells have been suggested by *in vitro* studies (99), little is known concerning their mode of action on carcinoma cells.

Recent advances in our knowledge of the actions of sex steroids in endometrial carcinoma seem to be divided into three categories: (a) estrogen production and metabolism in women with endometrial carcinoma or at high risk for endometrial carcinoma, (b) *in vitro* action of sex steroids on normal and carcinomatous endometrial cells, and (c) sex steroid receptors in endometrial carcinoma tissues. These will be briefly reviewed in the hope of providing further elucidation.

ESTROGEN PRODUCTION AND METABOLISM IN WOMEN WITH ENDOMETRIAL CARCINOMA OR AT HIGH RISK FOR ENDOMETRIAL CARCINOMA

Although endometrial carcinoma occurs most frequently in postmenopausal women, postmenopausal ovaries seem to make little or no contribution to estrogen production (5,52,97). Endogenous estrogen levels in postmenopausal women with endometrial hyperplasia or carcinoma have been reported to be higher than those in healthy postmenopausal women (6,105). Recently it has been determined that the principal estrogen formed in postmenopausal women is estrone and that the estrone is derived by peripheral aromatization of plasma androstenedione. Neither adrenal nor ovarian secretion of estrone or estradiol seems to contribute significantly to total estrogen production (28,71,76). As compared with healthy postmenopausal women, women with endometrial carcinoma were found to have significantly greater percentages of conversion of androstenedione to estrone by fat tissue *in vivo* (36) and *in vitro* (108). Plasma estrogen levels correlated significantly with obesity (1,53), which is one of the main risk factors for endometrial hyperplasia and carcinoma. Direct correlation between obesity and percentage of peripheral conversion of androstenedione to estrone was also reported (104).

Plasma estradiol and estrone levels have been reported to be elevated in patients with granulosa cell tumors of the ovary (50,124). High incidences of adenomatous hyperplasia and carcinoma, possibly under the stimulus of theca-granulosa cell tumors, have been reported by Gusberg and Kardon (33). McCormack and Riddick (82) studied hormonal function of granulosa cell tumors and found that grossly elevated levels of serum estradiol of primary ovarian origin decreased postoperatively within the first 24 hr, whereas estrone levels of both adrenal and ovarian origin fell more slowly and less completely. A recent report by MacDonald et al. (75) presented an interesting case of a postmenopausal woman who had complications of nonendocrine mucinous adenocarcinoma of the ovary and endometrial hyperplasia. The estrone production rate in this patient was five times higher than that normally expected for postmenopausal women; this was totally accounted for by extraglandular conversion of plasma androstenedione that was secreted by the hyperplastic stromal cells of the ovary. On the other hand, polycystic ovary (Stein-Leventhal) syndrome is also liable to complicate endometrial hyperplasia and carcinoma (10,48). Luteinizing hormone (LH) excretion (120) and plasma androstenedione levels (42) were reported to be elevated in patients with typical polycystic ovary syndrome. From these results, stimulation of androstenedione production by LH from the ovarian stroma is suspected (29).

A causal relationship between prolonged exogenous estrogen administration and the appearance of endometrial carcinoma was suggested by Gusberg and Hall (32). Endometrial carcinoma after stilbestrol therapy in women with gonadal dysgenesis has also been reported (15,126). An increase in the incidence of endometrial hyperplasia and carcinoma both in postmenopausal women (78,96,117,123,130) and in young women following long-term sequential oral contraception (74,116) has been pointed out retrospectively by recent epidemiological work; increasing use of estrogen preparations might be responsible for this increase in incidence. However, the questions of (a) a dose-response relationship for estrogens and endometrial carcinoma and (b) qualitative differences between synthetic and natural estrogens have not yet been fully elucidated (70). Recent work by Yen et al. (128) showed that a significant portion of orally administered estradiol was rapidly converted to estrone in postmenopausal women.

Thus recent extensive work on estrogen production and metabolism strongly suggests that the exclusive production of estrone by anovulatory subjects and unopposed exposure of endometrium to estrone may be the causal factor in the development of endometrial hyperplasia and carcinoma (115).

IN VITRO ACTION OF SEX STEROIDS ON NORMAL AND CARCINOMATOUS ENDOMETRIAL CELLS

An *in vitro* tissue culture system is necessary to avoid complex interactions among hormones on their target cells *in vivo.* Hardy et al. (34) and Kahn (55) were probably the first workers to suggest that estrogens act directly on their target cells; they reported that estrogens could produce cornification of rodent vaginal epithelia *in vitro.* It has also been reported that estrogens stimulate the mitosis of calf endometrium in organ culture (81) and human endometrial cells in monolayer culture (11,41). Katzenellenbogen and Gorski (56) reported that physiological concentrations (2 to 3×10^{-8} M) of estradiol added *in vitro* to immature rat uteri induced near maximal synthesis of a specific uterine protein. The magnitude of the protein induction closely corresponded to the amount of nuclear bound ^{3}H-estradiol. Other evidence for a direct stimulative action of estrogen on the uterus was reported by Pietras and Szego (94). Estradiol at a concentration of 10^{-9} M elicited significant increases in sodium and water contents of isolated endometrial cells of ovariectomized rats *in vitro* within 2 hr. These results indicate that estrogens act directly on their target cells and provoke gene expression.

Gerschenson et al. (24) described the antagonistic effects of stilbestrol and progesterone on the growth of rabbit endometrial cells *in vitro.* Addition of 10^{-7} M stilbestrol increased their growth, whereas the same concentration of progesterone inhibited growth. In the same tissue culture system of rabbit uterus, addition of 10^{-7} M stilbestrol had the effect of switching most of the nondividing or G_0 cells into the cell cycle and shortening the length of the cell cycle by shortening the G_1 and S phases. Progesterone had a reverse effect (25).

Sonnenschein et al. (118) reported the establishment of a cell line derived from endometrial tissue of a prepuberal rat; it was grown in a medium supplemented with estradiol at a concentration of 10^{-9} M. Clonal derivatives of this cell line produced tumors at the site of inoculation with histopathological features of adenocarcinoma of the endometrium. High-affinity and saturable binding proteins for estradiol were detected in the cells in tissue culture and in the tumor tissues *in vivo.* This report is the exception suggesting that estradiol might directly convert normal endometrial cells to malignant ones.

In addition to the growth-stimulating effects of estrogens, progestational effects in combination with estrogens on endometrium have been investigated *in vitro.* Ehrmann et al. (16) and Luginbuhl (73) found that human endometrial explants in organ culture showed secretory behavior in the absence of ovarian hormones, and they suggested that these hormones act *in vivo* by an indirect route. Figge (21) also did not find any morphological or histochemical changes in human endometrium following treatment with ovarian hormones in organ culture. In contrast to these early results, conversion of proliferative human endometrium maintained in organ culture to secretory endometrium by progesterone has been reported (14,44,62). These conflicting results might in part be due to the fact that variable levels of estrogens and progesterone are present in various mammalian sera that are essential constituents of culture media (17), and concentrations of hormone receptors in cells seem to decrease rapidly during their *in vitro* culture (107).

In addition to secretory induction by progesterone on endometrium *in vitro,* evidence of induction of avidin synthesis in cultured chick oviduct (92) and synthesis of blastokinin in cultured rabbit endometrium (125) suggests that progesterone or its metabolites also can interact with genetic materials of the target cells.

In analogy with these experimental designs, Nordqvist (90) reported cytotoxic effects of progesterone on human endometrial carcinoma tissues in an organ culture system. Marked regressive changes of the carcinoma tissue were seen after addition of progesterone at a concentration of 80 μg/ml. Progesterone at a concentration of 8 μg/ml produced a less marked effect. For progestagens, almost the same results were reported by Heckmann (38) and by Kohorn and

Tchao (61). Depression of ribonucleic acid (RNA) synthesis and deoxyribonucleic acid (DNA) synthesis in human endometrial carcinoma tissues has also been reported to occur in a dose-dependent manner (45,91). No hormonal effects were observed in nonendometrial carcinoma tissues, and the response was not correlated with morphological differentiation of tumor tissues (91).

Although an organ culture method is better for retaining structural integrity and functional activity than a monolayer culture, there are limitations with this technique, e.g., (a) interspecimen variability; (b) short finite life span; (c) difficulty of quantitative experiment. These defects of organ culture methods should be avoidable by the use of a steroid-sensitive cell line. Kuramoto et al. (64) recently established a permanent cell line (HEC-1) from a human endometrial adenocarcinoma that revealed original adenocarcinoma when transplanted into a cortisone-conditioned hamster cheek pouch. Progesterone at concentrations of 2.5 to 20 μg/ml directly suppressed RNA synthesis and DNA synthesis and mitotic activity of HEC-1 cells (65). Ishiwata et al. (47) established another cell line from a human endometrial adenocarcinoma and showed that progesterone at concentrations of 5 μg/ml or more produced a papillary cell arrangement consisting of cells morphologically more differentiated, as shown by optical and electron microscopic findings. Despite these results indicating that progesterone acts directly on uterine adenocarcinoma cells and induces morphological differentiation, the evidence for alteration of protein synthesis by estrogen or progesterone and the evidence for specific estrogen receptors in HEC-1 cells could not be confirmed (114). Merenda et al. (85) described the nonspecific effects of medroxyprogesterone on two established cell lines derived from human endometrial adenocarcinoma serially transplanted in nude mice.

We isolated two transplantable cloned cell lines from the same parent culture of dimethylbenz[*a*]anthracene-induced uterine adenocarcinoma of the rat *in vivo* (110,112). When they were treated with progesterone or estradiol at concentrations of 8 μg/ml or more *in vitro,* the colony forming rate was reduced as compared with controls grown in the same medium without the hormones, and the reduction was dose-dependent (111). One of these cloned cell lines, HTP/C1 culture, which did not display density-dependent inhibition of growth *in vitro,* easily adapted to grow in a culture medium containing progesterone (8 μg/ml). Compared with HTP/C1 cells, HTP/C1/P8 cells grown in the presence of progesterone were contact inhibited (Figs. 1 and 2), and morphological differentiation was observed in the tumor tissues that developed after inoculation of the cells into isologous newborn rats (Figs. 3 and 4). These actions of progesterone on uterine adenocarcinoma cells were completely reversed on removal of the hormone *in vitro* (109). Electron microscopic findings (Figs. 5 and 6) showed that, compared with HTP/C1 cells, HTP/C1/P8 cells were tightly connected with each other, and desmosomes were well developed. Other ultrastructural changes in the HTP/C1/P8 cells were increased numbers of organelles such as mitochondria, Golgi complexes, and rough endoplasmic reticulum, with relatively abundant lipid droplets in the cytoplasm (113), as found partly in primary

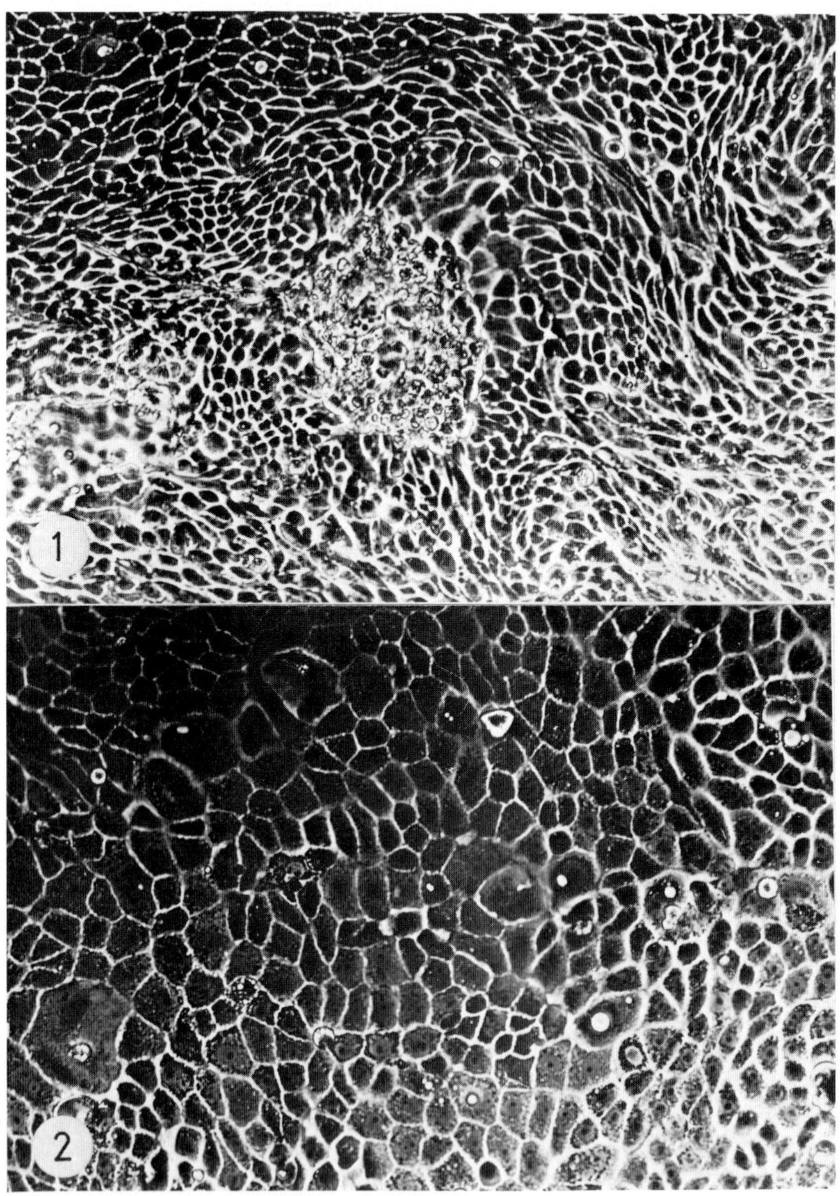

FIG. 1. HTP/C1 culture at confluent state. Note piling up of cells. Phase contrast, ×65.
FIG. 2. HTP/C1/P8 culture at confluent state. Piling up of cells was noticeably inhibited. Phase contrast, ×65.

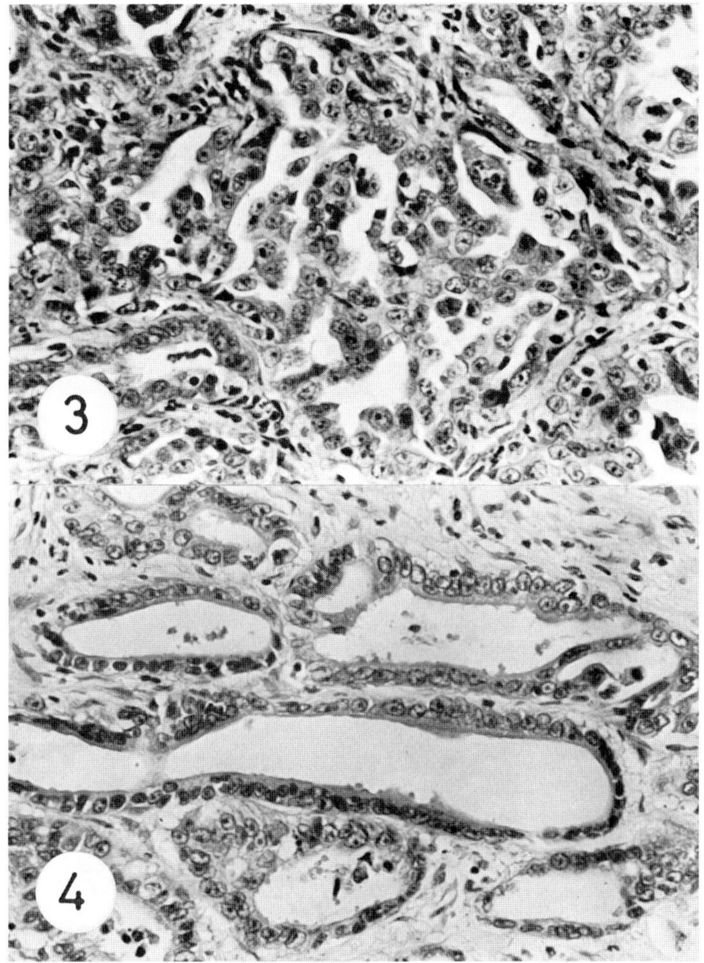

FIG. 3. Histological picture of tumor tissue 4 weeks after inoculation of 10^6 HTP/C1 cells into isologous newborn rat. H&E, ×85.
FIG. 4. Histological picture of tumor tissue 4 weeks after inoculation of 10^6 HTP/C1/P8 cells. Note marked glandular structure with proliferating stromal tissues. H&E, ×85.

rabbit uterine cell culture (7) and in human materials *in vivo* (37,103) after progesterone or progestagens treatment. These results indicate that the effect of progesterone on these uterine adenocarcinoma cells is different from the effects of other chemotherapeutic agents and radiation.

Although high-affinity, specific estrogen-binding proteins have been detected in the cytosol of hormone-responsive cell lines such as a rat pituitary tumor cell line (86), a stable cell line derived from pleural effusion from a breast cancer patient (9), and cloned mouse mammary cell lines (54), it is not yet

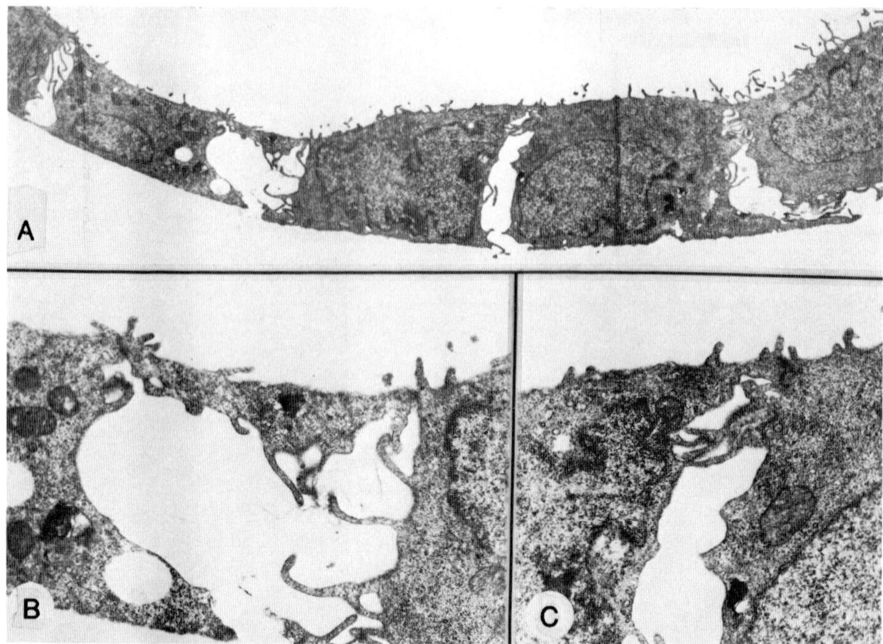

FIG. 5. A: Part of monolayer of HTP/C1 cells. Poorly formed cell contacts characterized by incomplete intracellular junctional complex are prominent. ×6,000. **B** and **C:** Intracellular junctions of HTP/C1 cells. Neither intermediate junctions nor desmosomes were observed. ×12,000.

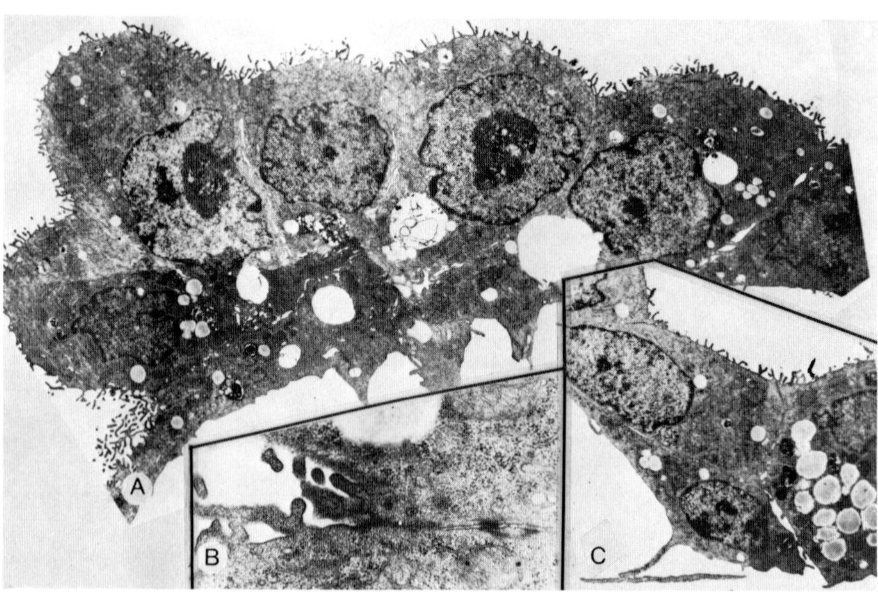

FIG. 6. A and **B:** Parts of HTP/C1/P8 monolayer are characterized by narrow intracellular spaces, abundant mitochondria, and rough endoplasmic reticula. Lipid droplets are also seen. ×6,000. **C:** Intracellular junction of HTP/C1/P8 cells. A desmosome is clearly evident. ×24,000.

clear if the previously described changes in uterine adenocarcinoma cells are provoked in a specific manner via intracellular receptors, since fairly high (pharmacological) dosages rather than physiological dosages of progesterone or progestagens have been required to initiate the effect.

SEX STEROID RECEPTORS IN ENDOMETRIAL CARCINOMA TISSUES

Recent extensive investigations have indicated that the actions of sex steroids are mediated at first by interaction of hormones with their normal target cells in which they form specific complexes with soluble cellular proteins called receptors (26,51,88,93). Although some differences in subcellular mechanisms of action may exist in detail among various steroid hormones, their modes of action on target cells are considered to be similar (68). Initially the steroid penetrates, possibly by free diffusion, into its target cells. In target cells, the first step in steroid hormone action is found to be intracellular binding of steroid to stereospecific cytoplasmic receptors; then this steroid-receptor protein complex undergoes temperature-dependent activation. At the second step, this modified complex migrates into the nucleus, where it interacts with chromatin, called the acceptor site. This interaction elicits as yet unknown changes in gene transcription (increased RNA synthesis, etc.) that ultimately lead to biological response, such as the induction of new proteins.

The estrogen-responsive or target tissues such as the uterus, vagina, anterior pituitary, and mammary gland in humans and in experimental animals contain estrogen receptors (2). Therefore, investigations into the variations of receptor levels from normal to pathological endometrium should be important in revealing hormone dependency, and the rationale for endocrine therapy is based on the hypothesis that certain tumor cells retain the ability to respond to the same hormonal control as their normal progenitor cells (69,102). Assay of estrogen receptors in mammary carcinoma in human and experimental animals is now being established as a method for differentiating between estrogen-dependent and autonomous lesions of the breast (84,127).

Terenius et al. (121) reported the presence of estradiol receptors in 7 of 9 endometrial adenocarcinoma tissues and in 3 of 26 cervical carcinoma tissues; this contrasted with malignant tumor tissues of non-target-tissue origin in which no receptor could be detected. Rubin et al. (106) detected estradiol receptors in about 32% of endometrial carcinomas. There seemed to be a correlation between the degree of morphological differentiation of tumor tissues and the estrogen-binding capacity, and highly differentiated tumors had high levels (18,121). In contrast, Pollow et al. (95) reported a high rate of binding in undifferentiated adenocarcinomas, whereas Taylor (119) and Crocker et al. (13) observed no such correlation. Thus the reports of correlation between the presence of estrogen receptors and morphological differentiation of endometrial carcinomas are contradictory among investigators up to the present time.

The presence of progesterone receptors has also been reported in the normal uterus in humans (27,35,46,98,122,129) and in experimental animals (20,63, 83,87). Haukkamaa et al. (35), Young and Cleary (129), and Rao et al. (98) each reported the absence of progesterone receptor in 2 cases of endometrial adenocarcinomas. However, a more recent report by MacLaughlin and Richardson (79) indicated that progesterone receptor was detected in 30 of 75 normal endometria, in 10 of 22 hyperplasias, and in 3 of 12 carcinomas. On the other hand, Collins (12) reported a case of endometrial adenocarcinoma that responded to progestagen following estrogen priming. This result may be supported by the finding that concentrations of progesterone receptor increase with estrogen priming in various mammalian uterine tissues (19,20,49,66,100).

Thus these fragmentary data seem to indicate that progesterone receptor is gradually lost during the process of malignant transformation of the endometrium.

REFERENCES

1. Aleem, F. A., Moukhtar, M. A., Hung, H. C., and Romney, S. L. (1976): Plasma estrogen in patients with endometrial hyperplasia and carcinoma. *Cancer,* 38:2101–2104.
2. Andre, J., and Rochefort, H. (1974): Estrogen receptors: Physiology and clinical application. *Eur. J. Obstet. Gynecol. Reprod. Biol.,* 4:67–81.
3. Andrews, W. C. (1961): Estrogens and endometrial carcinoma. *Obstet. Gynecol. Surv.,* 16:747–767.
4. Baba, N., and von Haam, E. (1967): Experimental carcinoma of the endometrium. *Prog. Exp. Tumor Res.,* 9:192–260.
5. Barlow, J. J., Emerson, K., Jr., and Saxena, B. N. (1969): Estradiol production after ovariectomy for carcinoma of the breast. Relevance to the treatment of menopausal women. *N. Engl. J. Med.,* 280:633–637.
6. Benjamin, F., and Deutsch, S. (1976): Plasma levels of fractioned estrogens and pituitary hormones in endometrial carcinoma. *Am. J. Obstet. Gynecol.,* 126:638–647.
7. Berliner, J. A., and Gerschenson, L. E. (1976): Sex steroid induced morphological changes in primary uterine cell culture. *J. Steroid Biochem.,* 7:153–158.
8. Bonte, J., Decoster, J. M., Ide, P., Wynants, P., and Billiet, G. (1974): Progestogens in endometrial cancer. In: *Recent Progress in Obstetrics and Gynecology,* edited by L. S. Persianinov, T. V. Chervakova, and J. Presl, pp. 285–297. Excerpta Medica, Amsterdam.
9. Brooks, S. C., Locke, E. R., and Soule, H. D. (1973): Estrogen receptor in a human cell line (MCF-7) from breast carcinoma. *J. Biol. Chem.,* 248:6251–6253.
10. Chamlian, D. L., and Taylor, H. B. (1970): Endometrial hyperplasia in young women. *Obstet. Gynecol.,* 659–666.
11. Chen, L., Lindner, H. R., and Lancet, M. (1973): Mitogenic action of oestradiol-17β on human myometrial and endometrial cells in long-term tissue cultures. *J. Endocrinol.,* 59:87–97.
12. Collins, J. (1973): Combined hormone therapy for recurrent adenocarcinoma of the endometrium. *Am. J. Obstet. Gynecol.,* 113:842–843.
13. Crocker, S. G., Milton, P. J. D., and King, R. J. B. (1974): Uptake of (6,7-^{3}H) oestradiol-17β by normal and abnormal human endometrium. *J. Endocrinol.,* 62:145–152.
14. Csermely, T., Demers, L. M., and Hughes, E. C. (1969): Organ culture of human endometrium. Effect of progesterone. *Obstet. Gynecol.,* 34:252–259.
15. Cutler, B. S., Forbes, A. P., Ingersoll, F. M., and Scully, R. E. (1972): Endometrial carcinoma after stilbestrol therapy in gonadal dysgenesis. *N. Engl. J. Med.,* 287:628–631.
16. Ehrmann, R. L., McKelvey, H. A., and Hertig, A. T. (1961): Secretory behavior of endometrium in tissue culture. *Obstet. Gynecol.,* 17:416–433.
17. Esber, H., Payne, I., and Bogden, A. (1973): Variability of hormone concentrations and ratios in commercial sera used for tissue culture. *J. Natl. Cancer Inst.,* 50:559–562.

18. Evans, L. H., Martin, J. D., and Hähnel, R. (1974): Estrogen receptor concentration in normal and pathological human uterine tissues. *J. Clin. Endocrinol. Metab.*, 38:23–32.
19. Faber, L. E., Sandmann, M. L., and Stavely, H. E. (1972): Progesterone-binding proteins of the rat and rabbit uterus. *J. Biol. Chem.*, 247:5648–5649.
20. Feil, P. D., Glasser, S. R., Toft, D. O., and O'Malley, B. W. (1972): Progesterone binding in the mouse and rat uterus. *Endocrinology*, 91:738–746.
21. Figge, D. C. (1963): The endocrine stimulation of *in vitro* endometrium. *Acta Cytol.*, 7:245–251.
22. Forsberg, J.-G. (1975): Late effects in the vaginal and cervical epithelia after injections of diethylstilbestrol into neonatal mice. *Am. J. Obstet. Gynecol.*, 121:101–104.
23. Gardner, W. U. (1944): Tumors in experimental animals receiving steroid hormone. *Surgery*, 16:8–32.
24. Gerschenson, L. E., Berliner, J., and Yang, J.-J. (1974): Diethylstilbestrol and progesterone regulation of cultured rabbit endometrial cell growth. *Cancer Res.*, 34:2873–2880.
25. Gerschenson, L. E., Conner, E., and Murai, J. T. (1977): Regulation of the cell cycle by diethylstilbestrol and progesterone in cultured endometrial cells. *Endocrinology*, 100:1468–1471.
26. Gorski, J., and Gannon, F. (1976): Current models of steroid hormone action: A critique. *Annu. Rev. Physiol.*, 38:425–450.
27. Grilli, S., Ferreri, A. M., Gola, G., Rocchetta, R., Orlandi, C., and Prodi, G. (1977): Cytoplasmic receptors for 17β-estradiol, 5α-dihydrotestosterone and progesterone in normal and abnormal human uterine tissues. *Cancer Letters*, 2:247–258.
28. Grodin, J. M., Siiteri, P. K., and MacDonald, P. C. (1973): Source of estrogen production in postmenopausal women. *J. Clin. Endocrinol. Metab.*, 36:207–214.
29. Gurpide, E. (1976): Hormones and gynecologic cancer. *Cancer*, 38:503–508.
30. Gusberg, S. B. (1967): Hormone-dependence of endometrial cancer. *Obstet. Gynecol.*, 30:287–293.
31. Gusberg, S. B. (1975): A strategy for the control of endometrial cancer. *Proc. R. Soc. Med.*, 68:163–168.
32. Gusberg, S. B., and Hall, R. E. (1961): Precursors of corpus cancer. III. The appearance of cancer of the endometrium in estrogenically conditioned patients. *Obstet. Gynecol.*, 17:397–412.
33. Gusberg, S. B., and Kardon, P. (1971): Proliferative endometrial response to theca-granulosa cell tumors. *Am. J. Obstet. Gynecol.*, 111:633–643.
34. Hardy, M. H., Biggers, J. D., and Claringbold, P. J. (1953): Vaginal cornification of mouse produced by oestrogens *in vitro. Nature*, 172:1196–1197.
35. Haukkamaa, M., Karjalainen, O., and Luukkainen, T. (1971): *In vitro* binding of progesterone by the human endometrium during the menstrual cycle and by hyperplastic, atrophic, and carcinomatous endometrium. *Am. J. Obstet. Gynecol.*, 111:205–210.
36. Hausknecht, R. U., and Gusberg, S. B. (1973): Estrogen metabolism in patients at high risk for endometrial carcinoma. II. The role of androstenedione as an estrogen precursor in post-menopausal women with endometrial carcinoma. *Am. J. Obstet. Gynecol.*, 116:981–984.
37. Hayakawa, K. (1969): Effects of dimethisterone on endometrial adenocarcinoma. Electron microscopic study. *Acta Obstet. Gynaecol. Jpn.*, 16:285–300.
38. Heckmann, U. (1966): The action of norhydroxyprogesterone capronate on endometrial carcinoma in tissue culture. *Obstet. Gynecol. Surv.*, 21:847.
39. Herbst, A. L., Ulfelder, H., and Poskanzer, D. C. (1971): Adenocarcinoma of the vagina. Association of maternal stilbestrol therapy with tumor appearance in young women. *N. Engl. J. Med.*, 284:878–881.
40. Hertz, R. (1976): The estrogen-cancer hypothesis. *Cancer*, 38:534–540.
41. Hiratsu, T. (1968): *In vitro* cultivation of human endometrium and influences of steroid hormones on a cell line derived from the endometrium. *Kobe J. Med. Sci.*, 14:29–48.
42. Horton, R., and Neisler, J. (1968): Plasma androgens in patients with polycystic ovary syndrome. *J. Clin. Endocrinol. Metab.*, 28:479–484.
43. Huggins, C. (1965): Two principles in endocrine therapy of cancers: Hormone deprival and hormone interference. *Cancer Res.*, 25:1163–1167.
44. Hughes, E. C., Demers, L. M., Csermely, T., and Jones, D. B. (1969): Organ culture of human endometrium. Effect of ovarian steroids. *Am. J. Obstet. Gynecol.*, 105:707–720.

45. Hustin, J. (1975): Effect of protein hormones and steroids on tissue cultures of endometrial carcinoma. *Br. J. Obstet. Gynaecol.*, 82:493–500.
46. Illingworth, D. V., Wood, G. P., Flickinger, G. L., and Kikhail, G. (1975): Progesterone receptor of the human myometrium. *J. Clin. Endocrinol. Metab.*, 40:1001–1008.
47. Ishiwata, I., Nozawa, S., Kiguchi, K., Taguchi, S., Tsutsui, F., Tamura, S., Kurihara, S., Okumura, H., and Komatsu, N. (1976): Effect of estradiol-17β and progesterone on cellular differentiation of human endometrial carcinoma *in vitro*. *J. Clin. Electron Microscopy (Osaka)*, 9:5–6.
48. Jackson, R. L., and Dockerty, M. B. (1957): The Stein-Leventhal syndrome; analysis of 43 cases with special reference to association with endometrial carcinoma. *Am. J. Obstet. Gynecol.*, 73:161–173.
49. Jänne, O., Kontula, K., Luukkainen, T., and Vihko, R. (1975): Oestrogen-induced progesterone receptor in human uterus. *J. Steroid Biochem.*, 6:501–509.
50. Jenner, M. R., Kelch, R. P., Kaplan, S. L., Grumbach, M. M. (1972): Hormonal changes in puberty. IV. Plasma estradiol, LH, and FSH in prepubertal children, pubertal female, and in precocious puberty, premature thelarche, hypogonadism, and in a child with feminizing ovarian tumor. *J. Clin. Endocrinol. Metab.*, 34:521–530.
51. Jensen, E. V., and DeSombre, E. (1972): Mechanism of action of the female sex hormones. *Annu. Rev. Biochem.*, 41:203–230.
52. Judd, H. L., Judd, G. E., Lucas, W. E., and Yen, S. S. C. (1974): Endocrine function of the postmenopausal ovary: Concentrations of androgens and estrogens in ovarian and peripheral vein blood. *J. Clin. Endocrinol. Metab.*, 39:1020–1024.
53. Judd, H. L., Lucas, W. E., and Yen, S. S. C. (1976): Serum 17β-estradiol and estrone levels in postmenopausal women with and without endometrial cancer. *J. Clin. Endocrinol. Metab.*, 43:272–278.
54. Jung-Testas, I., Desmond, W., and Baulieu, E.-E. (1976): Two sex steroid receptors in SC-115 mammary tumor cells. *Exp. Cell Res.*, 97:219–232.
55. Kahn, R. H. (1954): Effect of oestrogen and vitamin A on vaginal cornification in tissue culture. *Nature*, 174:317.
56. Katzenellenbogen, B. S., and Gorski, J. (1972): Estrogen action *in vitro*. Induction of the synthesis of a specific uterine protein. *J. Biol. Chem.*, 247:1299–1305.
57. Kelley, R. M., and Baker, W. H. (1965): The role of progesterone in human endometrial cancer. *Cancer Res.*, 25:1190–1192.
58. Kistner, R. W. (1959): Histological effects of progestins on hyperplasia and carcinoma in situ of the endometrium. *Cancer*, 12:1106–1122.
59. Kistner, R. W. (1976): Estrogen and endometrial cancer. *Obstet. Gynecol.*, 48:479–482.
60. Kistner, R. W., and Griffiths, C. T. (1968): Use of progestational agents in the management of metastatic carcinoma of the endometrium. *Clin. Obstet. Gynecol.*, 11:439–456.
61. Kohorn, E. I., and Tchao, R. (1968): The effect of hormones on endometrial carcinoma in organ culture. *J. Obstet. Gynaecol. Br. Commonw.*, 75:1262–1267.
62. Kohorn, E. I., and Tchao, R. (1969): Conversion of proliferative endometrium to secretory endometrium by progesterone in organ culture. *J. Endocrinol.*, 45:401–405.
63. Kontula, K., Jänne, O., Rajakoski, E., Tanhauanpää, E., and Vihko, R. (1974): Ligand specificity of progesterone-binding proteins in guinea pig and sheep. *J. Steroid Biochem.*, 5:39–44.
64. Kuramoto, H., Tamura, S., and Notake, Y. (1972): Establishment of a cell line of human endometrial adenocarcinoma *in vitro*. *Am. J. Obstet. Gynecol.*, 114:1012–1019.
65. Kuramoto, H., and Suzuki, K. (1976): Effects of progesterone on the growth kinetics and the morphology of a human endometrial cancer cell line. *Acta Obstet. Gynaecol. Jpn.*, 23:123–132.
66. Leavitt, W. W., Toft, D. O., Strott, C. A., and O'Malley, B. W. (1974): A specific progesterone receptor in the hamster uterus: Physiologic properties and regulation during estrous cycle. *Endocrinology*, 94:1041–1053.
67. Lerner, L. J. (1964): Hormone antagonists: Inhibitors of specific activities of estrogen and androgen. *Recent Prog. Hormone Res.*, 20:435–490.
68. Liao, S. (1975): Cellular receptors and mechanisms of action of steroid hormones. *Int. Rev. Cytol.*, 41:87–172.
69. Lippman, M. (1976): Steroid hormone receptors in human malignancy. *Life Sci.*, 18:143–152.
70. Lipsett, M. B. (1977): Estrogen use and cancer risk. *J.A.M.A.*, 237:1112–1115.

71. Longscope, C. (1971): Metabolic clearance and blood production rates of estrogens in postmenopausal women. *Am. J. Obstet. Gynecol.,* 111:778–781.
72. Lucas, W. E. (1974): Causal relationships between endocrine-metabolic variables in patients with endometrial carcinoma. *Obstet. Gynecol. Surv.,* 29:507–528.
73. Luginbuhl, W. H. (1968): Electron microscopic study of the effects of tissue culture on human endometrium. *Am. J. Obstet. Gynecol.,* 102:192–201.
74. Lyon, F. A., and Frisch, M. J. (1976): Endometrial abnormalities occurring in young women on long-term sequential oral contraception. *Obstet. Gynecol.,* 47:639–643.
75. MacDonald, P. C., Grodin, J. M., Edman, C. D., Vellios, F., and Siiteri, P. K. (1976): Origin of estrogen in a postmenopausal woman with a nonendocrine tumor of the ovary and endometrial hyperplasia. *Obstet. Gynecol.,* 47:644–650.
76. MacDonald, P. C., Rombaut, R. P., and Siiteri, P. K. (1967): Plasma precursors of estrogen. I. Extent of conversion of plasma Δ^4-androstenedione to estrone in normal males and nonpregnant normal, castrate, and adrenalectomized females. *J. Clin. Endocrinol. Metab.,* 27:1103–1111.
77. MacDonald, P. C., and Siiteri, P. K. (1974): The relationship between the extraglandular production of estrone and the occurrence of endometrial neoplasia. *Gynecol. Oncol.,* 2:259–263.
78. Mack, T. M., Pike, M. C., Henderson, B. E., Pfeffer, R. I., Gerkins, V. R., Arthur, M., and Brown, S. A. (1976): Estrogens and endometrial cancer in a retirement community. *N. Engl. J. Med.,* 294:1262–1267.
79. MacLaughlin, D. T., and Richardson, G. S. (1976): Progesterone binding by normal and abnormal human endometrium. *J. Clin. Endocrinol. Metab.,* 42:667–678.
80. MacMahon, B. (1974): Risk factors for endometrial cancer. *Gynecol. Oncol.,* 2:122–129.
81. Maurer, H. R., Rounds, D. E., and Raiborn, C. W. (1967): Effects of oestradiol on calf endometrial tissue *in vitro. Nature,* 213:182–183.
82. McCormack, T. P., and Riddick, D. H. (1976): Hormonal function of a granulosa cell tumor. *Obstet. Gynecol.,* 48(Suppl.):18s–21s.
83. McGuire, J. L., and DeDella, C. (1971): *In vitro* evidence for a progesterone receptor in the rat and rabbit uterus. *Endocrinology,* 88:1099–1103.
84. McGuire, W. L., Chamness, G. C., Costlow, M. E., and Shepherd, R. E. (1974): Subcellular biochemistry of estrogen in breast cancer. In: *Hormones and Cancer,* edited by K. W. McKerns, pp. 75–130. Academic Press, New York.
85. Merenda, C., Sordat, B., Mach, J. P., and Carrel, S. (1975): Human endometrial carcinomas serially transplanted in nude mice and established in continuous cell line. *Int. J. Cancer,* 16:559–570.
86. Mester, J., Brunelle, R., Jung, I., and Sonnenschein, C. (1973): Estrogen-sensitive cells. Hormone receptors in tumors and cells in culture. *Exp. Cell Res.,* 81:447–452.
87. Milgrom, E., and Baulieu, E.-E. (1970): Progesterone in uterus and plasma. I. Binding in rat uterus 105,000 g supernatant. *Endocrinology,* 87:276–287.
88. Milgrom, E., Thi, M. L., and Baulieu, E.-E. (1973): Control mechanisms of steroid hormone receptors in the reproductive tract. *Acta Endocrinol.* [*Suppl.*] *(Kbh),* 180:380–403.
89. Noble, R. L., Hochachka, B. C., and King, D. (1975): Spontaneous and estrogen-produced tumors in Nb rats and their behavior after transplantation. *Cancer Res.,* 35:766–780.
90. Nordqvist, R. S. B. (1964): Hormone effects on carcinoma of the human uterine body studied in organ culture. A preliminary report. *Acta Obstet. Gynecol. Scand.,* 43:296–307.
91. Nordqvist, R. S. B. (1970): The synthesis of DNA and RNA in human carcinomatous endometrium in short-term incubation *in vitro* and its response to estradiol and progesterone. *J. Endocrinol.,* 48:29–38.
92. O'Malley, B. W., and Kohler, P. O. (1967): Studies on steroid regulation of synthesis of a specific oviduct protein in a new monolayer culture system. *Proc. Natl. Acad. Sci. U.S.A.,* 58:2359–2366.
93. O'Malley, B. W., and Means, A. R. (1974): Female steroid hormones and target cell nuclei. *Science,* 183:610–620.
94. Pietras, R. J., and Szego, C. M. (1975): Steroid hormone-responsive, isolated endometrial cells. *Endocrinology,* 96:946–954.
95. Pollow, K., Lübbert, H., Bonquoi, E., Kreuzer, G., and Pollow, B. (1975): Characterization and comparison of receptors for 17β-estradiol and progesterone in human proliferative endometrium and endometrial carcinoma. *Endocrinology,* 96:319–328.

96. Quint, B. C. (1975): Changing patterns in endometrial adenocarcinoma. A study of 291 consecutive cases at large private hospital, 1960–1973. *Am. J. Obstet. Gynecol.,* 122:498–501.
97. Rader, M. D., Flickinger, G. L., DeVilla, G. O., Jr., Mikuta, J. J., and Mikhail, G. (1973): Plasma estrogens in postmenopausal women. *Am. J. Obstet. Gynecol.,* 116:1069–1073.
98. Rao, B. R., Wiest, W. G., and Allen, W. M. (1974): Progesterone "receptor" in human endometrium. *Endocrinology,* 95:1275–1281.
99. Reel, J. R. (1976): The mode of action of progestagens on endometrial carcinoma. In: *Steroid Hormone Action and Cancer,* edited by K. M. J. Menon and J. R. Reel, pp. 85–94. Plenum Press, New York.
100. Reel, J. R., and Shin, Y. (1975): Oestrogen-inducible uterine progesterone receptors. Characteristics in the ovariectomized immature and adult hamster. *Acta Endocrinol.,* 80:344–354.
101. Reifenstein, E. C., Jr. (1974): The treatment of advanced endometrial cancer with hydroxyprogesterone caproate. *Gynecol. Oncol.,* 2:377–414.
102. Richardson, G. S. (1972): Endometrial cancer as an estrogen-progesterone target. *N. Engl. J. Med.,* 286:645–647.
103. Richart, R. M., and Ferenczy, A. (1974): Endometrial morphologic response to hormonal environment. *Gynecol. Oncol.,* 2:180–197.
104. Rizkallah, T., Tovell, H. M., and Kelley, J. (1975): Production of estrone and fractional conversion of circulating androstenedione to estrone in women with endometrial carcinoma. *J. Clin. Endocrinol. Metab.,* 40:1045–1056.
105. Rome, M., Brown, J. B., Mason, T., Smith, M. A., Laverty, C., and Fortune, D. (1977): Oestrogen excretion and ovarian pathology in postmenopausal women with atypical hyperplasia, adenocarcinoma and mixed adenosquamous carcinoma of the endometrium. *Br. J. Obstet. Gynaecol.,* 84:88–97.
106. Rubin, B. L., Gusberg, S. B., Butterly, J., Han, T. C., and Maralit, M. (1972): A screening test for estrogen dependence of endometrial carcinoma. *Am. J. Obstet. Gynecol.,* 114:660–669.
107. Russell, S. L., and Thomas, G. H. (1972): Oestrogen metabolism and oestradiol-17β receptors in cultured uterus. *J. Endocrinol.,* 53:xxix.
108. Schindler, A. E., Ebert, A., and Friedrich, E. (1972): Conversion of androstenedione to estrone by human fat tissue. *J. Clin. Endocrinol. Metab.,* 35:627–630.
109. Sekiya, S., Kamiyama, M., and Takamizawa, H. (1975): Cellular differentiation of rat uterine adenocarcinoma cells by progesterone *in vitro. Cancer Res.,* 35:1713–1717.
110. Sekiya, S., Kikuchi, Y., and Takamizawa, H. (1973): High- and low-tumorigenic culture lines of rat uterine adenocarcinoma and their isozyme patterns of lactate dehydrogenase and hexokinase. *Cancer Res.,* 33:3324–3329.
111. Sekiya, S., Kikuchi, Y., and Takamizawa, H. (1974): The effects of hormones and chemotherapeutic agents on rat uterine adenocarcinoma cells in tissue culture. *Am. J. Obstet. Gynecol.,* 119:675–680.
112. Sekiya, S., Takamizawa, H., Wang, F., Takane, T., and Kuwata, T. (1972): *In vivo* and *in vitro* studies on uterine adenocarcinoma of the rat induced by 7,12-dimethylbenz[*a*]anthracene. *Am. J. Obstet. Gynecol.,* 113:691–695.
113. Sekiya, S., Takayama, N., and Takamizawa, H. (1976): Effects of progesterone on rat uterine adenocarcinoma cells *in vitro:* An electron microscopic study. *Eur. J. Cancer,* 12:493–496.
114. Shapiro, S. S., van der Schouw, M., and Hagerman, D. (1975): Failure of estrogen and progesterone to affect protein synthesis by an established endometrial cell line. *Am. J. Obstet. Gynecol.,* 121:570–572.
115. Siiteri, P. K., Schwarz, B., and MacDonald, P. (1974): Estrogen receptors and the estrone by hypothesis in relation to endometrial and breast cancer. *Gynecol. Oncol.,* 2:228–238.
116. Silverberg, S. G., and Makowski, E. L. (1975): Endometrial carcinoma in young women taking oral contraceptive agents. *Obstet. Gynecol.,* 46:503–506.
117. Smith, D. C., Prentice, R., Thompson, D. J., and Herrmann, W. L. (1975): Association of exogenous estrogen and endometrial carcinoma. *N. Engl. J. Med.,* 293:1164–1167.
118. Sonnenschein, C., Weiller, S., Farookhi, R., and Soto, A. M. (1974): Characterization of an estrogen-sensitive cell line established from normal rat endometrium. *Cancer Res.,* 34:3147–3154.
119. Taylor, R. W. (1973): The uptake of tritiated oestradiol by normal endometrium and by endometrial carcinoma. In: *Endometrial Cancer,* edited by M. G. Brush, R. W. Taylor, and D. C. William, pp. 161–164. William Heinemann, London.

120. Taymor, M. L., Clark, B. J., and Sturgis, S. H. (1963): The polycystic ovary. A clinical and laboratory study. *Am. J. Obstet. Gynecol.*, 86:188–196.
121. Terenius, L., Lindell, A., and Persson, B. H. (1971): Binding of estradiol-17β to human cancer tissue of the female genital tract. *Cancer Res.*, 31:1895–1898.
122. Verma, U., and Laumas, K. R. (1973): *In vitro* binding of progesterone to receptors in the human endometrium and the myometrium. *Biochim. Biophys. Acta*, 317:403–419.
123. Weiss, N. S., Szekely, D. R., and Austin, D. F. (1976): Increasing incidence of endometrial cancer in the United States. *N. Engl. J. Med.*, 294:1259–1262.
124. Wentz, A. C., and McCranie, W. M. (1976): Circulating hormone levels in a case of granulosa cell tumor. *Fertil. Steril.*, 27:167–170.
125. Whitson, G. L., and Murray, F. A. (1974): Cell culture of mammalian endometrium and synthesis of blastokinin *in vitro*. *Science*, 183:668–670.
126. Wilkinson, E. J., Friedrich, E. G., Jr., Mattingly, R. F., Regali, J. A., and Garancic, J. C. (1973): Turner's syndrome with endometrial adenocarcinoma and stilbestrol therapy. *Obstet. Gynecol.*, 42:193–200.
127. Wittliff, J. L. (1974): Specific receptors of the steroid hormones in breast cancer. *Semin. Oncol.*, 1:109–118.
128. Yen, S. S. C., Martin, P. L., Burnier, A. M., Czekala, N. M., Greaney, M. O., and Callatine, M. R. (1975): Circulating estradiol, estrone, and gonadotropin levels following the administration of orally active 17β-estradiol in postmenopausal women. *J. Clin. Endocrinol. Metab.*, 40:518–520.
129. Young, P. C. M., and Cleary, R. E. (1974): Characterization and properties of progesterone-binding components in human endometrium. *J. Clin. Endocrinol. Metab.*, 39:425–439.
130. Ziel, H. K., and Finkle, W. D. (1975): Increased risk of endometrial carcinoma among users of conjugated estrogens. *N. Engl. J. Med.*, 293:1167–1170.

Endocrine Control in Neoplasia, edited by
R. K. Sharma and W. E. Criss.
Raven Press, New York © 1978.

Molecular Aspects of Glucocorticoid Receptors

Dennis M. DiSorbo and Gerald Litwack

Fels Research Institute and Department of Biochemistry, Temple University School of Medicine, Philadelphia, Pennsylvania 19140

Glucocorticoids may be classified as ubiquitous hormones. Their effects on target tissues range from anabolic in liver to catabolic in thymus. Recent work on the mechanism of action of the glucocorticoids strongly suggests that biological responses to these steroids are mediated through intracellular receptors located in cellular cytoplasm of target tissues (7,23,41). These receptors are protein in nature and have high affinity for glucocorticoids. Thus the union of steroid with receptor sets into motion a series of events culminating in the tissues' response to the hormone (9,30,52).

The precise mechanism by which the steroid exerts its effect on a tissue is still not clear. The steroid is known to interact with the receptor of the soluble cytoplasm to form a complex. This complex, in an energy-dependent step, appears to be translocated into the nucleus and to bind to a nuclear acceptor site. The acceptor may be DNA or DNA modified by chromatin proteins, or proteins of chromatin. The result of this nuclear translocation is initiation of mRNA synthesis (16,19,26,51) coding for proteins, usually enzymes, whose effects bring about the phenotypic response of the tissue to the steroid.

Since numerous review articles have been written on the actions of the glucocorticoids (3,4,48,56), only a cursory background will be given here. We shall deal primarily with the accumulating evidence on receptor activation. A new model depicting steroid-receptor activation will be presented, and its possible significance in neoplastic cells will be emphasized.

METABOLIC EFFECTS OF GLUCOCORTICOIDS

Of the metabolic changes induced by adrenal glucocorticoids, those in protein and nucleic acid are among the earliest and most striking. Although extensive in magnitude, these changes are at the same time opposite in direction in two major anatomical loci, the liver and lymphoid tissue. Thus, shortly following the injection of cortisol into rats, there is acute stimulation of protein and nucleic acid synthesis in liver (15,21,25,60) and a similar early but diminished degree of formation of these macromolecular constituents in lymphoid tissue, notably the thymus (8,11,32,42).

Evidence for production of biochemical alterations in lymphoid cells by physiological concentrations of lymphocytolytic steroids added *in vitro* was first reported for thymocytes by Morita and Munck (38) and later by Makman et al. (33,34). Data presented in these reports indicate that cortisol added *in vitro* produces progressive inhibitory effects on glucose transport and on the incorporation of specific radioactive precursors into nucleic acids. Fox and Gabourel (10) observed a depression in RNA polymerase activity and RNA biosynthesis in lymphoid tissues that undergo dissolution following exposure to glucocorticoids, and Young (61) reported inhibition of incorporation of specific radioactive precursors into protein. Thus the early stimulation of protein and nucleic acid synthesis in thymus can be interpreted as the initiation of mRNA synthesis coding for a protein(s) that inhibits transport of glucose, amino acids, and nucleosides into the cell.

As was the case in lymphoid tissue, the liver has also been extensively characterized with respect to its response to glucocorticoid administration. Various enzymes that function in the metabolism of amino acids have been shown to be responsive to glucocorticoids. These include tryptophan oxygenase, tyrosine aminotransferase, and alanine aminotransferase. Significant increases in the activity of each of these enzymes have been demonstrated in the livers of rats treated with glucocorticoids.

Tryptophan oxygenase and tyrosine aminotransferase (TAT) have been studied by Knox et al. (24). The former enzyme can be induced in the livers of intact and adrenalectomized rats by both tryptophan and glucocorticoids. The other hepatic enzyme, TAT, showed a similar pattern of inducibility as tryptophan oxygenase, but it also showed notable differences (26). Adrenalectomy alone did not lower the level of this enzyme in liver, and when tyrosine was administered to adrenalectomized rats, the activity of the enzyme was not increased. Cortisol proved to be an effective inducer of TAT in both intact and adrenalectomized rats. Further proof that hydrocortisone was increasing the synthesis of new enzyme and not merely causing its activation was demonstrated by Kenney (20) for TAT and by Schimke et al. (53) for tryptophan oxygenase. These investigators, by use of a specific antiserum for the enzyme in question, showed that *in vivo* incorporation of isotopic amino acids into newly synthesized enzyme occurred after hydrocortisone administration.

After the pioneering work of Jensen and associates in 1957 on the estrogen receptor (18), researchers began to use radioactive steroids to investigate the mechanism of action of steroid hormones. The glucocorticoid receptor was characterized along similar lines.

The first clue that a glucocorticoid-binding protein existed was discovered in 1965 by Litwack et al. (28); they reported intracellular binding of [^{14}C]hydrocortisone to macromolecules in rat liver prior to enzymatic induction. The radioactive ligand was protein-bound and was found to accumulate in the cytoplasm, microsomes, and nucleus of the cell. These results led these investigators to conclude that the early binding of hydrocortisone to proteins was involved in the mechanism of enzyme induction. Subsequently, similar studies were reported by Beato et al. (5) who showed binding of cortisol to a cytoplasmic macromolecule in liver. After a 20-min injection of [^{3}H]cortisol, some of the counts were associated with nuclei. The implication was that cortisol was transported from the cytoplasm to the nucleus. How the receptor complex was involved in eliciting a biochemical response was still unclear.

To simplify studies of the effects of glucocorticoids on liver tissue, Tomkins and associates began to use a line of rat hepatoma tissue culture cells (HTC) that respond to cortisol in much the same way as rat liver (35,36). Preliminary data indicated that induction of TAT could be shown after incubation of HTC cells with either cortisol or dexamethasone (14). Later studies compared the behavior of the receptor in HTC cells and rat liver on ion-exchange chromatography, and the results suggested similar or identical proteins (55).

Munck and Brinck-Johnson (40) were the first investigators to report a specific binder in rat thymus tissue. Their initial work centered on equilibrium and kinetic studies of tritium-labeled steroids to intact thymus cells. These investigators reported that the steroid-receptor complex translocated into the nucleus in a temperature-dependent step.

The kinetics of this temperature-dependent step showed that after cells were warmed from 4°C to 37°C only 30 sec elapsed before the majority of counts appeared in the nucleus. This rapid migration into the nucleus correlated with *in vitro* data on inhibition of glucose transport (40,41). Within 10 min after the addition of cortisol to a thymus cell suspension, an inhibitory effect was observed on the transport of glucose into these cells. Young (63) reported that cortisol stimulates RNA synthesis within 6 min of exposure to hormone. Stimulation of RNA synthesis could lead to synthesis of a protein(s) that acts directly on the cell membrane to inhibit transport of glucose into the cells. If actinomycin D is added at the same time as cortisol, the glucocorticoid effect is blocked. However, if actinomycin D is added 5 min after cortisol, the blocking effect is not seen.

Subsequent experiments by Hallahan et al. (16) strengthened the argument for a specific glucocorticoid-induced protein involved in the inhibition of glucose transport into thymus cells. The results show that if protein synthesis is inhibited by either cycloheximide or puromycin, the effect of coritsol on glucose transport is also blocked.

GLUCOCORTICOID-RECEPTOR COMPLEX

In 1970 Samuels and Tomkins investigated the relationship of steroid structure to the induction of TAT in HTC cells as a means of studying the mechanism of steroid regulation of gene expression (50). On the basis of their results they postulated an allosteric system for the interaction between various steroids and a cytoplasmic receptor system (Fig. 1); this model later was extended by Rousseau et al. (49). The receptor was conceived to exist in equilibrium between two

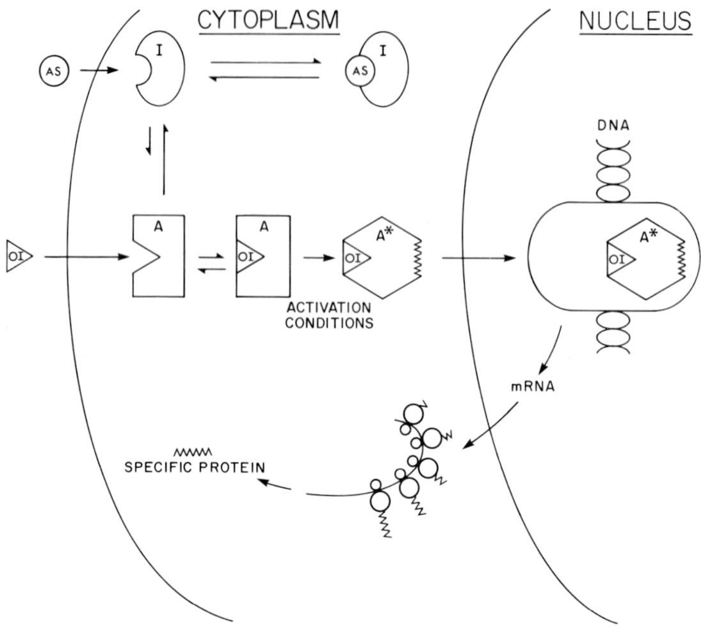

FIG. 1. Schematic representation of proposed allosteric model for interaction of steroids with glucocorticoid receptor. Two classes of steroids are illustrated, optimal inducers (OI) and antisteroids (AS). The receptor is shown in the inactive (I) and active (A) states.

conformational states: inactive (I) and active (A) forms. In the uninduced cell the equilibrium is shifted in favor of the inactive form, although a small percentage of receptors remain in the active state. When an optimal inducer (cortisol, dexamethasone) enters a target tissue it interacts with the A form, shifting the equilibrium in favor of the activated state. The newly formed complex can then undergo a conformational change that in a temperature-dependent step translocates into the nucleus. In the case of suboptimal inducers (11β-hydroxyprogesterone, deoxycorticosterone), the steroid has an affinity for both the I and A forms of the receptor. Since the equilibrium between either form is not greatly shifted (some intermediate ratio being reached), the induction of TAT is below that of an optimal inducer but elevated over the uninduced cell. Anti-inducers (progesterone, 17α-methyltestosterone) were considered to bind exclusively to the I form, thus keeping the receptors in an inactive state.

Support for this model has been obtained in studies with antisteroids. Turnell et al. (59) reported the competition of the antiglucocorticoid cortexolone with triamcinolone acetonide (TA) for binding to specific receptors in rat thymocytes, with subsequent nuclear uptake of the complex. This complex was shown to have an altered conformation (3.5S versus ~4S for [^{3}H]TA) and a low affinity for nuclear acceptor sites. In other studies the antimineralocorticoid spirolactone was shown to bind to the mineralocorticoid receptor, but the spirolactone-receptor complex did not bind to nuclear acceptor sites *in vivo* or *in vitro* (35).

In addition to the preceding experiments, numerous investigators have been studying the physical characteristics of the cytoplasmic receptor: Litwack et al. (29), Rees and Bell (47), Young et al. (64), Granberg and Ballard (13). The results indicate that the receptor has a molecular weight of 67,000 d, with a pI of 6.7. The K_D for dexamethasone was found to be about 6×10^{-10} M, and that for cortisol was in the range of 10^{-8} M. The addition of sulfhydryl-protecting agents (2-mercaptoethanol, dithiothreitol, thioglycerol) stabilized the receptor complex against inactivation. The receptor could be inactivated by incubation with chemical agents (*N*-ethylmaleimide, *p*-chloromercuriphenylsulfonic acid) capable of reacting with sulfhydryl groups on proteins. Consequently the binding of glucocorticoids to their cytoplasmic receptors may involve sulfhydryl groups at the ligand binding site or in close proximity to it.

MODULATOR: A NEW RECEPTOR MODEL

As was previously stated, the only model to explain the mechanism of activation of the receptor has been the allosteric model put forth by Rousseau et al. (49). However, more recent evidence requires modification of this model.

Experimental data from three laboratories indicate that there may be a cytoplasmic molecule that is associated with the receptor and that functions as a modulator of receptor activation. The theory and evidence for such a modulator will now be discussed.

In 1973, early events in glucocorticoid action occupied the attention of several research groups. Both Higgins et al. (17) and Milgrom et al. (37) observed that the glucocorticoid-receptor complex could be activated by several *in vitro* manipulations: dilution of the cytosol, increased ionic strength, or elevated temperature. Once the complex was activated, it could then bind to nuclei, chromatin, or DNA. Although the chemical nature of this activation remained obscure, it was observed that the activation caused an increase in positively charged groups on the surface of the molecule, which increased its affinity for DNA (37). Results of these studies led to the theory that activation was due to a conformational change of the steroid-receptor complex (37) or to disaggregation of the protein complex into subunits (17).

Research continued on the mechanism of action of the glucocorticoids, and in 1975 the first indication that there might be a cytoplasmic factor controlling activation was demonstrated (36). Milgrom and Atger, while studying interaction of the steroid-receptor complex with rat liver nuclei, observed that there was an inhibitor in the cytosol that prevented the receptor complex from translocating to the nucleus. Surprisingly, in a subsequent article on the kinetics of thermal activation of the glucocorticoid receptor complex, Atger and Milgrom reported that "thermal activation is a monomolecular reaction and gives strong evidence against mechanisms involving a polymerization or an interaction of receptor with another component of the cytosol" (1). Additional evidence to support an inhibitor of activation was provided by Simons et al. (54). These researchers reported that HTC cytosol contained a macromolecular factor that either inhibited activation or prevented the association of the steroid-receptor complex with isolated nuclei, chromatin, or DNA. During this same time period Cake et al. (6) demonstrated that the glucocorticoid receptor from rat liver could be activated at low temperatures by gel filtration. Gel filtration was considered to remove a component(s) from the cytosol that was involved in the activation mechanism. To further implicate the involvement of a low-molecular-weight component in the activation step, a minicolumn of Bio-Gel P-4 (10 ml bed volume) was equilibrated with the low-molecular-weight components of rat liver cytosol, followed by filtration of [^{3}H]dexamethasone-labeled cytosol. The results of the experiment can be seen in Fig. 2. When the minicolumn was buffer-equilibrated, the eluted steroid-receptor complex was activated, as demonstrated by its ability to bind to DNA-cellulose. However, the labeled cytosol that was passed through the column equilibrated with small molecules did not undergo activation. This implied that the receptor passing through the buffer-equilibrated

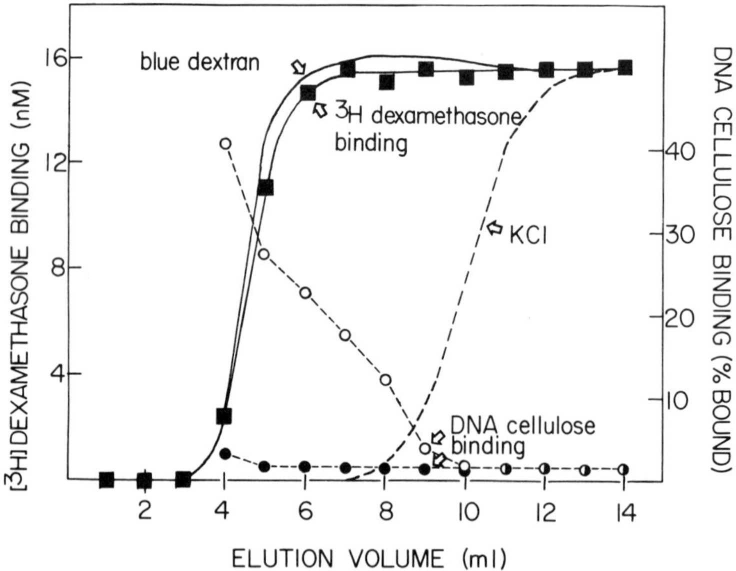

FIG. 2. Effect of gel filtration on glucocorticoid-receptor activation. [^{3}H]dexamethasone-labeled cytosol was applied to a Bio-Gel P-4 minicolumn equilibrated with either buffer or "small molecules," and 1.0-ml fractions were collected. Each fraction was assayed for [^{3}H]dexamethasone binding *(squares)* and ability to bind to DNA-cellulose: buffer-equilibrated *(open circles)*; "small-molecule"-equilibrated *(filled circles)*. The columns were characterized using a solution of blue dextran and KCl. These fractions were assayed for blue dextran by absorption at 625 nm and for salt by conductivity measurements. Each point represents the mean of two separate experiments. (From ref. 6 with permission.)

column became activated due to the separation of a small inhibitory component from the steroid-receptor complex.

Subsequently, the hepatic glucocorticoid receptor was activated by gel filtration on Sephadex G-15, G-25, and G-50 and Bio-Gel P-4. The fact that Sephadex G-15 caused activation suggested that the low-molecular-weight component involved in this activation process might have a molecular weight less than 1,500 d. Separate experiments showed that the inhibitor was not glutathione, pyridine nucleotides, or certain other commonly occurring biochemicals (M. H. Cake and G. Litwack, *unpublished observations*).

Bailly et al. (2) gave credence to the possibility that there might be a low-molecular-weight inhibitor in liver cytosol. These investigators showed that by dilution of rat liver cytosol (0° C) the glucocorticoid-receptor complex increased its affinity for nuclei. This enhanced binding to nuclei was found to be due to activation of the complex. The inhibitor was demonstrated to be of low molecular weight by dialysis, Sephadex G-25 chromatography, ammonium sulfate precipitation, and ultrafiltration. In a later report by Goidl et al. (12) the involvement of a small molecule in the activation step of the receptor was substantiated. The results of this study were in agreement with those of previous investigations and showed that activation by gel filtration was determined by factors other than a shift in pH of the eluent during chromatography.

Experimentation up to this time clearly indicated that there was an inhibitor in hepatic cytosol that was involved in some manner with activation of the receptor. Previous studies (6,12,37) made the possibility of a receptor-inhibitor complex attractive. Because of recent work by Parchman and Litwack (45), Parchman et al. (46), and Litwack and Cake (27), it was found that the glucocorticoid receptor could be resolved into two forms depending on its state of activation. The more acidic unactivated form required a very high salt concentration (0.6 M KCl) to be eluted from DEAE-Sephadex, whereas the less acidic form (activated) eluted at a lower salt concentration (0.18 M KCl) during rapid chromatography on DEAE-Sephadex minicolumns (Fig. 3). The less acidic activated form could bind to CM-Sephadex, indicating the presence of both positively and negatively charged regions on its surface.

A positively charged region on the surface of the activated receptor had been suggested by the work of Milgrom and Atger (37). The establishment of such a region by Parchman and Litwack (45) opened an area of investigation regarding the nature of the positive charges. Although the work in this area has only just begun, preliminary evidence indicates that basic amino acid residues may be partially responsible for the increased positive charges on activated receptor. Studies by Litwack and Cake (27) and Parchman et al. (44) showed that activation can be stimulated by basic amino acids (Table 1) or inhibited by exposure to pyridoxal phosphate (Table 2). Since a low-molecular-weight inhibitor is thought to be associated with the unactivated form of the receptor, the above data could be interpreted to mean that the basic amino acids compete with receptor for binding to the inhibitor. In net, the dissociation of the inhibitor

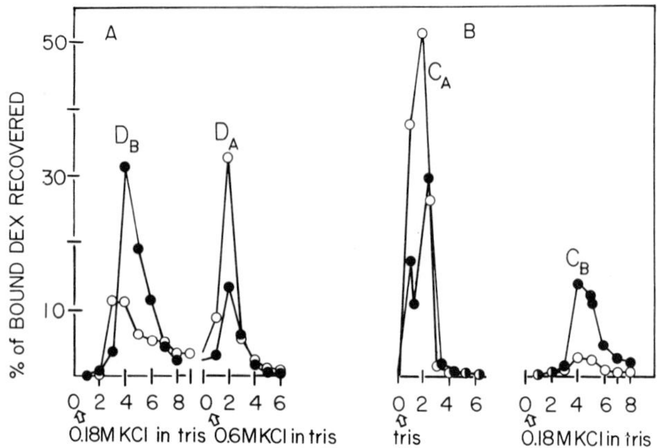

FIG. 3. Two-step chromatography. **A:** DEAE-Sephadex. Cytosol was incubated with 30 nM [^{3}H]dexamethasone for 90 min at 0°C. An aliquot was then heat-activated at 25°C for 30 min. Cytosol (0.5 ml) was applied to a minicolumn of DEAE-Sephadex and eluted in only two steps as indicated: D_A, acidic form; D_B, basic form. **B:** CM-Sephadex. One-half milliliter of the same cytosol as in A was applied to a minicolumn of CM-Sephadex and eluted in two steps as indicated: control cytosol *(open circles);* heat-activated cytosol *(filled circles);* C_A, acidic form; C_B, basic form. (From ref. 45 with permission.)

from the unactivated receptor would be favored. The mechanism to explain this reaction could be simply the formation of a Schiff base between the basic amine and a carbamoyl compound such as pyridoxal phosphate. In fact, pyridoxal phosphate is a good model for modulator. Because the rate of activation is greatly enhanced by Tris buffer at high pH (44) and Tris can form a Schiff base with pyridoxal-P, it is conjectured that the modulator may be bound to receptor through a Schiff base linkage.

More recent studies substantiate the involvement of basic amino acid residues in glucocorticoid-receptor activation. By using 1,2-cyclohexanedione, a compound known to react specifically with the guanidino group of arginine residues, it was shown that an arginine residue(s) was localized either at the ligand binding site or near it. Competition experiments between inhibitor and [^{3}H]TA showed that 1,2-cyclohexanedione was acting as a competitive inhibitor of ligand binding. Additional experiments using the activated receptor complex showed that 1,2-cyclohexanedione could also inhibit the binding of the receptor to DNA-cellulose (D. M. DiSorbo and G. Litwack, unpublished experiments). Thus the data suggest that an arginine residue(s) participates in both ligand binding to receptor and steroid-receptor binding to DNA.

Although the exact nature of receptor activation is still not clear, the accumulated evidence does suggest that the inactive receptor may be associated with a micromolecule and that dissociation of the two results in activation of the receptor. A model to explain this reaction is presented in Fig. 4. This model

TABLE 1. *Amino acid activation in PSM buffer*[a]

Sample	pH	Percentage of steroid-receptor complex bound to DNA-cellulose
Control	6.5	0.8
Control (after pH change)	7.3	2.4
+ Additions		
Alanine	7.3	2.4
Alanine (100 mM)	7.3	2.3
Monosodium glutamate	7.3	3.9
Lysine HCl	7.3	11
Arginine HCl	7.3	9.6
KCl	7.3	3.7
KCl (200 nM)	7.3	20

[a] Labeled PSM-buffered cytosol (pH 6.5) was adjusted to pH 7.3 with KOH. Additions were made as 1/10 volume dilutions of stock reagents giving final concentrations of 50 mM, except where indicated. Samples were assayed after 24 hr.

From ref. 44 with permission.

depicts passive transport of the steroid into the cell, where it associates with the inactive form of the receptor. The union of an active glucocorticoid (cortisol, TA) with receptor causes a conformational change in the complex (energy-dependent step), resulting in dissociation of modulator under activating conditions, with subsequent exposure of a positively charged region. The activated complex then translocates into the nucleus and binds to chromatin and/or DNA. Presumably the appearance of a group of positive charges on the surface of the steroid-receptor complex is sufficient to drive the translocation of the complex into the nucleus where a large number of negatively charged phosphate groups of DNA molecules could attract, by electrostatic forces, the activated steroid-receptor complex.

TABLE 2. *Inhibition of receptor binding to DNA-cellulose, nuclei, and phosphocellulose by pyridoxal 5′-phosphate*[a]

	DNA-cellulose	Nuclei	Phosphocellulose
Nonactivated	2.7 ± 0.4	1.0 ± 0.1	0.4 ± 0.2
Heat-activated	58.0 ± 2.8	25.9 ± 3.2	5.5 ± 0.6
Heat-activated + 10 mM PALP	4.0 ± 0.8	1.4 ± 0.5	1.3 ± 0.2
Inhibition by PALP (%)	97.6	98.4	82.4

[a] Rat liver cytosol (1 g liver + 1 ml BSM buffer) was incubated with 30 nM [^{3}H]dexamethasone for 3 hr at 0°C. A portion was incubated at 25°C for 45 min to heat-activate the steroid-receptor complexes. A portion of this was further incubated at 0°C for 30 min with 10 mM pyridoxal 5′-phosphate (PALP). Binding of these three fractions to DNA-cellulose, isolated rat liver nuclei, and phosphocellulose was determined. The results represent means ± SE of three separate experiments.

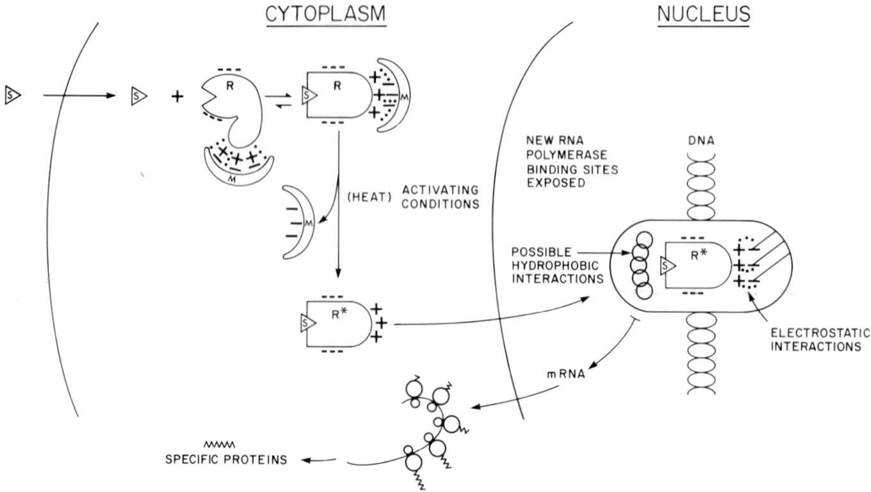

FIG. 4. Schematic representation of receptor-modulator model. Inactive receptor (R) is shown associated with modulator (M). Binding of an active glucocorticoid (S) to receptor induces a conformational change in the receptor (energy-dependent), with subsequent loss of modulator. The activated complex (R*) then has a region of positively charged groups that can interact with nuclear polyanions.

Although the evidence strongly favors the receptor-modulator model, conclusive proof for such a scheme ultimately depends on characterization of the modulator.

CONCLUSION

Studies on the mechanism of activation of the glucocorticoid-receptor complex have shown that liver cytosol contains a modulator that is associated with the receptor. Physiologically, the modulator could serve a dual role: (a) because of the binding of the modulator to receptor, the receptor would exist in a conformation readily able to interact with an active glucocorticoid; (b) the concentration of modulator in cytosol could control the rate of activation of the receptor. The implication of (a) is that ligand exchange should occur preferentially with the unactivated form of the steroid-receptor complex.

Since previous studies indicated that the steroid must be associated with receptor before the complex can be activated, evidence to substantiate the role of modulator in steroid-receptor interaction is not available. However, a recent report by Liu and Webb (31) does support the latter role for the modulator. These investigators compared the dexamethasone-receptor system of hepatic cells with Novikoff hepatoma cells. The levels of receptors were similar, but the *in vitro* translocation of the liver receptor complex into liver or hepatoma nuclei was three times greater than that of the receptor complex from the hepatoma. Further results were that the hepatoma cytosol contained an abnormally high concentration of a receptor translocation inhibitor and that possibily this elevated concentration of inhibitor could be responsible for the development of steroid resistance in some tumors.

It should be pointed out that the elevated levels of a receptor translocation inhibitor seen in the Novikoff hepatoma cells represent only one explanation for refractoriness to steroid treatment at the cellular level. Kenney et al. (22), using three lines of Morris hepatoma (7800, 9633, 9618A), showed that the non-responsiveness of hepatomas 9633 and 9618A to glucocorticoids was not due to either low receptor levels or inhibition of translocation of the receptor complex to the nucleus. Therefore the insensitivity of the hepatoma to glucocorticoids resides at the nuclear level and cannot be analyzed yet. This conclusion was reached in experiments on the developing rat (43).

The involvement of glucocorticoids in neoplastic tissue is a complex problem. Since other authors in this volume deal with this subject, we refer the reader to those chapters for more thorough treatment of the actions of glucocorticoids in neoplasms.

ACKNOWLEDGMENT

Research related to the material presented in this chapter in the authors' laboratory was supported by research grants AM-08350 and AM-13531 from the National Institute of Arthritis, Metabolism and Digestive Diseases and by CA-12227 from the National Cancer Institute to the Fels Research Institute.

REFERENCES

1. Atger, M., and Milgrom, E. (1976): Mechanism and kinetics of the thermal activation of glucocorticoid hormone receptor complex. *J. Biol. Chem.,* 251:4758–4762.
2. Bailly, A., Sallas, N., and Milgrom, E. (1977): A low molecular weight inhibition of steroid receptor activation. *J. Biol. Chem.,* 252:858–863.
3. Baxter, J. D. (1976): Glucocorticoid hormone action. *Pharmacol. Ther.* [*B*], 2:605–609.
4. Baxter, J. D., and Harris, A. W. (1975): Mechanism of glucocorticoid action: General features, with reference to steroid-mediated immunosuppression. *Transplant. Proc.,* 7:55–65.
5. Beato, M., Biesewig, D., Braendle, W., and Sekeris, C. E. (1969): On the mechanism of hormone action. XV. Subcellular distribution and binding of [1,2-^{3}H]cortisol in rat liver. *Biochim. Biophys. Acta,* 192:494–507.
6. Cake, M. H., Goidl, J. A., Parchman, L. G., and Litwack, G. (1976): Involvement of a low molecular weight component(s) in the mechanism of action of the glucocorticoid receptor. *Biochem. Biophys. Res. Commun.,* 71:45–52.
7. Cake, M., and Litwack, G. (1975): The glucocorticoid receptor. In: *Biochemical Actions of Hormones, Vol. 3,* edited by G. Litwack, pp. 319–386. Academic Press, New York.
8. Feigelson, M. (1964): Cortisone induced alterations in purine and RNA metabolism in liver and lymphoid tissues and their dependence on protein synthesis. *Fed. Proc.,* 23:481.
9. Feigelson, P., and Feigelson, M. (1964): Studies on the mechanism of cortisone action. In: *Actions of Hormones on Molecular Processes,* edited by G. Litwack and D. Kritchevsky, pp. 218–233. John Wiley & Sons, New York.

10. Fox, K. E., and Gabourel, J. D. (1967): Effect of cortisol on RNA polymerase system of rat thymus. *Mol. Pharmacol.,* 3:479.
11. Gabourel, J. D., and Fox, K. E. (1965): Effect of hydrocortisone on the size of rat thymus polysomes. *Biochim. Biophys. Res. Commun.,* 18:81–86.
12. Goidl, J. A., Cake, M. H., Dolan, K. P., Parchman, L. G., and Litwack, G. (1977): Activation of the rat liver glucocorticoid-receptor complex. *Biochemistry,* 16:2125–2130.
13. Granberg, J. P., and Ballard, P. L. (1977): The role of sulfhydryl groups in the binding of glucocorticoids by cytoplasmic receptors of lung and other mammalian tissues. *Endocrinology,* 100:1160–1168.
14. Granner, D. K., Hayashi, S., Thompson, E. B., and Tomkins, G. M. (1968): Stimulation of tyrosine aminotransferase synthesis by dexamethasone phosphate in cell culture. *J. Mol. Biol.,* 35:291–301.
15. Greenman, D. L., Wicks, W. D., and Kenney, F. T. (1965): Stimulation of ribonucleic acid synthesis by steroid hormones. II. High molecular weight components. *J. Biol. Chem.,* 240:4420–4426.
16. Hallahan, C., Young, D. A., and Munck, A. (1973): Time course of early events in the action of glucocorticoids on rat thymus cells *in vitro. J. Biol. Chem.,* 248:2922–2927.
17. Higgins, S. J., Rousseau, G. G., Baxter, J. D., and Tomkins, G. M. (1973): Early events in glucocorticoid action. Activation of the steroid receptor and its subsequent specific nuclear binding studied in a cell-free system. *J. Biol. Chem.,* 248:5866–5872.
18. Jensen, E. V. (1958): Studies of growth phenomena using tritium-labeled steroids. In: *Proceedings 4th International Congress on Biochemistry, Volume 15,* edited by O. Hoffmann-Ostenhof, p. 119. Pergamon Press, London.
19. Kenney, F. T. (1962): Induction of tyrosine α-ketoglutarate transaminase in rat liver. III. Immunochemical analysis. *J. Biol. Chem.,* 237:1610–1614.
20. Kenney, F. T. (1962): Induction of tyrosine α-ketoglutarate transaminase in rat liver. IV. Evidence for an increase in the rate of enzyme synthesis. *J. Biol. Chem.,* 237:3495–3498.
21. Kenney, F. T., and Kull, F. J. (1963): Hydrocortisone-stimulated synthesis of nuclear RNA in enzyme induction. *Proc. Natl. Acad. Sci. U.S.A.,* 50:493–499.
22. Kenney, F. T., Lane, S. E., Lee, K., and Ihle, J. N. (1976): Glucocorticoid control of gene expression. In: *Control Mechanisms in Cancer,* edited by W. E. Criss, T. Onto, and J. R. Sabine, pp. 25–35. Raven Press, New York.
23. King, R. J. B., and Mainwaring, W. I. P. (1974): Glucocorticoids. In: *Steroid-Cell Interactions,* pp. 102–161. University Park Press, Baltimore.
24. Knox, W. E., Auerbach, V. H., and Lin, E. C. C. (1956): Enzymatic and metabolic adaptations in animals. *Physiol. Rev.,* 36:164–254.
25. Korner, A. (1960): The role of the adrenal gland in the control of amino acid incorporation into protein of isolated rat liver microsomes. *J. Endocrinol.,* 21:177–189.
26. Lin, E. C. C., and Knox, W. E. (1957): Adaptation of the rat liver tyrosine α-ketoglutarate transaminase. *Biochim. Biophys. Acta,* 26:85–88.
27. Litwack, G., and Cake, M. H. (1977): DNA binding site of activated glucocorticoid receptor interaction with pyridoxal-P. *Fed. Proc.,* 36:911.
28. Litwack, G., Fiala, E. S., and Filosa, R. J. (1965): Intracellular binding of [^{14}C] hydrocortisone prior to enzymatic induction. *Biochim. Biophys. Acta,* 111:569–571.
29. Litwack, G., Filler, R., Rosenfield, S., Lichtash, N., Wishman, C., and Singer, S. (1973): Liver cytosol corticosteroid binder II, a hormone receptor. *J. Biol. Chem.,* 248:7481–7486.
30. Litwack, G., and Singer, S. (1972): Subcellular actions of glucocorticoids. In: *Biochemical Actions of Hormones, Vol. 2,* edited by G. Litwack, pp. 113–163. Academic Press, New York.
31. Liu, S. H., and Webb, T. E. (1977): Elevated concentration of a dexamethasone receptor translocation inhibitor in Novikoff hepatoma cells. *Cancer Res.,* 37:1763–1767.
32. Makman, M. H., Dvorkin, B., and White, A. (1966): Alterations in proteins and nucleic acid metabolism of thymocytes produced by adrenal steroids *in vitro. J. Biol. Chem.,* 241:1646–1648.
33. Makman, M. H., Dvorkin, B., and White, A. (1967): Studies of the mode of action of adrenal steroids on lymphocytes. *Recent Prog. Horm. Res.,* 23:195–227.
34. Makman, M. H., Dvorkin, B., and White, A. (1968): Influence of cortisol on the utilization of precursors of nucleic acids and protein by lymphoid cells *in vitro. J. Biol. Chem.,* 243:1485–1497.

35. Marver, D., Stewart, J., Funder, J. W., Feldman, D., and Edelman, I. S. (1974): Renal aldosterone receptors: Studies with [^{3}H]aldosterone and the antimineralocorticoid [^{3}H]spirolactone (SC-26304). *Proc. Natl. Acad. Sci. U.S.A.,* 71:1431–1435.
36. Milgrom, E., and Atger, M. (1975): Receptor translational inhibitor and apparent saturability of nuclear acceptor. *J. Steroid Biochem.,* 6:487–492.
37. Milgrom, E., Atger, M., and Baulieu, E. E. (1973): Acidophilic activation of steroid hormone receptors. *Biochemistry,* 12:5198–5205.
38. Morita, Y., and Munck, A. (1964): Effect of glucocorticoids *in vivo* and *in vitro* on net glucose uptake and amino acid incorporation by rat-thymus cells. *Biochim. Biophys. Acta,* 93:150–157.
39. Munck, A. (1968): Metabolic site and time course of cortisol action on glucose uptake, lactic acid output and glucose-6-phosphate levels of rat thymus cells *in vitro. J. Biol. Chem.,* 243:1039–1042.
40. Munck, A., and Brinck-Johnson, T. (1968): Specific and nonspecific physiochemical interactions of glucocorticoids and related steroids with rat thymus cells *in vitro. J. Biol. Chem.,* 243:5556–5565.
41. Munck, A., and Wira, C. (1971): Glucocorticoid receptors in rat thymus cells. In: *Advances in the Biosciences: Schering Workshop on Steroid Hormone Receptors, Vol. 7,* edited by G. Raspe, pp. 301–327. Pergamon Press, Oxford.
42. Nakagawa, S., and White, A. (1966): Acute decrease in RNA polymerase activity of rat thymus in response to cortisol injection. *Proc. Natl. Acad. Sci. U.S.A.,* 55:900–904.
43. Parchman, L. G., Cake, M. H., and Litwack, G. (1978): Glucocorticoid receptor in development. *Mech. Ageing Dev.,* 7:227–240.
44. Parchman, L. G., Goidl, J. A., and Litwack, G. (1977): Basic amino acids stimulate the activation of the glucocorticoid receptor complex. *F.E.B.S. Lett.,* 79:25–28.
45. Parchman, L. G., and Litwack, G. (1977): Resolution of activated and unactivated forms of the glucocorticoid receptor from rat liver. *Arch. Biochem. Biophys.,* 183:374–382.
46. Parchman, L. G., Markovic, R. D., and Litwack, G. (1977): Multiple forms of the glucocorticoid receptor determined by its state of activation. In: *Multiplicity of Steroid Hormone Receptors,* edited by M. K. Agarwal, pp. 1–15. Elsevier, Amsterdam.
47. Rees, A., and Bell, P. A. (1975): The involvement of receptor sulphydryl groups in the binding of steroids to the cytoplasmic glucocorticoid receptor from rat thymus. *Biochim. Biophys. Acta,* 411:121–132.
48. Rousseau, G. G. (1975): General review. Interaction of steroids with hepatoma cells. Molecular mechanisms of glucocorticoid hormone action. *J. Steroid Biochem.,* 6:75–89.
49. Rousseau, G. G., Baxter, J. D., and Tomkins, G. M. (1972): Glucocorticoid receptors: Relations between steroid binding and biological effects. *J. Mol. Biol.,* 67:99–115.
50. Samuels, H. H., and Tomkins, G. M. (1970): Relation of steroid structure to enzyme induction in hepatoma tissue culture cells. *J. Mol. Biol.,* 52:57–74.
51. Sarkar, P. K., and Lydigsen, J. (1976): Hydrocortisone receptors and their nuclear acceptor sites in the developing chick retina. *Biochem. Biophys. Res. Commun.,* 72:1084–1090.
52. Schimke, R. T., and Doyle, D. (1970): Control of enzyme levels in animal tissue. *Annu. Rev. Biochem.,* 30:929–976.
53. Schimke, R. T., Sweeney, E. W., and Berlin, C. M. (1965): The roles of synthesis and degradation in the control of rat liver tryptophan pyrrolase. *J. Biol. Chem.,* 240:322–331.
54. Simons, S. S., Jr., Martinez, H. M., Garcea, R. L., Baxter, J. D., and Tomkins, G. M. (1976): Interactions of glucocorticoid-steroid complexes with acceptor sites. *J. Biol. Chem.,* 251:334–343.
55. Singer, S., Becker, J. E., and Litwack, G. (1973): The principal glucocorticoid binding macromolecule in hepatoma cells in culture is similar to corticosteroid binder II of rat liver cytosol. *Biochem. Biophys. Res. Commun.,* 52:943–950.
56. Thompson, E. B., and Lippman, M. E. (1974): Progress in endocrinology and metabolism. Mechanism of action of glucocorticoids. *Metabolism,* 23:159–202.
57. Thompson, E. B., Tomkins, G. M., and Curran, J. F. (1966): Induction of tyrosine α-ketoglutarate transaminase by steroid hormones in a newly established tissue culture cell line. *Proc. Natl. Acad. Sci. U.S.A.,* 56:296–301.
58. Tomkins, G. M., Thompson, E. B., Hayashi, S., Gelehrter, T., Granner, D., and Peterkofsky, B. (1966): Tyrosine transaminase induction in mammalian cells in tissue culture. *Cold Spring Harbor Symp. Quant. Biol.,* 31:349–360.

59. Turnell, R. W., Kaiser, N., Milholland, R. J., and Rosen, F. (1974): Glucocorticoid receptors in rat thymocytes. Interactions with the antiglucocorticoid cortexolone and mechanism of its action. *J. Biol. Chem.*, 249:1133–1138.
60. White, A., and Dougherty, T. F. (1947): Role of the adrenal cortex and the thyroid in the mobilization of nitrogen from the tissues in fasting. *Endocrinology*, 41:230–242.
61. Young, D. A. (1969): Glucocorticoid action on rat thymus cells. Interrelationship between carbohydrate, protein and adenine nucleotide metabolism and cortisol effects in these functions *in vitro*. *J. Biol. Chem.*, 244:2210–2217.
62. Young, D. A. (1970): Glucocorticoid action on rat thymocytes. II. Interrelationship between ribonucleic acid and protein metabolism and between cortisol substrate effects on these metabolic parameters *in vitro*. *J. Biol. Chem.*, 245:2747–2752.
63. Young, D. A. (1970): 6-min stimulatory effects of cortisol *in vitro* on precursor incorporation into RNA and protein in rat thymus cells. *Fed. Proc.*, 29:778 (abstract).
64. Young, H. A., Parks, W. P., and Scolnick, E. M. (1975): Effect of chemical inactivating agents on glucocorticoid receptor proteins in mouse and hamster cells. *Proc. Natl. Acad. Sci. U.S.A.*, 72:3060–3064.

ADDENDUM

Since submission of this chapter, new evidence suggests that pyridoxal-P may be identical to the endogenous "modulator." Moreover, cytosols from pyridoxine-deficient, adrenalectomized rats show greater capacity of steroid-receptor complex to bind to DNA after heat activation than cytosols from adrenalectomized controls. Since heating is still required to activate receptor complexes in deficient cytosols, it appears that modulator binds to activated but not to unactivated steroid-receptor complex. In consequence, activation *in vitro* involves dissociation of modulator from activated receptor complexes as well as conversion of unactivated receptor complexes to a conformation enabling binding to DNA (D. M. DiSorbo, D. Phelps, and G. Litwack, *unpublished data*).

Endocrine Control in Neoplasia, edited by
R. K. Sharma and W. E. Criss.
Raven Press, New York © 1978.

Glucocorticoid Receptor Function in Leukemic Cells

Thomas J. Schmidt and E. Brad Thompson

Laboratory of Biochemistry, National Cancer Institute, National Institutes of Health, Bethesda, Maryland 20014

Although glucocorticoid hormones elicit a series of profound intracellular responses in lymphoid cells ultimately resulting in cytolysis, the exact mechanism(s) of this induced lysis is unknown. However, it is clear that most, if not all of these effects, are mediated through specific cytoplasmic glucocorticoid receptors which when complexed with active glucocorticoids, are translocated to the nucleus where they bind to chromatin. A transplantable mouse lymphoma (P1798), several mouse lymphoid cell lines (S49, W7), and recently, a human leukemic cell line (CEM) have been used as *in vitro* model systems to study the function of glucocorticoid receptors in mediating lymphocytolysis and the genetics of steroid resistance. From the results with these cells, it is clear that resistance is often correlated with loss of receptor sites. No clone of cells lacking receptors or showing abnormal nuclear transfer has to date been shown to be sensitive to glucocorticoids. On the other hand, it has been shown in these and other cells that receptor presence and normal nuclear transfer can be associated with steroid resistance. Although mitogen stimulation of normal human lymphocytes increases the concentration of glucocorticoid receptors, macromolecular synthesis in both stimulated and unstimulated normal lymphocytes is inhibited by glucocorticoids.

Using whole-cell and cell-free techniques, several laboratories have quantified and partially characterized the saturable, high-affinity, specific glucocorticoid receptors in a variety of human leukemias, including adult and childhood lymphoblastic leukemia, adult myelogenous leukemia, chronic lymphocytic leukemia, and the Sézary syndrome. The presence of receptors in some of these leukemias, particularly those of T-cell origin, has been correlated with *in vitro* inhibitory responses to glucocorticoids. Thus measurement of functional receptor levels may serve as a useful tool in predicting the responsiveness of leukemia patients to glucocorticoid therapy and may enable one to avoid the possible side effects of unnecessary steroid treatment.

INTRODUCTION

Although it has been over 40 years since the inhibitory effects of adrenal hormones on lymphoid tissues were first described (65,90), the exact mechanism by which these effects are elicited remains unknown (5,17,104). Despite this lack of thorough understanding concerning their mode of action, the ability of glucocorticoids to inhibit the growth of lymphoid tissues has found important practical applications in the treatment of certain leukemias (17,31). Although steroids are now used in combination with other drugs, results obtained during the single-drug era indicate that whereas certain leukemic cell populations are rapidly killed by steroids, others are resistant (57). It was also found that many leukemic patients who initially responded to glucocorticoid therapy later became unresponsive (108), which suggests that sensitive leukemic cells eventually become resistant or are replaced by resistant cells.

Despite the fact that modern treatment schedules with glucocorticoids usually are designed to minimize undesirable side effects which may include gastric ulcers, Cushing's syndrome, suppression of immune responsiveness, heightened risk of infection, psychosis, and others (48), these side effects may occasionally occur; in any case, the omission of a potentially harmful drug from the therapeutic regimen remains a desirable goal. Various tests have been applied to ascertain the cytotoxicity of glucocorticoids on leukemic lymphocytes *in vitro,* but these tests have proved to be of only limited value (18,20). Numerous studies have shown that quantitation of estrogen receptors in tumor cells from breast cancer patients is very useful in predicting the effectiveness of therapeutic endocrine manipulations (64). Encouraged by these results, several laboratories have attempted analogous studies on glucocorticoid receptors in human leukemic cells in the hope of finding a correlation with clinical responsiveness to glucocorticoids. In this chapter, we shall review the published reports dealing with quantitation and function of glucocorticoid receptors in various types of human leukemia and in appropriate *in vitro* model systems.

MODE OF ACTION OF GLUCOCORTICOIDS

Biochemical studies on the mode of action of glucocorticoids, as well as steroids in general, have suggested the following sequence of events: diffusion of glucocorticoids into the responsive cell, binding to specific cytoplasmic receptor proteins, "activation" of the receptor-hormone complex, entry of the activated complex into the cell nucleus, and subsequent association with DNA-containing nuclear binding sites (7,34,45,69). The exact mechanism(s) beyond this nuclear binding by which glucocorticoids kill lymphoid cells is not known. Based on experiments using inhibitors of RNA (63,66,67) and protein (63,82) synthesis, it has been suggested that specific RNA(s) and/or protein(s) are induced by glucocorticoids (32,62,100). Clearly this model relies heavily on analogy with the more thoroughly documented increases in specific mRNAs and proteins in inducible, non-inhibited, nonlymphoid target tissues in response to a variety of steroids (9,14, 61,75,76,80,88). Through this putative initial protein induction, glucocorticoids ultimately exert inhibitory effects *in vivo* and *in vitro* on a number of biosynthetic and transport functions in lymphoid tissues, resulting in cytolysis. Some of the basic responses noted in lymphoid tissues following exposure to glucocorticoids include inhibition of growth and DNA synthesis (35,36), inhibition of RNA (77) and protein synthesis (44,82), and decreased uptake of amino acids (3), nucleic acid precursors (77,82), and glucose (67,82,102), resulting in inhibition of ATP generation. Unlike these processes, glucocorticoid-induced inhibition of RNA polymerase activity does not require prior protein synthesis (63). However, since the induced protein(s) that is believed to be responsible for the majority of the glucocorticoid-induced inhibitory effects has not been specifically detected, and since these effects are numerous, it has not been possible to assign a primary role to any one of these responses. Several other effects have also been postulated as alternative mechanisms of glucocorticoid-induced cytolysis. Giddings and Young (30) reported a glucocorticoid-induced increase in nuclear fragility that does not require a carbohydrate energy source to become apparent. It has also been suggested that enhanced Ca^{2+} uptake (41) and increased acid ribonuclease activity (2,60) are partially responsible for the lytic effect. Behrens and Hollander (8) detected a decrease in the negative charge of sialoglycoproteins on the surface of sensitive lymphosarcoma cells exposed to glucocorticoids that may or may not be related to the subsequent lysis. Turnell and Burton (107) concluded that cell lysis is attributable to the release of free fatty acids that damage the nuclear membrane, resulting in karyorrhexis and cytolysis. Although these investigators speculated that this increased release of fatty acids from triglycerides may be modulated by a glucocorticoid-sensitive lipase that responds either directly to glucocorticoids or indirectly through glucocorticoid-induced protein synthesis, such a sensitive lipase has not been demonstrated.

Thus it is still not clear exactly how glucocorticoids cause lymphocytolysis, despite the fact that they evoke a number of profound intracellular responses. It is also unclear whether some effects are responsible for a cascade of other effects or whether they are all induced coordinately by some basic interaction of glucocorticoids with lymphoid cells. Despite this uncertainty, it is clear that many, if not all, of these responses to glucocorticoids are mediated through specific intracellular receptors.

MODEL SYSTEMS

Rodent Cell Lines and Transplantable Tumors

Several mouse lymphoma cell lines have been used to study the mechanism(s) of glucocorticoid-induced cytolysis and the genetics of glucocorticoid resistance. Both solid and ascitic forms of the P1798 tumor, which originated in the thymus of a BALB/c mouse after administration of diethylstilbestrol (59), have been used to study the biochemistry and genetics of steroid action. Rosen and his colleagues extensively studied both glucocorticoid-sensitive and -insensitive sublines developed from this cell line and showed that *in vitro* exposure of the cells to pharmacological doses of glucocorticoids produces significant inhibition of DNA, RNA, and protein metabolism (81,82,84) and glucose uptake (81–83) in glucocorticoid-sensitive tumors. These inhibitory effects of glucocorticoids were also correlated with growth inhibition, regression, and eventual dissolution of sensitive tumors *in vivo.*

Other studies have concentrated on the isolation, characterization, and quantitation of specific glucocorticoid receptors in sensitive and resistant lines of this same tumor. Analysis of binding of glucocorticoids in P1798 tumors was initiated by Hollander and Chiu (37), who demonstrated that the concentration of glucocorticoid binding sites in the sensitive subline was twice that found in the resistant subline. The physiochemical properties of these receptors were elucidated by Kirkpatrick et al. (46,47) and Kaiser et al. (42) and were found to be similar to those of receptors in normal lymphoid tissues. When tumor cells from both sensitive and resistant lines were incubated with radiolabeled triamcinolone at 0° C, extracted with a buffer containing 0.15 M KCl, and analyzed on sucrose gradients, a complex sedimenting at 4S to 5S was identified. Under low-salt conditions, bound radioactivity sedimented at 7S to 8S (42). Although the receptor complexes from the resistant cell lines showed small but statistically significant differences in their sedimentation coefficients, no differences in equilibrium dissociation constants between the glucocorticoid-sensitive and -resistant lines were found. Although these authors favored the view that the receptors in the resistant cells were functional, they recognized that the altered sedimentation coefficients could reflect some subtle but significant change. Their experiments designed to study the *in vivo* effects of glucocorticoids on the number of binding sites in the various tumors suggested that the resistant tumors consisted of a mixture of cells and that when the cortisol-sensitive cells were eliminated, resistance was more clearly associated with decreased receptor concentration.

The S49 line of established mouse lymphoma cells that are normally killed by glucocorticoids (40) has been used to study the possible mechanisms of steroid resistance. Using a single-step selection procedure, Sibley and Tomkins (96,97) were able to isolate a number of steroid-resistant clones that were classified as r^- (deficient in specific cytoplasmic receptors for steroid binding), nt^- (incapable of transferring the normal amount of receptor-steroid complex into the nucleus), or d^- (deathless, i.e., deficient in the reactions subsequent to nuclear localization of the complex). Later, a subcategory of d^- was reclassified as nt^i (increased nuclear transfer of steroid-receptor complex) (111). When the relative proportions of these variants were determined in a steady-state population, 80% were found to be r^-, and the remaining were equally divided between nt^- and d^-. These results are consistent with the concept that formation of the hormone-receptor complex is required for glucocorticoid action, since those cells that lacked receptors were insensitive. The existence of nt^- cells that contain receptors also indicates that nuclear uptake is required for glucocorticoid-induced lysis. However, the presence of d^- cells, in which nuclear binding occurs without causing lysis, suggests that binding of steroid-receptor complex in the nucleus, although necessary, is not sufficient for hormone action.

Gehring and Tomkins (29) continued to study the resistant mutants defective in the nuclear transfer reaction (nt$^-$). Their studies showed that dexamethasone bound to the specific cytoplasmic receptors of these mutant cells with the same affinity as to the receptors of sensitive parental cells. The activated dexamethasone-receptor complex from these sensitive cells bound to isolated nuclei from either sensitive or resistant cells, whereas the complex from the resistant cells failed to bind to nuclei from either source. The complex from the resistant cells also displayed reduced binding affinity for isolated homologous and heterologous DNA. These results suggest that the normal glucocorticoid receptor may consist of two active domains, one for steroid binding and the other for interaction with nuclear acceptor sites, and that the receptors of nt$^-$ cells may be defective only in the latter activity.

In addition to studying the nt$^-$-resistant S49 mutants, Yamamoto et al. (111) further studied the resistant mutants that demonstrated increased nuclear transfer (nt^i) relative to the parental line. They found that receptors of the nt^i cells showed higher DNA-binding affinity than receptors from the sensitive parental cells and that both nt$^-$ and nt^i receptor complexes showed altered sedimentation properties on sucrose gradients. These workers postulated that lymphocytolysis requires binding of steroid-receptor complexes to a limited number of specific DNA sites and that the increased nuclear binding of the nt^i receptors is the result of increased affinity for nonspecific DNA binding sites. The net effect is thus paradoxical: increased total nuclear binding masking loss of specific binding. Further analysis of the d$^-$ class of resistant cells has not been presented. Thus the major groups of resistant cells have been shown to have reduced numbers or altered characteristics of their receptors.

Bourgeois and Newby (10) recently compared another glucocorticoid-sensitive mouse thymoma line, W7, with the S49 cell line. They found that the receptors of both cell lines had the same affinity for dexamethasone ($K_d = 1.3 \pm 0.3 \times 10^{-8}$ M) but that the W7 cells contained twice as many receptors and were sensitive to lower concentrations of dexamethasone. When placed in 10^{-6} M dexamethasone, W7 cells gave rise to resistant clones very rarely ($< 3 \times 10^{-9}$/cell/generation). However, by first selecting for resistance to much lower concentrations of steroids, they were able to isolate derivatives of W7 that were similar to the S49 cells, i.e., with higher resistance than the parental W7 line and approximately half the receptor content. Like the S49 cell line, the partially resistant W7 variants gave rise to fully resistant derivatives at a high rate (2×10^{-6}/cell/generation). They interpreted these experiments as suggesting that in lymphoid cells, the inactivation of glucocorticoid receptor leading to resistance to high concentrations of steroid may proceed in two steps:

$$r^{+/+} \rightarrow r^{+/-} \rightarrow r^{-/-}$$

Each step would thus correspond to inactivation of one of the two functional alleles, r$^+$, of a gene coding for the receptor, or a functional receptor subunit. Since the probability of each allele being damaged was assumed to be constant and independent, the development of the $r^{-/-}$ state would require two genetic events and thus would occur with a low frequency in diploid cells. The semiresistant $r^{+/-}$ heterozygotes would contain half the receptors present in the wild type, as would be expected from a gene dosage effect. Bourgeois and Newby further concluded from these results that the receptor gene, r, is autosomal and that inactivation of the gene is a recessive genetic event. It was pointed out by these investigators that although this inactivation could result from recessive mutations, it could also occur by chromosome loss or translocation. Although nothing is known concerning the frequency of translocation in these cells, the karyotypes of three of the W7 derivative lines failed to reveal any obvious loss of chromosomes.

Human Leukemic Cells in Culture

Most recently, Norman and Thompson (72) characterized a glucocorticoid-sensitive human leukemic T-cell line, CEM, originally isolated from a young female patient with acute lymphoblastic leukemia (25,48). Uncloned CEM cells were obtained from two sources. Those obtained from the American Type Culture Collection contained receptors but were completely unresponsive to glucocorticoids (55). However, CEM cells obtained from Dr. Dean Mann of the National Cancer Institute showed some growth inhibition by glucocorticoids (72). Since these latter cells had been grown continuously for many years, ample time had passed for the accumulation of resistant mutants. Norman and Thompson (72) therefore cloned this partially sensitive cell line and isolated a number of sensitive clones. The growth of a typical sensitive clone, CEM C7, was shown to be completely blocked by 2 to 3 days of exposure to 10^{-6} M dexamethasone, and after 4 to 5 days, these cells became pyknotic and lysed. Polysome profiles of CEM C7 cells were analyzed after exposure to dexamethasone (Fig. 1). After 24 hr, there was a marked loss of polyribosomal ribosomes, as compared with controls, whereas monomeric ribosomes were increasing. After 48 hr, the conversion of polyribosomal ribosomes to monomers was complete. These changes in sedimentation pattern are consistent with either defective initiation of protein synthesis or decreased availability of mRNA. Since ribonuclease damage to polysomes would produce a different pattern characterized by an increased proportion of small polysomes (71), it is unlikely that activation of ribonuclease was responsible for this effect of glucocorticoids on CEM cells.

Cytosol and whole-cell receptor analyses comparing sensitive with resistant clones demonstrated the presence in the sensitive CEM C7 cells of specific glucocorticoid receptors with a dissociation constant for dexamethasone of about 1.3×10^{-8} M. The specificity of these receptors was further verified through competition studies in which it was shown that only biologically active glucocorticoids were capable of displacing radiolabeled dexamethasone from the receptors

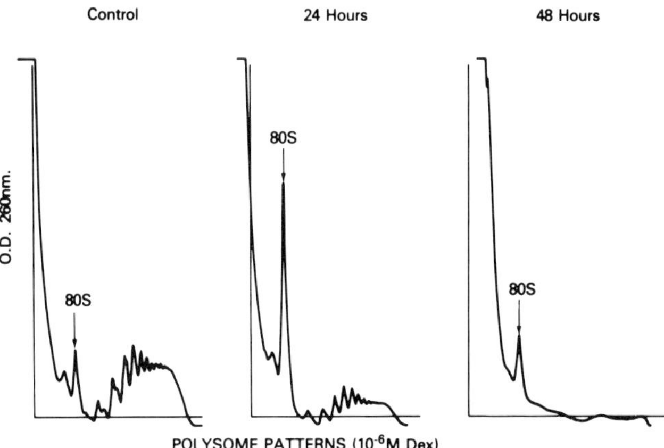

FIG. 1. Effect of dexamethasone on polysome profiles obtained from CEM cells (clone C7). Monomeric ribosomes are marked 80S. **Left:** Control cells. **Center:** 24-hr treatment with 10^{-6} M dexamethasone. **Right:** 48-hr treatment with 10^{-6} M dexamethasone. (From Norman and Thompson, ref. 72, with permission.)

or inhibiting cloning of the sensitive cells in agarose. The synthetic glucocorticoid dexamethasone was found to be a potent inhibitor when the CEM C7 cells were cloned in agarose, showing a substantial effect at a concentration of 7×10^{-9} M (Fig. 2).

The potential usefulness of this human cell line for future studies concerning the function of glucocorticoid receptors in leukemic cells is clear. Not only are there differences between the leukemias of humans and rodents, there are also species differences in the sensitivity of normal lymphoid cells to glucocorticoids (17). One difference already noted between CEM cells and the mouse lines is that whereas the CEM cells develop resistance to 10^{-6} M dexamethasone at a rate of about 8×10^{-6}/cell/generation (similar to the presumptive haploid mouse lines), they contain about 25,000 receptor sites per cell (J. M. Harmon and E. B. Thompson, unpublished results), a concentration much like that of the presumptive diploid W7 mouse line. Various possibilities may explain this observation. The quantitative correlations between receptor content and steroid sensitivity may not be identical in the two species. Human diploid cells may contain 50,000 sites/cell, or still other mechanisms may be involved in establishing cell receptor levels. Whatever the explanation, it appears that CEM cells have high receptor levels and also develop resistance at a high rate. Thus it is possible that factors other than simple ploidy of the receptor gene may influence the development of resistance in human cells. The CEM cell line is therefore being used to study the genetics of steroid resistance as well as the potency of several chemotherapeutic drugs used as single agents or in combination with glucocorticoids (M. R. Norman and associates, unpublished data).

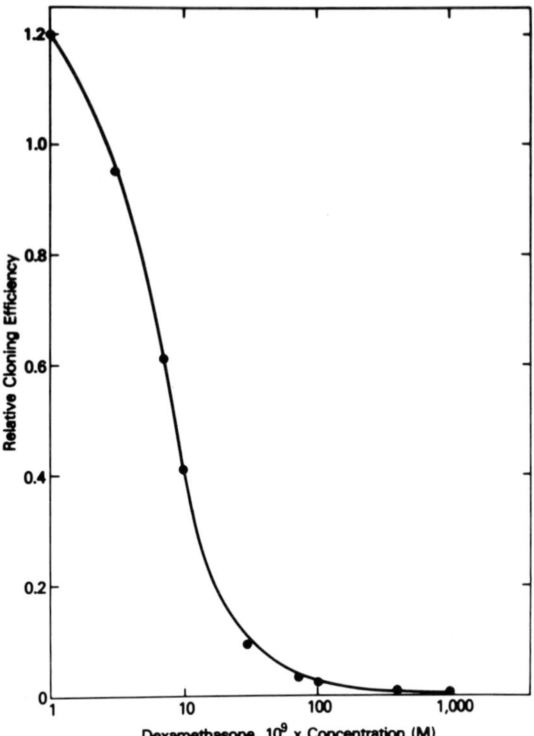

FIG. 2. Effects of dexamethasone on cloning efficiency of CEM cells (clone C7) in agarose gels. Relative cloning efficiency refers to cloning efficiency of treated cells divided by that of untreated cells. In the absence of steroid, cells cloned with an efficiency of 37%. For each steroid concentration, the number of cells plated was adjusted to give between 10 and 100 colonies. Each point represents the mean of four plates. (From Norman and Thompson, ref. 72, with permission.)

GLUCOCORTICOID RECEPTORS IN NORMAL HUMAN LYMPHOCYTES

Since glucocorticoids are known to exert suppressive effects on certain lymphocytes of most species (17), it is appropriate that a brief discussion of the role of glucocorticoid receptors in mitogen-stimulated and unstimulated human lymphocytes precede a discussion of human leukemias. It will become clear in the following discussion that most investigators agree that mitogen stimulation increases the concentration of glucocorticoid receptors per cell and that macromolecular biosynthesis in both stimulated and unstimulated lymphocytes is inhibited by glucocorticoids.

Prior to receptor studies it became clear that glucocorticoid sensitivity, in addition to varying with the state of lymphocyte differentiation and maturation, also varies with the state of antigen- or mitogen-induced activation. Nowell

(73) showed *in vitro* that prednisolone 21-phosphate reduced the number of mitoses induced in human peripheral blood lymphocytes by phytohemagglutinin (PHA). He also showed that this inhibition required the presence of glucocorticoids during the first 24 hr of exposure to PHA. These results were confirmed by Tormey et al. (105), who showed that prednisolone 21-phosphate inhibited incorporation of radiolabeled thymine and cytidine into PHA-stimulated lymphocytes and that delayed addition of glucocorticoids reduced this inhibition. These and other studies contributed to the basic concept that glucocorticoid sensitivity varies with the state of immunological activation of the cell. According to this model, lymphocytes are believed to be insensitive until they are stimulated by a specific antigen or mitogen, which induces an early glucocorticoid-sensitive phase before resistance again predominates during morphologic blast transformation and mitosis (5,17).

Contrary to this general model, however, Smith et al. (98) recently reported that cultured human lymphocytes are sensitive to dexamethasone-mediated metabolic inhibition regardless of their state of activation. They also demonstrated that blastic transformation is associated with a striking increase in the number of receptor sites per cell. Although PHA produced the greatest increase (over sixfold), other mitogens also increased the number of binding sites (Table 1). Steroid competition studies and the time course of nuclear binding at 37°C also indicated that the glucocorticoid receptors in the mitogen-stimulated lymphocytes were similar to receptors in normal lymphocytes (68) and different from those in unstimulated cells only by their greater number. Adler et al. (1) reported similar changes in receptor content in PHA-stimulated human lymphocytes. However, Smith et al. (98) found that the inhibitory effects of glucocorticoids did not require prior exposure of lymphocytes to mitogenic stimuli. Thus, although incorporation of radiolabeled uridine and thymidine was significantly depressed if dexamethasone (10^{-7}M) was added after exposure to

TABLE 1. *Effects of mitogenic stimuli on nuclear dexamethasone binding sites*[a]

		Dexamethasone binding sites per cell		
Stimulus	Number of experiments	Unstimulated	Stimulated	Stimulated/ unstimulated
Con A	7	3151 ± 726[b]	9,483 ± 1,513[b]	3.79 ± 0.71
PHA	1	1640	10,300	6.28
PWM	1	2490	6,750	2.71
MLC	2	1,541; 4,070[c]	3,248; 11,160[c]	2.11; 2.71[c]

[a] Human lymphocytes were obtained from defibrinated fresh blood by discontinuous density-gradient separation over Ficoll-Hypaque, and monocytes were removed by incubation on plastic for 18 hr. Nuclear binding of dexamethasone was determined as described by Smith et al. (98).

[b] Mean ± SEM.

[c] Values shown are ranges for first and second subjects, respectively, taken from Smith et al. (98).

conconavalin A (Con A) for 6 or 19 hr, unstimulated human lymphocytes cultured with or without dexamethasone (10^{-10} to 10^{-6} M) also revealed dose-dependent suppression of incorporation of radiolabeled uridine and leucine measured after 24, 48, and 72 hr of culture. Dexamethasone was also found to decrease glucose uptake by approximately the same absolute amount in both Con-A-stimulated and unstimulated lymphocytes. Thus, these results indicate that human lymphocytes are equally sensitive to glucocorticoid suppression at all stages of activation, despite the large increase in receptor concentration following mitogen stimulation. These workers believed that the increase in receptor concentration they observed after stimulation might reflect variations in receptor number with phases of the cell cycle, since acute stimulation with mitogen might result in a degree of synchronization. This appears to be possible, since Cidlowski and Michaels (16) reported that in synchronized HeLa cultures there is doubling of the receptor number per cell as the cells pass through late G_1, followed by a return to the original number after mitosis.

Neifeld et al. (70) also reported that PHA stimulation of normal human lymphocytes results in a twofold to threefold increase (normal lymphocytes contained approximately 2,700 sites per cell) in glucocorticoid receptor activity within 16 hr of culture. As expected, significant competition for radiolabeled dexamethasone binding in these cells was not observed with steroids lacking glucocorticoid activity. Their studies with cycloheximide and actinomycin D also suggested that this PHA stimulation of receptors probably is not a direct activation of preexisting receptors, since RNA synthesis and protein synthesis are required. However, since these antibiotics also block mitogen-induced blastic transformation, the exact mechanism of mitogen regulation of receptors remains unclear. Although in this study Neifeld et al. did not measure the sensitivity of normal peripheral lymphocytes to glucocorticoids, they speculated that the quantitative increase in binding sites following addition of mitogen might correlate with increased inhibition of protein and RNA synthesis. This conclusion agreed with an earlier report showing that unstimulated human lynphocytes had a basal level of RNA synthesis that was not affected by glucocorticoids, although hydrocortisone completely inhibited PHA-induced RNA synthesis (74). More recently, however, Lippman and Barr (52) clearly showed that *in vitro* nucleoside incorporation into purified unstimulated human T and non-T lymphocytes is significantly inhibited by glucocorticoids. Whether mitogen stimulation would result in a further increase in sensitivity was not ascertained.

Obviously one important factor that must be considered when comparing receptor contents and sensitivities of stimulated and unstimulated cells is the purity of the lymphocyte preparations used. In an earlier study Homo et al. (38), using a whole-cell binding assay, found that normal human lymphocytes contain glucocorticoid receptors, although dose-response relationships and specificity were not ascertained. These investigators used Ficoll-Hypaque (11) to separate mononuclear cells, but such preparations may contain up to 10% monocytes as well as a significant number of granulocytes. Since Lippman and Barr

(52) have recently shown that monocytes may contain about 8,000 glucocorticoid binding sites per cell, it is obvious that thorough characterization of the cell population being studied may be critical. In the previously discussed report, Smith et al. (98) obtained mononuclear cells by discontinuous density-gradient separation over Ficoll-Hypaque, and monocytes were removed by incubation on plastic for 18 hr, leaving a cell population consisting of 94% or more lymphocytes. However, Neifeld and colleagues separated lymphocytes using a glass-wool column technique modified after the method of Rabinowitz (79), and the resultant cell population consisted of over 99.5% small lymphocytes (T cells 65 to 75%; B cells 20 to 30%), as verified by differential cell counts on Wright-stained smears. As was noted previously, both stimulated and unstimulated lymphocytes isolated using this improved procedure contained glucocorticoid receptors.

GLUCOCORTICOID RECEPTORS IN HUMAN LEUKEMIC LYMPHOBLASTS

Acute Lymphocytic Leukemia

Shortly after their introduction as chemotherapeutic agents, corticosteroids were found to be effective against acute lymphocytic leukemia (ALL). During this single-drug era it was shown that steroids alone used daily in the first course of treatment produced a complete remission rate between 45 and 65% (57), although when steroids were used a second time after the patient had suffered a relapse, the rate of remission induction fell to about 25% (108). In subsequent years, it was shown that glucocorticoids used in combination with other agents were superior to single drugs in the treatment of ALL. The most successful early combination proved to be prednisone plus vincristine, a combination that induced remissions in more than 80% of affected children (33); this combination of drugs is still a standard regimen for initial remission induction. Today other drugs such as daunorubicin, methotrexate, mercaptopurine, and L-asparaginase have also been added to some protocols, and with such multiple-agent protocols the rate of remission induction may rise to 88% or even 100% (26,31,33).

Because cytoplasmic receptors seem to be essential for lymphocytolysis in rodent cells (as discussed previously), and because it would be desirable to omit any ineffective drug from combination therapy, Lippman et al. (53,54) decided to examine cells from ALL patients for glucocorticoid receptors to determine if their presence correlated with a favorable clinical response to glucocorticoids. Using a modified competitive binding assay (4,85) they detected, quantified, and partially characterized glucocorticoid receptors in cytosols prepared from human lymphoblastic leukemic blasts obtained by leukapheresis. Using either radiolabeled cortisol or dexamethasone (because of its negligible affinity for human serum corticosteroid-binding globulin) they found specific

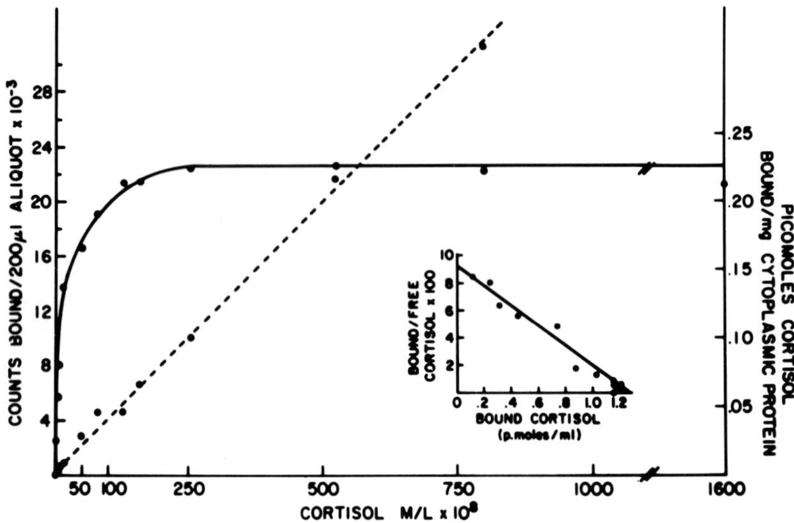

FIG. 3. Specific binding of ^{3}H-cortisol at 4°C to cytoplasmic extract from lymphoblasts of an untreated ALL patient. Solid line shows specifically bound ^{3}H-cortisol; dotted line shows non-specifically bound cortisol. Inset shows a Scatchard plot of specific binding curve. (From Lippman et al., ref. 53, with permission.)

glucocorticoid receptors in most of the cytosols that were analyzed. In these studies, 20% glycerol was added to the binding buffer (20 mM Tris, 2 mM $CaCl_2$, 1 mM $MgCl_2$, pH 7.4, mercaptoethanol as reducing agent) because this addition was found to increase the sensitivity of the assay at low protein concentrations, probably by stabilizing the binding protein. Figure 3 shows a typical binding curve for increasing concentrations of radiolabeled cortisol in the cytoplasmic extract prepared from the cells of one patient. These data demonstrate both total and specific (competable) binding, and the inset (Fig. 3) shows a Scatchard plot (87) of the specific binding data. In the experiment depicted, 0.26 pmoles of cortisol were specifically bound per milligram of cytoplasmic protein; assuming one steroid molecule bound per receptor, the receptor concentration was 2.5×10^{-9} M. Since there was approximately 1×10^{-8} mg of cytoplasmic protein per cell, this corresponds to approximately 1,500 receptors per cell (the originally published value of 1.5×10^5 receptors per cell was a typographical error). From the intercepts of the Scatchard plot in similar experiments using radiolabeled dexamethasone, a dissociation constant of 7×10^{-9} M was obtained for that steroid. The receptors were saturated at about 2.5×10^{-7} M, a concentration that could easily be achieved in the serum following a parenteral dose of 5 mg of dexamethasone (15,17). The specificity of these receptors was also examined by testing the ability of a variety of steroids (100-fold excess) to compete with radiolabeled dexamethasone in the binding assay. These studies demonstrated that active glucocorticoids such as prednisolone, dexamethasone, hydrocortisone, and triamcinolone competed well; inactive glucocorticoids such

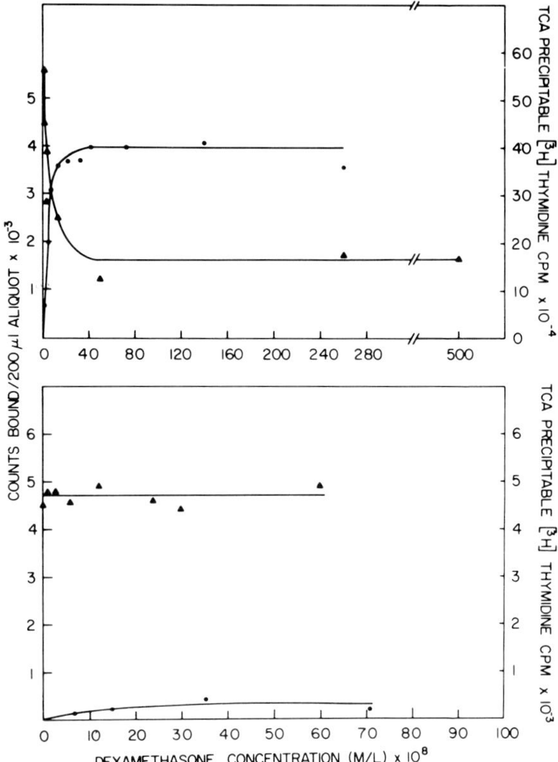

FIG. 4. Top: Comparison of specific binding of ³H-dexamethasone to cytoplasmic receptors at 4°C *(filled circles)* with inhibition of ³H-thymidine incorporation at 37°C *(triangles)* as a function of dexamethasone concentration. Data are for lymphoblasts from a patient with untreated ALL. **Bottom:** Comparison similar to top panel, except that lymphoblasts were from a patient with ALL who was clinically resistant to glucocorticoids. (From Lippman et al., ref. 53, with permission.)

as prednisone, cortisone, and tetrahydrocortisol competed poorly. Both progesterone and cortexolone, which are inactive as glucocorticoids but act as anti-inducers in rodent lymphoid cells (69,6), were effective competitors for binding. Preincubation of the cytosols with trypsin, chymotrypsin, papain, or protease completely destroyed all binding activity, whereas deoxyribonuclease, ribonuclease, and phospholipase A, C, and D had no effect on the receptor proteins. Since inhibition of incorporation of nucleoside precursors into nucleic acids has also been shown to be an early effect of steroids in glucocorticoid-inhibited cells (78,101), uptake of ³H-thymidine by ALL lymphoblasts in short-term tissue culture in the presence of glucocorticoids was also measured. These experiments indicated that the concentration of dexamethasone that was sufficient to saturate the cytoplasmic receptors in cytosols prepared from untreated patients also produced maximal inhibition of ³H-thymidine incorporation (Fig. 4). Those blasts

TABLE 2. *Glucocorticoid receptor levels in cytoplasm of lymphoblasts from patients with acute lymphoblastic leukemia*

Clinical status (number of patients)	Receptor concentration (pmoles dexamethasone specifically bound per milligram cytoplasmic protein, mean + SD)
Untreated ALL (22)	0.31 ± 0.1
Previously treated, still sensitive to combined therapy including glucocorticoids (6)	0.30 ± 0.12
Previously treated, now resistant (6)	0.015 ± 0.0095
Normal volunteers (16)	0.03 ± 0.025

From data reported by Lippman et al. (53).

that lacked receptors showed no inhibition of incorporation of nucleoside precursor at any steroid concentration studied. These results showed a strong correlation between receptor occupancy by glucocorticoids and inhibition of vital cell processes in human ALL blasts.

Retrospective clinical correlations in these patients further suggested that measurement of glucocorticoid receptors might be useful in predicting therapeutic response (Table 2). Twenty-two previously untreated patients with ALL were found to have significant levels of cytoplasmic glucocorticoid receptors (0.1–0.6 pmoles/mg protein). Six patients in relapse who subsequently responded to the same therapy also had cells with receptor levels in the same range. Six other patients in relapse whose lymphoblasts showed very low receptor levels failed to respond to the same therapy. Thus in this study the presence of receptors in leukemic blasts correlated with *in vitro* responsiveness of cells to the inhibitory effects of glucocorticoids and with clinical remission following combination therapy. Likewise, absence of receptors correlated with nonresponsiveness both *in vivo* and *in vitro.*

More recent studies have dealt with quantitation of glucocorticoid receptors in different cell subpopulations of ALL, a disease that may vary in cell types in different patients. Approximately one-fifth of ALL patients have lymphoblasts that form spontaneous rosettes with sheep erythrocytes (T-derived lymphoblasts); in general, these patients have a more aggressive form of the disease (43,91,106). The majority of patients have lymphoblasts that lack identifiable surface markers (null cells). Konior et al. (50) correlated surface markers, receptor content, and steroid responsiveness in childhood ALL lymphoblasts. In addition to identifying T lymphoblasts and null lymphoblasts, they further subdivided the latter on the basis of their ability to stimulate allogeneic donors in mixed lymphocyte culture (MLC), since lack of stimulation in MLC is a characteristic of T cells. The levels of glucocorticoid receptors in these different subcategories determined in whole-cell binding assays are summarized in Table 3. It is clear that the

TABLE 3. *Glucocorticoid receptors in subcategories of childhood acute lymphocytic leukemia*

Surface markers (number of patients)	Glucocorticoid receptors (sites/cell), mean (range)
Null (MLC+) (18)	10,117 (4,096–21,869)
Null (MLC−) (9)	6,729 (2,936–16,469)
T (9)	2,538 (0–5,887)

From data reported by Konior et al. (50).

highest concentration of receptors was detected in the null lymphoblasts that stimulated in MLC (mean = 10,117 sites/cell), whereas the lowest concentration of receptors was detected in T lymphoblasts (mean = 2,538 sites/cell). Glucocorticoid receptors in both the null and T blasts were saturated at 0.8×10^{-8} M dexamethasone, and Scatchard analyses of the binding data revealed parallel straight lines, indicating identical dissociation constants of 3.9×10^{-9} M for the high-affinity receptors in each (Fig. 5). The binding in each was also shown to be specific through competition studies. Although biologically active steroids such as dexamethasone and 11β-hydroxycortisol competed for binding sites,

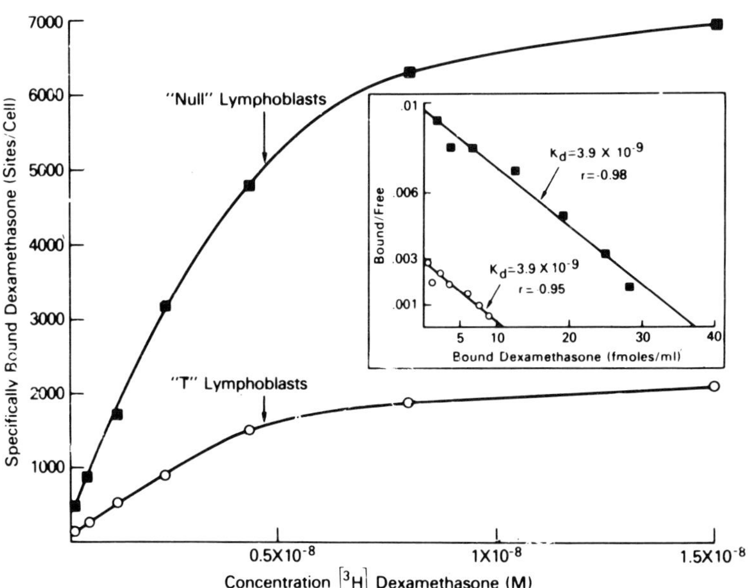

FIG. 5. Specific binding of ^{3}H-dexamethasone to specific glucocorticoid receptors in representative T and null lymphoblasts (childhood ALL) at varying steroid concentrations. Inset shows a Scatchard plot of specific binding curve. (From Konior et al., ref. 50, with permission.)

TABLE 4. *Glucocorticoid receptors and complete remission duration in subcategories of childhood acute lymphocytic leukemia*

Surface markers	Glucocorticoid receptors (sites/cell)	Median complete remission duration (months)
T	<2,500	7.6
T	2,501–<6,000	18.5
Null	2,501–<6,000	22.7
Null	>6,000	>26.0

From Konior et al. (49), with permission.

inactive glucocorticoids such as tetrahydrocortisol and 11α-hydrocortisol and the sex steroids were very poor competitors.

Konior and colleagues (49) subsequently assayed viable lymphoblasts from 45 children with ALL for glucocorticoid receptors and for duration of complete remission (Table 4). Patients with T-cell ALL and low levels of glucocorticoid receptors had short durations of complete remission, whereas patients with T-cell and null-cell ALL and intermediate receptor levels had similar intermediate durations of complete remission. The longest complete remission duration was in null-cell ALL with high levels of glucocorticoid receptors. Data on 21 of these patients are summarized in Table 5 with respect to median age, white blood cell count, and complete remission duration. As can be seen, although both null groups were of the same age and had the same white blood cell count, those with less than 6,000 receptor sites per cell responded as poorly as those with T-cell ALL. These results suggest that glucocorticoid receptor levels have clinical significance that is independent of age, white blood cell count, and cell type, and these levels may be very useful in designing therapeutic regimens for different subcategories of ALL.

Acute Myelogenous Leukemia

Acute myelogenous leukemia (AML) is a disease in which there is frequently little or no response to glucocorticoid therapy, although partial or complete remissions are induced in 20% or less of childhood cases (51,94) and in 15%

TABLE 5. *Glucocorticoid receptors and complete remission duration in subcategories of childhood acute lymphocytic leukemia with respect to age and WBC*

Surface markers	Glucocorticoid receptors	Age	WBC (×10⁻³)	Median complete remission duration (months)
T	<6,000	13.8	80	8.0
Null	<6,000	5.0	84	8.0
Null	>6,000	4.5	67	25.0

From Konior et al. (49), with permission.

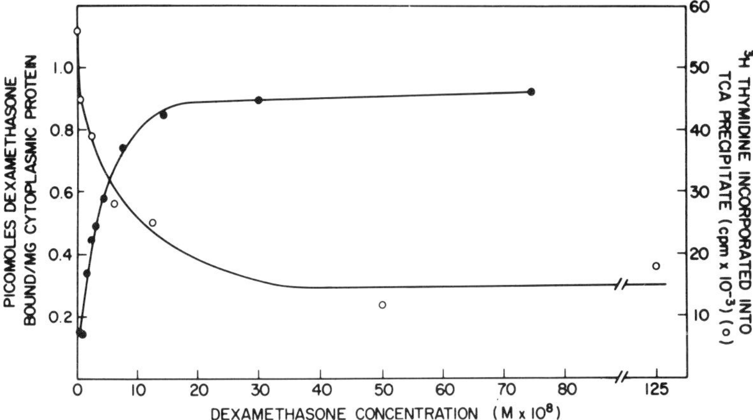

FIG. 6. Correlation between saturation of glucocorticoid receptors and inhibition of DNA synthesis in receptor-rich leukemic blasts from a patient with AML. Binding of ^{3}H-dexamethasone to specific cytosol sites *(filled circles)* and ^{3}H-thymidine incorporation into trichloroacetic-acid-precipitable material *(open circles)* are shown. (From Lippman et al., ref. 56, with permission.)

or less of adult cases (33). Because of this relative ineffectiveness of steroid therapy, Lippman and his colleagues (56) examined the myeloblasts of 16 adult patients with untreated AML for specific glucocorticoid-binding proteins. Using either activated charcoal (53) or filtration through DEAE filter paper (86), they detected high-affinity receptors in only 3 of 16 patients, a ratio that agrees with the proportion of adult AML patients who normally respond to glucocorticoid therapy. In a study involving fewer patients, Gailiani et al. (28) detected cytoplasmic glucocorticoid receptor activity in 2 of 6 AML patients. In the 3 receptor-positive patients studied by Lippman et al. (56), there appeared to be good correlation between the concentration of glucocorticoid required to saturate the receptors and the concentration that inhibited macromolecular synthesis (Fig. 6). These same 3 patients also responded clinically to a drug combination that included glucocorticoids by achieving complete or partial remissions. Very low receptor levels (1/15 that seen in 3 receptor-positive patients) were detected in the remaining 13 patients. In these cases no distinction could be made between a homogeneous population of myeloblasts with little binding activity, a heterogeneous population containing some receptor-positive myeloblasts, and a myeloblast population contaminated by a small number of receptor-positive nonmyeloid cells. Whatever the exact nature of this population, this relative lack of receptor activity in 6 untreated AML patients was correlated with lack of significant glucocorticoid inhibition of nucleic acid synthesis. Likewise, glucocorticoids at high concentrations (2×10^{-6} M dexamethasone) also failed to inhibit glucose uptake in 4 patients whose cells lacked receptor activity. By use of biologically active and inactive glucocorticoids in competition studies, the specificity of the receptors detected in the positive patients was verified. This study thus suggested a relationship between cytoplasmic receptor levels in AML and *in vitro* inhibitory responses to glucocorticoids.

Chronic Lymphocytic Leukemia

Glucocorticoids are often used in the treatment of chronic lymphocytic leukemia (CLL) in an attempt to reduce lymphoid mass (19). These steroids are particularly useful as primary therapy under two circumstances: (a) when the disease is resistant to alkylating agents and (b) when the marrow is densely packed with lymphocytes and complicating granulocytopenia or thrombocytopenia exists. In these situations, glucocorticoids exert a lympholytic effect with minimal myelosuppression (27,95). Although the glucocorticoids are lympholytic, initiation of therapy may be associated with a transient increase in the peripheral lymphocyte count, but this leukocytosis occurs at a time when the central lymphoid tissues are shrinking (95). In this regard, Dighiero et al. (22) studied the peripheral lymphocyte count prior to and 4 hr after injection of hydrocortisone in 43 CLL patients and found variable responses: decrease, no change, or increase. These workers showed that there was a correlation between a decrease in lymphocyte count and the clinical staging of the disease. Thus those patients with involvement restricted to blood and marrow often showed a drop in count. It was also shown that the percentage of T lymphoblasts was higher in those patients whose peripheral lymphocyte counts decreased.

Several reports dealing with quantitation of glucocorticoid receptors in CLL have appeared relatively recently. In one of the first studies, Gailiani et al. (28) failed to detect receptor activity in any of 8 CLL patients studied. Their assay technique included homogenization of cell pellets (0.1 M Tris buffer lacking thio-protective agents) in the presence of radiolabeled triamcinolone with or without excess nonradiolabeled cortisol, centrifugation at 27,000 × *g* for 1 hr, and subsequent analysis of the supernatants on Sephadex G-25 columns. Homo et al. (38), using a whole-cell binding technique, later demonstrated glucocorticoid receptors in 19 cases of CLL, although the receptor levels were generally lower than in normal lymphocytes. In this study no correlation between receptor level and response to any previous or current treatment was shown. More recently, Terenius et al. (103) analyzed cells from 27 unselected CLL patients for several parameters, including the following: specific cytoplasmic glucocorticoid receptors; cell surface immunoglobulin; complement and sheep red blood cell receptors; Con A agglutinability; proliferative activity measured by direct uptake of radiolabeled thymidine or by autoradiography. Their results showed that most of the CLL cases (26 of 27) were of B-lymphocyte origin, which agrees with data in the literature (89). Using a cytosol assay in 0.01 M Tris buffer supplemented with 0.25 M sucrose, 15 mM EDTA, and 0.01 M dithiothreitol as the reducing agent, they detected glucocorticoid receptors in 17 patients. The mean apparent dissociation constant for these receptor-positive cells was $K_d = 3 \times 10^{-8}$ M. Again the specificity of binding was that expected for glucocorticoid receptors. Those patients lacking glucocorticoid receptors generally showed no disease progression and a comparatively low labeling index. In 6 patients, all of whose lymphoblasts contained receptors, the progress of the disease was such that glucocorticoid therapy was started. A positive clinical response and a reduction in DNA synthesis were observed in 4 of 6 cases, while 2 cases showed only a reduction in DNA synthesis (determined by autoradiography). One patient was subject to serial sampling on nine different occasions while on prednisolone therapy. In each treatment session a clinical response and a reduction in labeling index were observed, whereas the level of glucocorticoid receptors remained relatively constant. Although this study suggested a correlation between receptor level and clinical response to glucocorticoids, further studies involving larger numbers of CLL patients are needed.

Most recently, Homo et al. (39) examined lymphocytes from 27 CLL patients (about half of whom were being treated with chlorambucil) at different stages for glucocorticoid receptors and steroid-induced inhibition of incorporation of nucleic acid precursors. Their results failed to demonstrate any correlation between receptor level and stage of the disease, and in the majority of patients the receptor levels fell within the limits of normal lymphocytes. However, they did find that the levels of spontaneous incorporation of ^{3}H-thymidine and ^{3}H-uridine and the percentages of steroid-induced inhibition increase significantly from stage 0 to stage III/IV of the disease. These results may be simply a reflection of the presence of an increasing proportion of circulating proliferative cells in the latter stages of the disease. No attempts were made in this study to ascertain whether the leukemic blasts were of T- or B-cell origin.

Sézary Syndrome

The Sézary syndrome, which was first described in 1938 (92,93), is a rare and frequently lethal chronic leukemia that is characterized by atypical circulating malignant lymphocytes (21) and cutaneous infiltration. The prime symptom of this leukemia is intensely pruritic generalized erythrodermia, with formation of plaques; lymphadenopathy and hepatosplenomegaly are also common (110). Lutzner et al. (58) have reviewed the evidence that suggests that the Sézary syndrome represents merely the leukemic phase of mycosis fungoides and that these lymphoproliferative disorders may be grouped together as cutaneous T-cell lymphomas. The distinguishing abnormal circulating lymphocyte seen in Sézary syndrome is typically a large cell with a voluminous convoluted nucleus that is surrounded by a thin rim of cytoplasm (23,58). Several investigators (23,58,112) have shown that the membrane characteristics of Sézary cells are those of T lymphocytes. Broder et al. (12) have presented data suggesting that Sézary cells originate from a subset of T cells programmed exclusively for helper-like interactions with B cells in their production of immunoglobulin molecules.

Although mycosis fungoides and the Sézary syndrome do not always respond to conventional therapy, alkylating agents such as chlorambucil and cyclophos-

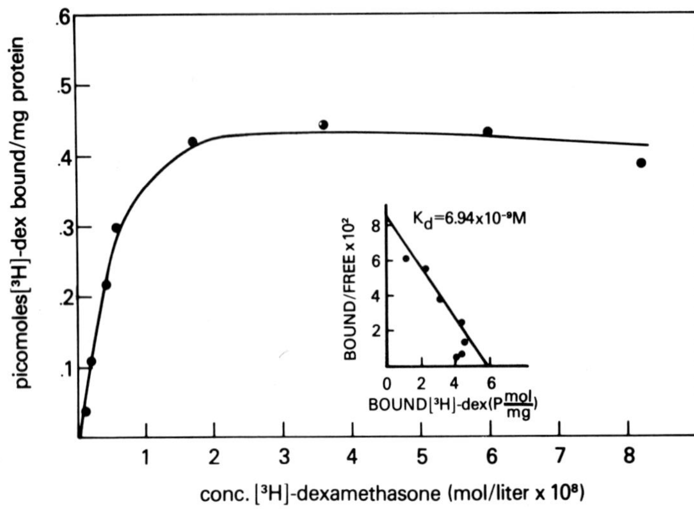

FIG. 7. Specific binding of ^{3}H-dexamethasone at 4°C to cytoplasmic extract prepared from lymphoblasts of a Sézary patient. Binding incubation was for 6 hr, and specific binding was assayed using a 100-fold molar excess of nonradioactive dexamethasone and adsorption of unbound steroid with dextran-coated charcoal. Inset shows a Scatchard plot of specific binding data.

phamide and antimetabolites such as methotrexate often have prolonged palliative effects (24). In many cases much of the edema and erythema associated with the Sézary syndrome can be improved by local corticosteroid therapy, and often the systemic use of corticosteroids can further reduce these symptoms, as well as the pruritus (109). Dighiero et al. (22) reported a 59% decrease in the peripheral lymphocyte count of a Sézary patient within 4 hr after a single intravenous injection of hydrocortisone. Combined chemotherapy including chlorambucil and prednisolone has also been shown to result in freedom from pruritus, followed by partial resolution of the erythroderma and histological disappearance of Sézary cells in many patients (109). Since pre-Sézary syndrome, Sézary syndrome, and Sézary syndrome with lymphoma can now be recognized, the strategy of the therapy must be determined by the staging procedure (109). Since most Sézary patients live an average of 5 years following the onset of symptoms (13), it would be beneficial to determine at which specific stage(s) the malignant lymphocytes are most sensitive to systemic glucocorticoids. Omission of glucocorticoids from the therapy of resistant patients would reduce immunosuppression and render these patients less susceptible to infections.

Preliminary results from our laboratory (T. J. Schmidt and E. B. Thompson, *unpublished data*) demonstrate that malignant lymphocytes from some Sézary patients contain specific glucocorticoid receptors. Using a cytosol assay (0.01 M Tris, 0.0015 mM EDTA, 5 mM dithiothreitol, 20% glycerol, pH 7.5), we detected glucocorticoid receptors in the lymphocytes of 2 patients with elevated white blood cell counts who underwent leukapheresis. Figure 7 shows a binding

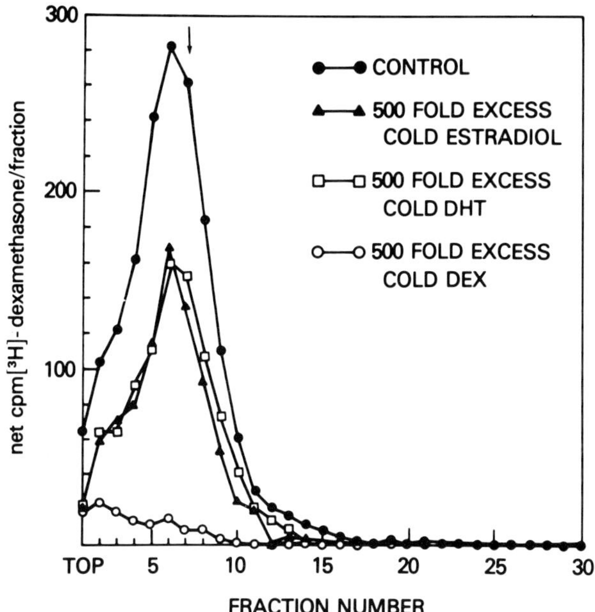

FIG. 8. Sucrose density-gradient analysis of ³H-dexamethasone binding in cytoplasmic extract prepared from lymphoblasts of a Sézary patient. Following 6-hr incubation with appropriate competing steroid, unbound steroid was adsorbed with dextran-coated charcoal, and 0.3-ml aliquots (0.9 mg protein) from each treatment were layered onto linear 5–20% sucrose gradients (prepared in appropriate Tris buffer containing 10% glycerol and 0.4 M KCl). Gradients were centrifuged at 149,000 × *g* for 18 hr in the SW 50.1 rotor of a Beckman L5-65 ultracentrifuge. Thirty fractions (0.18 ml each) were then collected and assayed for radioactivity.

curve for increasing concentrations of radiolabeled dexamethasone in cytosol prepared from lymphocytes of a patient who demonstrated marked clinical improvement while receiving glucocorticoid therapy. As can be seen from the binding curve, approximately 0.42 pmole of dexamethasone was specifically bound per milligram of cytoplasmic protein, and the Scatchard analysis (inset, Figure 7) revealed a dissociation constant of $K_d = 6.9 \times 10^{-9}$ M for a homogeneous population of receptors. This binding affinity agrees with that previously mentioned for adult lymphoblastic leukemias (53). The functionality of these receptors was also demonstrated by the dexamethasone-induced decrease in uptake of radiolabeled thymidine and uridine by the lymphocytes maintained in short-term tissue culture. Cytosol competition studies demonstrated the specificity of these receptors. The active glucocorticoids dexamethasone and prednisolone completely blocked the specific binding of radiolabeled dexamethasone when present at a 50-fold molar excess; prednisone, the less active precursor of prednisolone, and cortexolone were less effective. Other steroids such as estradiol and 5α-dihydrotestosterone showed considerable competition, but only when present at a 500-fold molar excess, as demonstrated by sucrose density-gradient analysis (Fig. 8). Whether these steroids are competing directly for glucocorticoid binding sites or are exerting their effects entirely via an allosteric mechanism is unclear.

Problems in Methodology

From a review of the literature it is apparent that quantitation of receptors in a particular cell type varies somewhat between laboratories. Some of this variation may be partially due to the different techniques (i.e., preparation of cytoplasmic extracts) and experimental conditions (i.e., buffer components) used to measure receptors. When using either the whole-cell binding assay or cytosol binding assay, one must be conscious of endogenous glucocorticoids and of those administered as part of the therapeutic regimen, since they may partially occupy receptors and thereby reduce the binding of radiolabeled hormone in the assay. Although cytosol preparations have been used to quantitate a variety of steroid receptors, including those for glucocorticoids, there are inherent problems associated with this technique. Since lymphocytes, both normal and leukemic, contain a very thin rim of cytoplasm, one must be aware of the efficiency of the homogenization procedure employed. Alternative procedures for preparing cytoplasmic extracts such as repeated freeze-thawing or sonication may produce a cytosol fraction containing less contamination by nuclear material. Possible breakage of lysosomes and release of proteolytic enzymes that partially inactivate cytoplasmic receptors must also be considered. Since functional sulfhydryl groups are required for glucocorticoid binding to its receptors, one must be careful to include sulfhydryl-protective agents in the appropriate buffer. Since unbound glucocorticoid receptors may be sequestered in the nuclei of lymphocytes, cytoplasmic assays may result in underestimation of the total cellular receptor content. By using a whole-cell binding assay, one can overcome some of these problems and measure total (cytoplasmic plus nuclear) receptors in the appropriate cells. However, one major technical problem associated with this technique is the difficulty of distinguishing between free radiolabeled glucocorticoid and nonspecifically bound steroid after cell washes. Thus the optimal number of washes required to remove free steroid without affecting bound steroid is highly dependent on the conditions surrounding the procedure and must be carefully determined. As was evident in the preceding discussion on human leukemias, most laboratories have employed either the whole-cell or cytosol assay. Obviously a thorough comparison of quantitation of glucocorticoid receptors in leukemic cells using both of these techniques would be valuable.

CONCLUSIONS

A long sequence of experiments has led to the conclusion that many types of lymphoid cells possess specific glucocorticoid receptors. Careful correlations have been made in normal rodent thymocytes linking receptor occupancy and nuclear accumulation with inhibition by glucocorticoids of a variety of biochemical events. In transformed rodent lymphoid tissue culture cell lines, development of resistance to the lethal effects of corticosteroids has been shown to be associated with outright loss or altered function of receptors. Recently similar correlations have also been made in a corticosteroid-sensitive human leukemic cell line (CEM). Use of this cell line and development of additional human *in vitro* model systems will be helpful in studying the mechanisms by which steroid resistance develops and the possible mechanisms of steroid-induced lymphocytolysis.

The retrospective clinical studies that we have reviewed in this chapter suggest that quantitation of glucocorticoid receptors and measurement of their function may reflect the glucocorticoid sensitivity of certain forms of leukemia, particularly those of T-cell origin such as ALL. One fact that has become clear from these studies is that those leukemic cells that lack receptors fail to show any of the typical intracellular responses to glucocorticoids. Obviously, however, further prospective studies comparing receptor content with response to glucocorticoids will be required to determine if receptor levels can provide an accurate prediction of the clinical response to glucocorticoid therapy. The fact that many of the responsive patients studied thus far have received other chemotherapeutic drugs in addition to glucocorticoids has made it impossible to ascribe clinical remissions solely to the administered steroids.

A number of areas remain in which future research will be most beneficial in clarifying unresolved questions concerning the role of glucocorticoid receptors. In light of the known examples of glucocorticoid-resistant mutants that contain cytoplasmic receptors, the necessity of coupling receptor quantitation with functional assays such as inhibition of glucose uptake or incorporation of nucleic acid precursors is clear. The development of additional functional specific markers for functional receptors would obviously be valuable. Studies focusing on the differential sensitivity of normal human T and B lymphocytes and on the unresolved question whether or not the increase in receptor content following stimulation of normal lymphocytes corresponds to an increase in sensitivity are also needed. It is hoped that a more thorough understanding of the factors that control receptor levels and glucocorticoid sensitivity in subpopulations of normal human lymphocytes will aid our understanding of the role of glucocorticoid receptors in leukemic cells.

ACKNOWLEDGMENTS

T. Schmidt is the recipient of an NIH postdoctoral fellowship (1 F32 CA05447–01) awarded by the National Cancer Institute, DHEW. The authors would like to express their appreciation to those colleagues and publishers of medical journals who gave their permission to reproduce the tables and figures appearing in this chapter.

REFERENCES

1. Adler, V. V., Ioannesyants, I. A., Dmitreeva, L. A., Kadagidze, Z. G., and Shapot, V. S. (1976): Action of dexamethasone on RNA synthesis in blood lymphocytes stimulated by phytohemagglutinin. *Bull. Exp. Biol. Med.,* 81:850–853.
2. Ambellan, E., and Roth, J. S. (1967): Steroid effects on rat thymus acid ribonuclease. *Biochem. Biophys. Res. Commun.,* 28:244–248.
3. Baran, D. T., Lichtman, M. A., and Peck, W. A. (1972): Alpha-aminoisobutyric acid transport in human leukemic lymphocytes: *In vitro* characteristics and inhibition by cortisol and cycloheximide. *J. Clin. Invest.,* 51:2181–2189.
4. Baxter, J. D. (1971): Specific cytoplasmic glucocorticoid hormone receptors in hepatoma tissue culture. *Proc. Natl. Acad. Sci. U.S.A.,* 68:932–937.
5. Baxter, J. D., and Harris, A. W. (1975): Mechanism of glucocorticoid action: General features with reference to steroid-mediated immunosuppression. *Transplant. Proc.,* 7:55–65.
6. Baxter, J. D., Harris, A. W., Tomkins, G. M., and Cohn, M. (1971): Glucocorticoid receptors in lymphoma cells in culture: Relationship to glucocorticoid killing activity. *Science,* 171:189–191.
7. Baxter, J. D., Rousseau, G. G., Higgins, S. J., and Tomkins, G. M. (1973): In: *The Biochemistry of Gene Expression in Higher Organisms,* edited by J. K. Pollack and J. W. Lee, p. 206. D. Reidel Publishing, Boston.
8. Behrens, U. J., and Hollander, V. P. (1976): Cell membrane sialoglycopeptides of corticoid-sensitive and -resistant lymphosarcoma P1798. *Cancer Res.,* 36:172–180.
9. Bergink, E. W., and Wallace, R. A. (1974): Estrogen-induced synthesis of yolk protein in roosters. *Am. Zool.,* 14:1177–1193.
10. Bourgeois, S., and Newby, R. F. (1977): Diploid and haploid states of the glucocorticoid receptor gene of mouse lymphoid cell lines. *Cell,* 11:423–430.
11. Böyum, A. (1968): Isolation of mononuclear cells and granulocytes from human blood. *Scand. J. Clin. Lab. Invest.,* 21(Suppl. 97):77–89.
12. Broder, S., Edelson, R., Lutzner, M. A., Nelson, D. L., MacDermott, R. P., Durm, M. E., Goldman, C. K., Meade, B. D., and Waldmann, T. A. (1976): The Sézary syndrome. A malignant proliferation of helper cells. *J. Clin. Invest.,* 58:1297–1306.
13. Brody, J. I., Cypress, E., Kimball, S. G., and McKenzie, D. (1962): The Sézary syndrome. *Arch. Intern. Med.,* 110:205–210.
14. Chan, L., Means, A. R., and O'Malley, B. W. (1973): Rates of induction of specific translatable messenger RNAs for ovalbumin and avidin by steroid hormones. *Proc. Natl. Acad. Sci. U.S.A.,* 70:1870–1874.
15. Chard, R. J., Smith, E. K., and Hartman, J. R. (1966): Metabolic studies on prednisone in previously untreated acute leukemia of childhood. *Proc. Am. Assoc. Cancer Res.,* 7:13.
16. Cidlowski, J. A., and Michaels, G. A. (1977): Alteration in glucocorticoid binding site number during the cell cycle in HeLa cells. *Nature,* 266:643–645.
17. Claman, H. N. (1972): Corticosteroids and lymphoid cells. *N. Engl. J. Med.,* 287:388–397.
18. Cline, M. J. (1967): Prediction of *in vivo* cytotoxicity of chemotherapeutic agents by their effect on malignant leukocytes *in vitro. Blood,* 30:176–188.
19. Cline, M. J. (1975): Adrenal steroids in hematologic malignancies. In: *Steroid Therapy,* edited by D. L. Azarnoff, p. 114. W. B. Saunders, Philadelphia.
20. Cline, M. J., and Rosenbaum, E. (1968): Prediction of *in vivo* cytotoxicity of chemotherapeutic agents by their *in vitro* effect on leukocytes from patients with acute leukemia. *Cancer Res.,* 28:2516–2521.
21. Crossen, P. E., Mellor, J. E. L., Ravich, R. B. M., Vincent, P. C., and Gunz, F. W. (1971): The Sézary syndrome. Cytogenetic studies and identification of the Sézary cell as an abnormal lymphocyte. *Am. J. Med.,* 50:24–34.
22. Dighiero, G., Vaugier, G., Charron, D., d'Athis, P., and Binet, J.-L. (1977): Variations in lymphocyte counts four hours after administration of hydrocortisone in patients with chronic lymphocytic leukemia. *Blood,* 49:719–728.
23. Edelson, R. L., Lutzner, M. A., Kirkpatrick, C. H., Shevach, E. M., and Green, I. (1974): Morphologic and functional properties of the atypical T lymphocytes of the Sézary syndrome. *Mayo Clin. Proc.,* 49:558–566.
24. Epstein, E. H., Jr., Levin, D. L., Croft, J. D., Jr., and Lutzner, M. A. (1972): Mycosis fungoides:

Survival, prognostic features, response to therapy and autopsy findings. *Medicine,* 15:61–72.
25. Foley, G., Lazarus, H., Farber, S., Uzman, B. G., Boone, B., and McCarthy, R. (1965): Continuous culture of human lymphoblasts from peripheral blood of a child with acute leukemia. *Cancer,* 18:522–529.
26. Freireich, E. J., Henderson, E. S., Karon, M., and Frei, E., III (1968): The treatment of acute leukemia considered with respect to cell population kinetics. In: *The Proliferation and Spread of Neoplastic Cells,* p. 441. Williams & Wilkins, Baltimore.
27. Freymann, J. G., Vander, J. B., Marler, E. A., and Meyer, D. G. (1960): Prolonged corticosteroid therapy of chronic lymphocytic leukemia and closely allied malignant lymphomas. *Br. J. Haematol.,* 6:303–323.
28. Gailiani, S., Minowada, J., Silvernail, P., Nussbaum, A., Kaiser, N., Rosen, F., and Shimaoka, K. (1973): Specific glucocorticoid binding in human hemopoietic cell lines and neoplastic tissue. *Cancer Res.,* 33:2653–2657.
29. Gehring, U., and Tomkins, G. M. (1974): A new mechanism for steroid unresponsiveness: Loss of nuclear binding activity of a steroid hormone receptor. *Cell,* 3:301–306.
30. Giddings, S. J., and Young, D. A. (1974): An *in vitro* effect of physiological levels of cortisol and related steroids on the structural integrity of the nucleus in rat thymic lymphocytes as measured by resistance to lysis. *J. Steroid Biochem.,* 5:587–595.
31. Goldin, A., Sandberg, J., Henderson, E., Newman, J., Frei, E., and Holland, J. (1971): The chemotherapy of human and animal acute leukemia. *Cancer Chemother. Rep.,* 55:309–507.
32. Hallahan, C., Young, D. A., and Munck, A. (1973): Time course of early events in the action of glucocorticoids on rat thymus cells *in vitro.* Synthesis and turnover of a hypothetical cortisol-induced protein inhibitor of glucose metabolism and of a presumed ribonucleic acid. *J. Biol. Chem.,* 248:2922–2927.
33. Henderson, E. S. (1969): Treatment of acute leukemia. *Semin. Hematol.,* 6:271–319.
34. Higgins, S. J., Rousseau, G. G., Baxter, J. D., and Tomkins, G. M. (1973): Early events in glucocorticoid action. Activation of the steroid receptor and its subsequent specific nuclear binding studied in a cell-free system. *J. Biol. Chem.,* 248:5866–5872.
35. Hofert, J. F., and White, A. (1968): Effect of a single injection of cortisol on the incorporation of ^{3}H-thymidine and ^{3}H-deoxycytidine into lymphatic tissue DNA of adrenalectomized rats. *Endocrinology,* 82:767–776.
36. Hofert, J. F., and White, A. (1968): Inhibitory effect of a liver extract on the incorporation of ^{3}H-deoxycytidine into thymus DNA of adrenalectomized and adrenalectomized-hepatectomized rats. *Endocrinology,* 82:777–785.
37. Hollander, N., and Chiu, J.-W. (1966): *In vitro* binding of cortisol-1,2-^{3}H by a substance in the supernatant fraction of P1798 mouse lymphosarcoma. *Biochem. Biophys. Res. Commun.,* 25:291–297.
38. Homo, F., Duval, D., and Meyer, P. (1975): Étude de la liaison de la dexamethasone tritiée dans les lymphocytes de sujets normaux et leuchémiques. *C. R. Acad. Sci.* [*D*] *(Paris),* 280:1923–1926.
39. Homo, F., Duval, D., Meyer, P., Belas, F., Debre, P., and Binet, J.-L. (1977): Chronic lymphocytic leukemia: Cellular effects of glucocorticoids *in vitro. Br. J. Haematol., (in press).*
40. Horibata, K., and Harris, A. W. (1970): Mouse myelomas and lymphomas in culture. *Exp. Cell Res.,* 60:61–77.
41. Kaiser, N., and Edelman, I. S. (1977): Calcium dependence of glucocorticoid-induced lymphocytolysis. *Proc. Natl. Acad. Sci. U.S.A.,* 74:638–642.
42. Kaiser, N., Milholland, R. J., and Rosen, F. (1974): Glucocorticoid receptors and mechanism of resistance in the cortisol-sensitive and -resistant lines of lymphosarcoma P 1798. *Cancer Res.,* 34:621–626.
43. Kersey, J., Nesbit, M., Hallgren, H., Sabad, A., Yunis, E., and Gajl-Peczalsaka, K. (1975): Evidence for the origin of certain childhood acute lymphoblastic leukemias and lymphosarcomas in thymus-derived lymphocytes. *Cancer,* 36:1348–1352.
44. Kidson, C. (1967): Cortisol in the regulation of RNA and protein synthesis. *Nature,* 213:779–782.
45. King, R. J. B., and Mainwaring, W. I. P. (1974): *Steroid-Cell Interactions.* University Park Press, Baltimore.
46. Kirkpatrick, A. F., Kaiser, N., Milholland, R. J., and Rosen, F. (1972): Glucocorticoid-binding macromolecules in normal tissues and tumors. *J. Biol. Chem.,* 247:70–74.
47. Kirkpatrick, A. F., Milholland, R. J., and Rosen, F. (1971): Stereospecific glucocorticoid

binding to subcellular fractions of the sensitive and resistant lymphosarcoma P1798. *Nature* [*New Biol.*], 232:216–218.
48. Kjellstrand, C. M. (1975): Side effects of steroids and their treatment. *Transplant. Proc.*, 7:123–129.
49. Konior, G. S., Lippman, M. E., Johnson, G. E., and Leventhal, B. G. (1977): Correlation of glucocorticoid receptor (GR) levels and complete remission duration (CRD) in "poor prognosis" acute lymphocytic leukemia (ALL). *Proc. Am. Soc. Clin. Oncol.* 18:353.
50. Konior, G. S., Lippman, M. E., Johnson, G. E., and Leventhal, B. G. (1977): Glucocorticoid receptors in subpopulations of childhood acute lymphocytic leukemia. *Cancer Res.*, 37:2688–2695.
51. Leiken, S. L., Brubaker, C., Hartman, J. R., Murphy, M. L., Wolff, J. A., and Perrin, E. (1968): Varying prednisone dosage in remission induction of previously untreated childhood leukemia. *Cancer*, 21:346–351.
52. Lippman, M. E., and Barr, R. (1977): Glucocorticoid receptors in purified subpopulations of human peripheral blood lymphocytes. *J. Immunol.*, 118:1977–2003.
53. Lippman, M. E., Halterman, R. H., Leventhal, B. G., Perry, S., and Thompson, E. B. (1973): Glucocorticoid-binding proteins in acute lymphoblastic leukemic blast cells. *J. Clin. Invest.*, 52:1715–1725.
54. Lippman, M. E., Halterman, R., Perry, S., Leventhal, B., and Thompson, E. B. (1973): Glucocorticoid binding proteins in human leukemic lymphoblasts. *Nature* [*New Biol.*], 242:157–158.
55. Lippman, M. E., Perry, S., and Thompson, E. B. (1974): Cytoplasmic glucocorticoid-binding proteins in glucocorticoid-unresponsive human and mouse leukemic cell lines. *Cancer Res.*, 34:1572–1576.
56. Lippman, M. E., Perry, S., and Thompson, E. B. (1975): Glucocorticoid binding proteins in myeloblasts of acute myelogenous leukemia. *Am. J. Med.*, 59:224–227.
57. Livingston, R. B., and Carter, S. K. (editors) (1970): *Single Agents in Cancer Chemotherapy.* Plenum Press, New York.
58. Lutzner, M., Edelson, R., Schein, P., Green, I., Kirkpatrick, C., and Ahmed, A. (1975): Cutaneous T-cell lymphomas: The Sézary syndrome, mycosis fungoides and related disorders. *Ann. Intern. Med.*, 83:534–552.
59. MacLampkin, J., and Potter, M. (1958): Response to cortisone and development of cortisone resistance in a cortisone-sensitive lymphosarcoma of the mouse. *J. Natl. Cancer Inst.*, 20:1091–1111.
60. MacLeod, R. M., King, C. E., and Hollander, V. P. (1963): Effect of corticosteroids on ribonuclease and nucleic acid content in lymphosarcoma P1798. *Cancer Res.*, 23:1045–1050.
61. Mainwaring, W. I. P., Mangan, F. R., Irving, R. A., and Jones, D. A. (1974): Specific changes in the messenger ribonucleic acid content of the rat ventral prostate after androgenic stimulation. Evidence for the synthesis of aldolase messenger ribonucleic acid. *Biochem. J.*, 144:413–426.
62. Makman, M. H., Dvorkin, B., and White, A. (1971): Evidence for induction by cortisol *in vitro* of a protein inhibitor of transport and phosphorylation process in rat thymocytes. *Proc. Natl. Acad. Sci. U.S.A.*, 68:1269–1273.
63. Makman, M. H., Nakagawa, S., Dvorkin, B., and White, A. (1970): Inhibitory effects of cortisol and antibiotics on substrate entry and ribonucleic acid synthesis in rat thymocytes *in vitro. J. Biol. Chem.*, 245:2556–2563.
64. McGuire, W. L., Carbone, P. P., and Vollmer, E. P. (editors) (1975): *Estrogen Receptors in Human Breast Cancer.* Raven Press, New York.
65. Moon, H. (1937): Inhibition of somatic growth in castrate rats with pituitary extract. *Proc. Soc. Exp. Biol. Med.*, 37:34–36.
66. Mosher, K. M., Young, D. A., and Munck, A. (1971): Evidence for irreversible, actinomycin D-sensitive and temperature-sensitive steps following binding of cortisol to glucocorticoid receptors and preceding effects on glucose metabolism in rat thymus cells. *J. Biol. Chem.*, 246:654–659.
67. Munck, A. (1971): Glucocorticoid inhibition of glucose uptake by peripheral tissues. Old and new evidence, molecular mechanisms and physiological significance. *Prospect. Biol. Med.*, 14:265–269.
68. Munck, A., and Wira, C. (1975): Methods for assessing hormone-receptor kinetics with cells in suspension: Receptor-bound and nonspecifically bound hormone; cytoplasmic-nuclear translocation. *Methods Enzymol.*, Part A: 36:255–264.

69. Munck, A., Wira, C., Young, D. A., Mosher, K. M., Hallahan, C., and Bell, P. A. (1972): Glucocorticoid-receptor complexes and the earliest steps in the action of glucocorticoids on thymus cells. *J. Steroid Biochem.*, 3:567–578.
70. Neifeld, J. P., Lippman, M. E., and Tormey, D. C. (1977): Steroid hormone receptors in normal human lymphocytes. Induction of glucocorticoid receptor activity by phytohemagglutinin stimulation. *J. Biol. Chem.*, 254:2972–2977.
71. Noll, H. (1969): Polysomes: Analysis of structure and function. In: *Techniques in Protein Biosynthesis*, edited by J. R. Sargent, pp. 101–179. Academic Press, New York.
72. Norman, M. R., and Thompson, E. B. (1977): Characterization of a glucocorticoid-sensitive human lymphoid cell line. *Cancer Res.*, 37:3785–3791.
73. Nowell, P. C. (1961): Inhibition of human leukocyte mitosis by prednisolone *in vitro*. *Cancer Res.*, 21:1518–1521.
74. Ono, T., Terayama, H., Takatu, F., and Nakao, K. (1968): Inhibitory effects of hydrocortisone upon the phytohemagglutinin-induced RNA-synthesis in human lymphocytes. *Biochim. Biophys. Acta*, 161:361–367.
75. Osawa, S., and Tomino, S. (1977): Regulation of androgen mRNA level for the major urinary protein complex in mouse liver. *Biochem. Biophys. Res. Commun.*, 77:628–633.
76. Palmiter, R. D. (1973): Ovalbumin messenger ribonucleic acid translation. Comparable rates of polypeptide initiation and elongation on ovalbumin and globin messenger ribonucleic acid in a rabbit reticulocyte lysate. *J. Biol. Chem.*, 248:2095–2106.
77. Peck, W. A., Messinger, K., Brandt, J., and Carpenter, J. (1969): Impaired accumulation of ribonucleic acid precursors and depletion of ribonucleic acid in glucocorticoid treated bone cells. *J. Biol. Chem.*, 244:4174–4184.
78. Pratt, W. B., and Aronow, L. (1966): The effect of glucocorticoids on protein and nucleic acid synthesis in mouse fibroblasts growing *in vitro*. *J. Biol. Chem.*, 241:5244–5250.
79. Rabinowitz, Y. (1964): Separation of lymphocytes, polymorphonuclear leukocytes and monocytes on glass columns, including tissue culture observations. *Blood*, 23:811–828.
80. Roewekamp, W. G., Hofer, E., and Sekeris, C. E. (1976): Translation of mRNA from rat-liver polysomes into tyrosine aminotransferase and tryptophan oxygenase in a protein-synthesizing system from wheat germ. *Eur. J. Biochem.*, 70:259–268.
81. Rosen, J. M., Fina, J. J., Milholland, R. J., and Rosen, F. (1970): Inhibition of glucose uptake in lymphosarcoma P1798 by cortisol and its relationship to the biosynthesis of deoxyribonucleic acid. *J. Biol. Chem.*, 245:2074–2080.
82. Rosen, J. M., Fina, J. J., Milholland, R. J., and Rosen, F. (1972): Inhibitory effect of cortisol *in vitro* on 2-deoxyglucose uptake and RNA and protein metabolism in lymphosarcoma P1798. *Cancer Res.*, 32:350–355.
83. Rosen, J. M., Milholland, R. J., and Rosen, F. (1970): A comparison of the effect of glucocorticoids on glucose uptake and hexokinase activity in lymphosarcoma P1798. *Biochim. Biophys. Acta*, 219:447–454.
84. Rosen, J. M., Rosen, F., Milholland, R. J., and Nichol, C. A. (1970): Effects of cortisol on DNA metabolism in the sensitive and resistant lines of mouse lymphoma P1798. *Cancer Res.*, 30:1129–1136.
85. Rousseau, G. G., Baxter, J. D., and Tomkins, G. M. (1972): Glucocorticoid receptors: Relations between steroid binding and biologic effects. *J. Mol. Biol.*, 67:99–115.
86. Santi, D. V., Sibley, C., Perriard, E., Tomkins, G. M., and Baxter, J. E. (1973): A filter assay for steroid hormone receptors. *Biochemistry*, 12:2412–2416.
87. Scatchard, G. (1949): The attractions of proteins for small molecules and ions. *Ann. N.Y. Acad. Sci.*, 51:660–675.
88. Schutz, G., Killewich, L., Chen, G., and Feigelson, P. (1975): Control of the mRNA for hepatic tryptophan oxygenase during hormonal and substrate induction. *Proc. Natl. Acad. Sci. U.S.A.*, 72:1017–1020.
89. Seligmann, M., Preud'Homme, J.-L., and Brouet, J.-C. (1973): B and T cell markers in human proliferative blood diseases and primary immunodeficiencies, with special reference to membrane bound immunoglobulins. *Transplant. Rev.*, 16:85–113.
90. Selye, H. (1937): Studies on adaptation. *Endocrinology*, 21:169–188.
91. Sen, L., and Borella, L. (1975): Clinical importance of lymphoblasts with T markers in childhood acute leukemia. *N. Engl. J. Med.*, 292:828–832.
92. Sézary, A., and Bouvrain, Y. (1938): Erythrodermie avec presence de cellules monstrueuses dans le derme et les sang circulant. *Bull. Soc. Fr. Dermatol. Syphiligr.*, 45:254–260.

93. Sézary, A., Horowitz, A., and Maschas, H. (1938): Erythrodermie avec presence de cellules monstrueses dans le derme et dans le sang circulant (second cas.). *Bull. Soc. Fr. Dermatol. Syphiligr.*, 45:395–400.
94. Shanbrom, E., and Miller, S. (1962): Critical evaluation of massive steroid therapy of acute leukemia. *N. Engl. J. Med.*, 226:1354–1358.
95. Shaw, R. K., Boggs, D. R., Silberman, H. R., and Frei, E. (1961): A study of prednisone therapy in chronic lymphocytic leukemia. *Blood*, 17:182–195.
96. Sibley, C. H., and Tomkins, G. M. (1974): Isolation of lymphoma cell variants resistant to killing by glucocorticoids. *Cell*, 2:213–220.
97. Sibley, C. H., and Tomkins, G. M. (1974): Mechanisms of steroid resistance. *Cell*, 2:221–227.
98. Smith, K. A., Crabtree, G. R., Kennedy, S. J., and Munck, A. U. (1977): Glucocorticoid receptors and glucocorticoid sensitivity of mitogen stimulated and unstimulated human lymphocytes. *Nature*, 267:523–526.
99. Smith, R. W., Blaese, R. M., Hathcock, K. R., Buell, D. N., Edelson, R. L., and Lutzner, M. A. (1974): T and B lymphocyte markers in lymphoid cell research in human disease. In: *Lymphocyte Recognition and Effector Mechanisms*, edited by K. Lindahl-Kiessling and D. Osaba, pp. 127–146. Academic Press, New York.
100. Stevens, W., Bedke, C., and Dougherty, T. F. (1967): Effects of cortisol acetate on various aspects of cellular metabolism in mouse lymphatic tissues. *J. Reticuloendothel. Soc.*, 4:254–285.
101. Stevens, W., Colissides, C., and Dougherty, T. F. (1966): A time study on the effect of cortisol on the incorporation of thymidine-2-C^{14} into nucleic acids of mouse lymphatic tissues. *Endocrinology*, 78:600–604.
102. Stuart, J. J., and Ingram, M. (1971): The effect of cortisol on viability and glucose uptake in rat thymocytes *in vitro. Proc. Soc. Exp. Biol. Med.*, 136:1146–1150.
103. Terenius, L., Simonsson, B., and Nilsson, K. (1976): Glucocorticoid receptors, DNA synthesis, membrane antigens and their relation to disease activity in chronic lymphatic leukemia. *J. Steroid Biochem.*, 7:905–909.
104. Thompson, E. B., and Lippman, M. E. (1974): Mechanism of action of glucocorticoids. *Metabolism*, 23:159–202.
105. Tormey, D. C., Fudenberg, H. H., and Kamin, R. M. (1967): Effect of prednisolone on synthesis of DNA and RNA by human lymphocytes *in vitro. Nature*, 213:281–282.
106. Tsukimoto, I., Wong, K. Y., and Lampkin, B. C. (1976): Surface markers and prognostic factors in acute lymphoblastic leukemia. *N. Engl. J. Med.*, 294:245–248.
107. Turnell, R. W., and Burton, A. F. (1975): Glucocorticoid receptors and lymphocytolysis in normal and neoplastic lymphocytes. *Mol. Cell. Biochem.*, 9:175–189.
108. Vietti, T. J., Sullivan, M. P., Berry, D. H., Hardy, T., Haggard, M., and Blattner, R. (1965): The response of acute childhood leukemia to an initial and a second course of prednisolone. *J. Pediatr.*, 66:18–26.
109. Winkelmann, R. K., Perry, H. O., Muller, S. A., Schroeter, A. L., Jordan, R. E., and Rogers, R. S. (1974): Treatment of the Sézary syndrome. *Mayo Clin. Proc.*, 49:590–592.
110. Wintrobe, M. M. (editor) (1974): *Clinical Hematology* (7th edition), p. 1589. Lea & Febiger, Philadelphia.
111. Yamamoto, K. R., Stampfer, M. R., and Tomkins, G. M. (1974): Receptors from glucocorticoid-sensitive lymphoma cells and two classes of insensitive clones: Physical and DNA-binding properties. *Proc. Natl. Acad. Sci. U.S.A.*, 71:3901–3905.
112. Zuckler-Franklin, D., Melton, J. W., III, and Quagliata, F. (1974): Ultrastructural, immunologic and functional studies on Sézary cells. *Proc. Natl. Acad. Sci. U.S.A.*, 71:1877–1881.

Endocrine Control in Neoplasia, edited by
R. K. Sharma and W. E. Criss.
Raven Press, New York © 1978.

Androgen and Androgen Receptors in Prostatic Cancer

Walter Voigt and Albert Castro

Department of Pathology, University of Miami School of Medicine, Miami, Florida 33152

Androgen metabolism in carcinoma tissue of human prostate will be compared with that in normal and hypertrophic tissue. Although androgens are known to be important in the etiology of prostate carcinoma and hypertrophy, no evidence has yet been reported that these diseases are caused by androgens. A review of recent developments in the study of the relationship between androgen metabolism and prostate carcinoma may facilitate an understanding of the importance of androgens in prostatic disease.

Studies on metabolism of testosterone in human prostate reported by Djoseland et al. (14) showed that metabolism of testosterone to dihydrotestosterone (DHT) was significantly lower in cancerous tissue than in normal and hypertrophic tissue. The most extensive metabolism of testosterone was seen in the tissue of benign nodular prostatic hyperplasia. Only very small amounts were further metabolized to 3α- and 3β-androstanediols, of which 95% was the 3α isomer. Conversely, some metabolites of testosterone such as 4-androstenedione have been shown to be converted into testosterone and DHT by cancerous tissue of the human prostate. DiSilverio et al. postulated that metabolites produced in adrenal cortex can actively be converted into steroids with strong androgenic activity. Prostatic tissue specimens removed at biopsy from 6 patients with prostatic carcinoma were able to convert dihydroepiandrosterone sulfate into dihydroandrosterone, which possesses about 20% of the testosterone activity. The results strongly suggested the possibility that other androgens produced by the adrenal cortex might be converted not only into testosterone but also into DHT. Although many investigators have indicated the importance of androgens in the etiology of prostate carcinoma, it has never been produced by steroid administration. Carcinoma of the prostate can be produced in rats only by direct application of chemical carcinogens to the gland. However, the induction of prostatic adenocarcinoma in the Nb strain of rats by prolonged administration of sex hormone was reported recently for the first time (40). The report showed that the low spontaneous incidence (0.45%) of grossly recognizable adenocarcinoma of the prostate in the Nb rats was increased to 20% by prolonged treatment with testosterone propionate pellets. These results emphasized the possibility of a hormonal etiology of prostate carcinoma in humans. We have also reviewed the experimental data showing binding of the androgens by receptor proteins in prostatic cytosol.

Although various methods have been used, many of these fail to discriminate effectively against binding by sex-hormone-binding globulin (SHBG), a serum contaminant in human tissues. Among the most promising techniques are density-gradient ultracentrifugation used in conjunction with other procedures such as gel electrophoresis or protamine sulfate precipitation. Nevertheless, it seems certain that specific DHT-binding proteins occur in some but not all samples of benign prostatic hypertrophy (BPH) and cancerous prostate.

A major characteristic of the prostate gland is its susceptibility to hypertrophy and neoplasia in aging man, as compared to other accessory reproductive glands. The need to understand the biochemical factors in these diseases has been stimulated by suggestions from a number of investigators that an endocrine imbalance in the aging male might be causal in this process (25,41).

The presence of androgens in the human prostate is important for its normal development and maturation (26). When subjects have been castrated in later life, hypertrophy of this gland has not occurred (6,26), which indicates that androgens may be involved in hypertrophy of the prostate. However, no evidence has yet been found that benign prostatic hypertrophy is caused by changes in the total hormonal status of the patient (8,44), although local factors within the prostate may be involved.

Although it has been shown that androgens are important in the etiology of prostate neoplasia, their relationship to the development of prostatic carcinoma is unclear, and the biochemical mechanisms involved are still poorly understood.

Therefore we would like to review briefly the recent findings concerning the relationship between androgen metabolism and prostatic carcinoma and compare it with those of normal and hypertrophic tissues.

METABOLISM OF TESTOSTERONE IN HUMAN PROSTATE

The metabolic pathway of testosterone in the prostate was studied previously, and it was found that the 5α reduction of ring A commonly yields 5α-DHT (3,7,9,11,20,43). Moreover, it has been suggested by many workers that the importance of these 5α-reduced metabolites of testosterone is as mediators of androgenic action (50).

In an attempt to examine possible metabolic differences between normal tissue and hyperplastic or neoplastic tissue, Djoseland et al. (14) recently compared the ability of normal human prostatic tissue to metabolize ^{3}H-testosterone *in vitro* with that of hyperplastic and cancerous prostatic tissue. In these studies, approximately 60% of the radioactivity in normal prostatic tissue was identified as nonmetabolized testosterone when prostatic tissue was incubated with ^{3}H-testosterone, whereas 30 to 35% of the radioactivity was identified as DHT. Only very small quantities were further metabolized to 3α- and 3β-androstanediols, of which 95% was the 3α isomer. The formation of oxidative metabolites, such as androstanedione, was demonstrated to be due to the presence of a 17β-hydroxy steroid dehydrogenase.

When the radiolabeled testosterone was incubated with equal amounts of prostatic carcinoma tissue, the same metabolites that were formed by normal prostatic tissue were also found. However, there were distinctive quantitative differences. Only about 25% of the testosterone was metabolized by the carcinoma tissue, in contrast to 40 to 50% conversion by the normal tissue, probably mainly due to reduced formation of DHT. The other metabolites were formed to about the same extent as in the normal prostatic tissue.

The most extensive testosterone metabolism was found in tissue obtained from benign nodular hyperplasia. About 6% of the incubated radiolabeled testosterone was shown to be metabolized, of which 49% was identified as DHT and 8% as 5α-androstanediols. The amount of testosterone metabolized was thus significantly greater than that of normal and cancerous tissue. Even though this investigation suggested that DHT might be causally related to the development of human prostatic hyperplasia and that a relatively restricted capacity to form 5α-reduced metabolites (i.e., the amount of DHT formed by the carcinomatous tissue being significantly lower than that of normal and hyperplastic tissue) might be caused by the transformation of normal cells to the less well differentiated cancer cells, no possible correlation of etiological significance between the prostatic cancer and observed metabolic difference was suggested.

METABOLISM OF ANDROGENIC HORMONES IN CANCEROUS TISSUE OF PROSTATE

It has been shown by some investigators (1,12) that 4-androstenedione can be converted into testosterone and dihydrotestosterone by cancerous prostatic tissue. DiSilverio et al. (13) recently postulated that some metabolites such as dehydroepiandrosterone sulfate, produced in large quantities in the adrenal cortex, may be actively metabolized at the prostatic level and converted into steroids with strong androgenic activity.

Specimens of prostatic tissue removed at biopsy were obtained from 6 patients with prostatic adenocarcinoma (of these, 3 patients received no treatment, 2 patients were treated with diethylstilbestrol, and 1 patient received cyproterone acetate therapy). These specimens were minced in the cold room at 4° C and incubated at 37° C with ^{3}H-dehydroepiandrosterone sulfate in a substrate : tissue ratio of 1 : 1,000,000 (w/w). Incubation was stopped by adding acetone, and specimens were stored overnight at 4° C. Following addition of several standard steroids and extraction with ether, extracts were separated by paper chromatography and then by thin-layer chromatography.

The results indicated the conversion of dehydroepiandrosterone sulfate into dehydroepiandrosterone in fairly large quantities in neoplastic prostatic tissue, but only into minute quantities of testosterone and dihydrotestosterone. Patients receiving no diethylstilbestrol or cyproterone acetate therapy were not significantly different from the treated group in converting dehydroepiandrosterone sulfate into testosterone and dihydrotestosterone.

These studies thus indicated the possibility that 3β-ol-dehydrogenase and 5α-reductase activity in neoplastic tissue is very low or completely absent.

PROSTATIC ADENOCARCINOMA CAUSED BY PROLONGED HORMONE ADMINISTRATION IN RATS

Induction of prostatic carcinoma has been known to be extremely difficult to duplicate in mice and rats. It has never been produced by steroid treatment. Prostatic cancer may be produced in rats only by the direct application of chemical carcinogens to the gland (15,21,28,34,38). The lack of confirmative experimental evidence to implicate hormones as the cause of prostatic carcinoma has led some investigators to an intensified search for environmental or other carcinogenic factors of etiological importance in man.

Recently the induction of prostatic adenocarcinoma in the Nb strain of rats by prolonged administration of sex hormone was reported for the first time (40). The report showed that the low spontaneous incidence (0.45%) of grossly recognizable adenocarcinoma of the prostate in Nb rats was increased to 20% by prolonged treatment with testosterone propionate pellets. It indicated that the success of these experiments was related to the pellet form of hormone administration. The results also indicated that tumors appeared at a younger age when treatment was combined with estrogen, which raised the speculation that concomitant treatment with estrogen, an antagonizing hormone, resulted in exaggerated hormone fluctuation and thus accelerated malignant change. However, pretreatment for some months with estrogen may make tumors of the prostate less frequent on subsequent treatment with testosterone. A unique adenoma of the prostate that developed following the removal of estrogen treatment is probably due to constant stimulation by endogenous androgen leading to malignant change. The results presented emphasized the possible hormonal etiology of cancer of the prostate and offered a new experimental approach for study of the cause and treatment of this condition. It emphasized the possibility that a hormonal etiology of the condition in humans should be seriously reconsidered.

The enzyme catalyzing the transformation of testosterone to DHT, i.e., 5α-reductase, is found to be localized in both cytoplasmic and nuclear membranes of prostate cells (30). This enzyme has been shown to be influenced by various agents such as estrogens (13,18), Estracyt (29), 4-androsten-3-one-17-carboxylic acid (47), gestagens (2), dexamethasone (46), and desoxycorticosterone (45). If the transformation of testosterone to DHT is causally related to the development and maintenance of prostatic disease, substances capable of reducing 5α-reductase activity may prove useful in the treatment of prostatic neoplasms.

As was mentioned previously, Djoseland et al. (14) have shown that there is significant conversion of testosterone to DHT by hypertrophic tissue. It was also found that the concentration of DHT is much higher in the inner zone than in the outer zone of the prostate. Since hyperplasia usually develops in the inner mass of the prostate, this finding may indicate that DHT is causally related to the development of human prostatic hyperplasia.

On the other hand, restricted capacity to form 5α-reduced metabolites of testosterone was seen in prostatic carcinoma tissue. The amount of DHT formed by the carcinomatous tissue was significantly lower than that of normal and hyperplastic tissue. It was speculated, therefore, that the transformation of normal cells to the less well differentiated cancer cells is associated with reduction or loss of the 5α-reductase activity. However, it is important to correlate the histological grading of the tumor with determinations of the 5α-reductase activity, as was done recently by Morfin et al. (39). To determine if tumors with different histological gradings also exhibit differences in steroid metabolism, it is necessary to examine a large series of patients. Moreover, the possibility of using 5α-reduction of testosterone as an indicator of endocrine-sensitive prostatic tumors may require further investigation. The recent finding that prolonged administration of testosterone to the Nb strain of rats induces a high incidence of prostatic carcinoma (40) may provide a new experimental approach for investigating such a possibility.

ANDROGEN RECEPTORS

The mechanism of action of androgens in target tissues is generally accepted to include two important steps. One is the reduction of testosterone to 5α-dihydrotestosterone on entering the target cell; the second is binding of DHT to soluble receptor proteins and subsequent transport of the steroid-receptor complex into the nucleus of the cell. A great deal of work has been done on the importance of DHT as a mediator of testosterone action. The reader can refer to the comprehensive review of the subject by Wilson (50). Work from our laboratories has contributed to confirmation of the importance of DHT mediation; we obtained antiandrogenic effects on administration of inhibitors of 5α-reductase to female hamster flank organs stimulated with testosterone topically (47). That this antiandrogenic effect is due to decreased conversion of testosterone to DHT was demonstrated by failure to obtain similar results when exogenous DHT was used instead of testosterone.

In the next step after testosterone is metabolized to DHT, this "activated" androgen molecule is bound to receptor proteins that transport the steroid into the nucleus in a temperature-dependent process. The presence of DHT-binding proteins in prostatic cells has been demonstrated by many investigators. Bruchovsky and Wilson (10) extracted from rat ventral prostate a nuclear protein containing labeled DHT following the injection of ^{3}H-testosterone to the animals. Similar results were obtained by Mainwaring (31), who demonstrated noncovalent binding of DHT to acidic nuclear proteins, and by Fang and Liao (17), who demonstrated cytoplasmic DHT-binding proteins and called them β proteins.

These investigations have in general found high-affinity binding, with a K_d of the order of 10^{-8} to 10^{-9} M. Liao's group has postulated a two-step mechanism by which DHT is first bound to a 3.5S cytoplasmic protein, and complex is then translocated into the nucleus where a new steroid-protein moiety with a 3S sedimentation constant is formed (16). The nuclear receptor can be retained tightly only if it is bound to DHT (8).

ANDROGEN RECEPTORS IN HUMAN PROSTATE

Studies on androgen receptors have also been carried out in human prostatic tissue, both normal and neoplastic. However, most of these studies have been done in BPH rather than in cancerous tissue. This is probably a reflection of the greater availability of BPH tissues from transurethral resection scrapings.

These studies have been hampered by the presence in human tissues of SHBG, also called testosterone-binding globulin (TBG). This serum protein, which is not present in the rat, binds DHT also with high affinity (49) and has a 4.5S sedimentation constant according to Menon et al. (33). These authors stated that tissue contamination with as little as 4% SHBG would represent 2,000 to 3,000 fmoles of high-affinity binding protein per gram of tissue. In breast cancer studies of estrogen receptors, contamination with SHBG has been a lesser problem because the affinity of estradiol for cytoplasmic receptors ($K_d = 2 \times 10^{-10}$ M) is one to two orders of magnitude higher than the affinity of DHT for its receptors. Therefore useful methods to estimate androgen receptors in human prostatic tissue must take in consideration the binding contributed by SHBG and thus must be able to discriminate it effectively.

Following is a description of the varying results of measurements of androgen receptor obtained with various methods.

CHARCOAL SEPARATION

Mobbs et al. extracted human pathological prostatic tissues and incubated them with various amounts of ^{3}H-DHT with cold DHT added as competitor for saturable sites (35). Unbound steroid was separated by the addition of 0.5% charcoal and 0.05% dextran in Tris-HCl buffer. Although measurable binding was observed, the authors concluded that the steroid specificity reflected that of SHBG more than the specificity of androgen binding in rat ventral prostate.

SEPHADEX GEL FILTRATION

Sephadex filtration has been used by several authors. Hannson et al. (22) incubated slices of BPH with ^{3}H-testosterone, and a $105{,}000 \times g$ supernatant fraction was run in a Sephadex G-100. Androphilic proteins containing radioactivity were found in the excluded volume. Similar results were found after incubation of prostatic cytosol directly with ^{3}H-DHT. In a later publication, Attramadal et al. (5) used Sephadex G-200 to separate the labeled supernatant. They observed two peaks of radioactivity. The one in the void volume was heat-sensitive but nondisplaceable, whereas the retained androgen-protein complex having a distribution coefficient (K_{av}) similar to that of SHBG was easily displaced. Mainwaring and Milroy (32) also used Sephadex G-200 to analyze cytoplasmic extracts of human prostatic tissue. They found two peaks of radioactivity. The more rapidly eluted peak represented high-affinity binding, since in the presence of a 100-fold excess of cold DHT the peak was severely reduced. This was not the case with the second peak.

AMMONIUM SULFATE PRECIPITATION

Geller and Worthman (19) incubated slices of prostatic tissue with ^{3}H-testosterone. A 100,000 × *g* supernatant fraction was obtained and fractionated by successive addition of 33%, 55%, and 70% ammonium sulfate. The 33% precipitate, shown by double-label studies to be free of SHBG (which precipitates between 34 and 55% ammonium sulfate), was redissolved and filtered on Sephadex G-50. A labeled protein peak was found in the excluded volume. The radioactivity was later identified as mostly DHT. Hsu et al. (24) also used ammonium sulfate fractionation followed by DEAE cellulose chromatography. They found that SHBG was eluted with 0.04 M phosphate and the receptor in 0.4 M phosphate.

GEL ELECTROPHORESIS

By using agar gel electrophoresis, Steins et al. (44) observed three peaks of radioactivity both in plasma and in BPH tissue that had been incubated with ^{3}H-testosterone. The authors stated that the peak at the cathode side represents free unbound steroid; the second peak is typical for SHBG; the third small anodal peak probably represents albumin-bound steroid. Similar data were obtained with DHT and 17β-estradiol. Wagner et al. (48) claimed that by using agar gel electrophoresis at low temperature, good separation was obtained between DHT receptors and SHBG. With these techniques they showed DHT and estradiol receptors in samples of normal BPH and cancerous prostate tissue.

Attramadal et al. (5) used polyacrylamide gel electrophoresis to separate androgen-binding components from human prostate cancer. Tissue was incubated with 4 nM ^{3}H-DHT, and the 105,000 × *g* supernatant fraction was analyzed. Two peaks were found, one moving with the same mobility as SHBG and one moving slower.

PROTAMINE PRECIPITATION

Mobbs et al. (36) used protamine precipitation to show receptors for DHT in BPH and cancerous prostatic tissue. They claimed that interference by other androgen-binding proteins was eliminated and that the steroid specificity was similar to that in the rat ventral prostate. No high-affinity binding was demonstrated in nontarget tissues. They found low DHT binding to receptors in nontreated subjects (0–0.64 fmoles/mg tissue). These results were higher in estrogen-treated or orchiectomized patients (0.23–3.58 fmoles/mg tissue).

CYPROTERONE ACETATE

Taking advantage of the fact that cyproterone acetate competes much more strongly with ^{3}H-DHT for androgen receptors than for SHBG, Mobbs et al. (37) measured androgen receptors in patients with BPH and prostate cancer. The results, expressed as cyproterone-inhibitable binding, are similar to those reported by these authors with protamine sulfate.

DENSITY GRADIENTS

Density-gradient ultracentrifugation offers one of the best ways of separating the radioactivity bound to SHBG from that bound to the true androgen receptors. Using 5 to 20% sucrose gradients, Mainwaring and Milroy (32) demonstrated two peaks of radioactivity in both normal and adenomatous prostate tissue. Using ^{3}H-DHT, one peak had an 8S sedimentation constant, and the other was a 4S. The 8S peak could be abolished by addition of a 100-fold excess of nonradioactive DHT or a 1,000-fold excess of cyproterone acetate. When tritiated testosterone, estradiol-17β, or cortisol was used instead of ^{3}H-DHT, only the 4S peak was observed. It is to be noted that not all adenomatous prostate samples contained the 8S peak. These authors also showed that in incubations containing 0.5 M KCl, the 8S peak was decreased.

Steins et al. (44), using sucrose density centrifugation of BPH tissue and plasma, demonstrated two peaks also of about 8S and 4S when ^{3}H-DHT was incubated. When ^{3}H-testosterone was incubated, binding was observed only in the plasma. The effects of various androgens on DHT binding show comparable displacements of radioactivity in plasma BPH samples. Attramadal et al. (5) showed by sucrose density ultracentrifugation peaks sedimenting at 8S and 4S in samples of prostatic cancer. The 8S peak was heat-sensitive and was displaceable by unlabeled DHT and cyproterone acetate. Similar results were obtained by Jung-Testas et al. (27) using glycerol gradients. One 8S to 10S component and another of 4S to 5S were shown by steroid binding experiments to correspond to androgen receptor protein and SHBG, respectively.

Similarly, Menon et al. (33) showed a 9S and a 4.6S when BPH cytosols were incubated with ^{3}H-DHT and analyzed by sucrose density centrifugation. These peaks were displaceable by excess unlabeled DHT. The 9S peak was not seen when tritiated testosterone, 3α-androstanediol, or 17β-estradiol was incubated instead of ^{3}H-DHT. However, a 4.6S peak was seen with these steroids, suggesting SHBG. Also, heating to 45°C for 1 hr destroyed the 9S peak but minimally affected the 4.6S peak.

Perhaps the most useful information can be derived when sucrose density-gradient experiments are combined with other methods. Hawkins et al. (23) analyzed a cytosol from a cervical lymph node containing metastatic prostatic tissue and reported both 8S and 4S forms of high-affinity binding of ^{3}H-DHT. When agar gel electrophoresis was performed on samples from these regions, anodally migrating steroids were found only in the 8S peak, whereas the 4S peak contained radioligand bound to cathodically directed SHBG. However, in other tissue samples showing only the 4S peak, electrophoresis of this region uncovered both anodically and cathodically migrating components. Interestingly, these authors found no anodal binding from any of 25 BPH samples.

Recently methyltrienolone (R 1881) has been proposed as a new ligand for an androgen receptor (4). This compound has little affinity for SHBG, and thus binding can be attributed only to the true receptor. However, in BPH studies with R 1881 the binding specificity differed from that in rat ventral prostate in that it more closely resembled the specificity of a progestin receptor. The authors suggested the presence of atypical androgen receptors in BPH cytosol.

From the preceding discussion it is obvious that no clear-cut method exists today for fast and accurate measurement of androgen receptors in human prostatic tissue. Perhaps the most practical one is density ultracentrifugation, because of the nondestructive characteristic of the process. However, it is time-consuming. Another obstacle in measuring androgen receptors in prostate cancer is the relatively large amount of tissue needed with the existing methods. Often only tissue in needle biopsy quantities is available, and this is not enough. It is hoped that a fast and sensitive assay will be developed that will allow classification of prostatic cancers as endocrine-responsive or not. This will allow an early decision for the most promising therapy.

ACKNOWLEDGMENTS

This work was supported in part by a National Cancer Institute grant (CA-12990) and by grant 884-M from the Council for Tobacco Research, U.S.A., Inc.

We would like to thank Nobuo Monji for his help with this manuscript.

REFERENCES

1. Acevedo, E. F., and Goldzieher, J. W. (1965): Further studies on the metabolism of ^{14}C-androstene-3,17-dione by normal and pathological human prostate tissue. *Biochim. Biophys. Acta,* 97:564–570.
2. Altwein, J. E., Rubin, A., Klose, K., Krapstein, P., and Orestano, F. (1974): Kinetic der 5-alpha-reductase in prostataadenom in gegenwart von oestradiol, diathyl-stilbostrol, progesteron und gestonoron capronat. *Urologe,* A13:41–46.

3. Anderson, K. M., and Liao, S. (1968): Selective retention of dihydrotestosterone by prostatic nuclei. *Nature,* 219:277–279.
4. Asselin, J., Labrie, F., Gourdeau, Y., Boune, C., and Raynaud, J. (1976): Binding of ^{3}H-methyltrienolone (R-1881) in rat prostate and human benign hypertrophy (BPH). *Steroids,* 28:449–459.
5. Attramadal, A., Tveter, K. J., Weddington, S. C., Djoseland, O., Naess, O., Hanson, V., and Torgersen, O. (1975): Androgen binding and metabolism in the human prostate. *Vitam. Horm.,* 33:247–264.
6. Balogh, F., and Szendroi, Z. (1968): In: *Cancer of the Prostate.* Akademi Kiado, Budapest, p. 37.
7. Baulieu, E. E., Lasnitzki, I., and Robel, P. (1968): Metabolism of testosterone and action of metabolites on prostate glands grown in organic culture. *Nature,* 219:1155–1156.
8. Becker, H., Kaufman, J., Klozterhalfen, H., and Voigt, K. D. (1972): In vivo uptake and metabolism of ^{3}H-5α-dihydrotestosterone by human benign prostatic hypertrophy. *Acta Endocrinol. (Kbh),* 71:589–599.
9. Bruchovsky, N., and Wilson, J. D. (1968): The conversion of testosterone to 5α-androstan-17β-ol-3-one by rat prostate in vivo and in vitro. *J. Biol. Chem.,* 243:2012–2021.
10. Bruchovsky, N., and Wilson, J. D. (1968): The intranuclear binding of testosterone and 5α-androstan-17β-ol-3-one by rat prostate. *J. Biol. Chem.,* 243:5953–5960.
11. Buric, I., Becker, H., Peterson, C., and Voigt, K. D. (1972): Metabolism and mode of action of androgens in target tissue of male rats. I. Metabolism of testosterone and 5α-dihydrotestosterone in target organs and peripheral tissues. *Acta Endocrinol. (Kbh),* 69:153–164.
12. Collins, W. P., Koullapis, E. N., Bridges, C. E., and Sommerville, I. F. (1970): Studies on steroid metabolism in human prostatic tissue. *J. Steroid Biochem.,* 1:195–206.
13. diSilverio, F., Gagliardi, V., Sorcini, G., and Sciarra, F. (1976): Biosynthesis and metabolism of androgenic hormone in cancer of the prostate. *Invest. Urol.,* 13:286–288.
14. Djoseland, D., Tveter, K. J., Attramadal, A., Hansson, V., Hangen, H. N., and Mathisen, W. (1977): Metabolism of testosterone in the human prostate and seminal vesicles. *Scand. J. Urol. Nephrol.,* 11:1–6.
15. Dunning, W. F., Curtis, M. R., and Segaloff, A. (1946): Methylcholanthrene squamous cell carcinoma of the rat prostate with skeletal metastases and failure of the rat liver to respond to the same carcinogen. *Cancer Res.,* 6:256–262.
16. Fang, S., Anderson, K. M., and Liao, S. (1969): Receptor proteins for androgens. *J. Biol. Chem.,* 244:6584–6598.
17. Fang, S., and Liao, S. (1971): Androgen receptor. *J. Biol. Chem.,* 246:16–24.
18. Farnsworth, W. E. (1969): A direct effect of estrogens on prostatic metabolism of testosterone. *Invest. Urol.,* 6:423–427.
19. Geller, J., and Worthman, C. (1973): Characterization of a human prostate cytosol receptor protein. *Acta Endocrinol.* [*Suppl. 177*] *(Kbh),* p. 4.
20. Giorgi, E. P., Stewart, J. C., Grant, J. K., and Scott, K. (1971): Androgens dynamics in vitro in the normal and hyperplastic human prostate gland. *Biochem. J.,* 123:41–55.
21. Gupta, S. K., Mathur, I. S., and Kar, A. B. (1971): Chemical induction of prostatic tumours in random-bred rats. *J. Exp. Biol.,* 9:296–297.
22. Hannson, V., Tveter, K. J., Attramadal, A., and Torgersen, O. (1971): Androgenic receptors in human benign nodular hyperplasia. *Acta Endocrinol. (Kbh),* 68:79–88.
23. Hawkins, E. F., Nijs, M., and Brassinne, C. (1977): Steroid receptors in human prostate. Detection of tissue specific androgen binding in prostate cancer. *Clin. Chim. Acta,* 75:303–312.
24. Hsu, R. S., Middleton, R. C., and Fang, S. (1975): Androgen receptors in human prostate. In: *Normal and Abnormal Growth of the Prostate Gland,* edited by M. Goland, pp. 663–675. Charles C Thomas, Springfield, Ill.
25. Huggins, C. (1947): The etiology of benign prostatic hypertrophy. *Bull. N.Y. Acad. Med.,* 23:696–704.
26. Huggins, C., and Clark, P. J. (1940): Quantitative studies of prostatic secretion. II. The effect of castration and of estrogen injection on the normal and on the hyperplastic prostate glands of dogs. *J. Exp. Med.,* 72:747–762.
27. Jung-Testas, I., Mercier-Boudard, C., and Robel, P. (1976): Androgen binding proteins in human prostate. *Ann. Endocrinol. (Paris),* 37:97–98.
28. Kallen, B., and Rohl, L. (1960): Tissue culture studies on a rat-prostatic cancer, induced with 20-methylcholanthrene. *Acta Pathol. Microbiol. Scand.,* 50:283–290.

29. Kirdani, R. Y., Muntzing, J., Varkarakis, M. J., Murphy, G. P., and Sandberg, A. A. (1974): Studies on the antiprostatic action of Estracyt®, a nitrogen mustard of estradiol. *Cancer Res.,* 34:1031–1037.
30. Liao, S. (1975): Cellular receptors and mechanisms of action of steroid hormones. *Int. Rev. Cytol.,* 41:87–112.
31. Mainwaring, W. I. P. (1969): The binding of [1,2-^{3}H]testosterone within nuclei of rat prostate. *J. Endocrinol.,* 44:323–333.
32. Mainwaring, W. I. P., and Milroy, E. J. G. (1973): Characterization of the specific androgen receptors in the human prostate gland. *J. Endocrinol.,* 57:371–384.
33. Menon, M., Tananis, C. E., McLoughlin, M. G., Lippman, M. E., and Walsh, P. E. (1977): The measurement of androgen receptors in human prostatic tissue utilizing sucrose density centrifugation and a protamine precipitation assay. *J. Urol.,* 117:309–312.
34. Mirand, E. A. (1956): Experimental induction of prostatic neoplasms in rats. *Cancer Res.,* 2:134.
35. Mobbs, B. G., Johnson, I. E., and Connolly, J. G. (1975): In vitro assay of androgen binding by human prostate. *J. Steroid Biochem.,* 6:453–458.
36. Mobbs, B. G., Johnson, I. E., and Connolly, J. G. (1976): In vitro assay of androgen receptors in human prostate. *Clin. Res.,* 24:660A.
37. Mobbs, B. G., Johnson, I. E., and Connolly, J. G. (1976): High affinity binding of androgen by human prostate. *Proc. Am. Assoc. Cancer Res.,* 17:9.
38. Moore, R. A., and Melchionna, R. H. (1937): Production of tumors of the prostate of the white rat with 1 : 2-benzprene. *Am. J. Cancer,* 30:731–741.
39. Morfin, R. F., Leav, I., Charles, J. F., Cavazos, L. F., Ofner, P., and Floch, H. H. (1977): Correlative study of the morphology and C_{19}-steroid metabolism of benign and cancerous human prostatic tissue. *Cancer,* 39:1517–1534.
40. Noble, R. L. (1977): The development of prostatic adenocarcinoma in Nb rats following prolonged sex hormone administration. *Cancer Res.,* 37:1929–1933.
41. Ofner, P. (1968): Effect and metabolism of hormones in normal and neoplastic tissue. *Vitam. Horm.,* 26:237–291.
42. Roy, A. B. (1971): The steroid 5α-reductase activity of rat liver and prostate. *Biochimie,* 53:1031–1040.
43. Shimazaki, J., Kurihara, H., Ito, Y., and Shida, K. (1965): Testosterone metabolism in prostate: Formation of androstan-7β-ol-3-one and androst-4-ene-3,17-dione, and inhibitory effect of natural and synthetic estrogens. *Gunma J. Med. Sci.,* 14:313–325.
44. Steins, P., Krieg, M., Hollman, H. J., and Voigt, K. D. (1974): In vitro studies of testosterone and 5α-dihydrotestosterone binding in benign prostatic hypertrophy. *Acta Endocrinol. (Kbh),* 75:773–784.
45. Tan, S. V., Antonipillai, J., and Murphy, B. E. P. (1974): Inhibition of testosterone metabolism in the human prostate. *J. Clin. Endocrinol. Metab.,* 39:936–941.
46. Varkarakis, M. J., Williams, P. D., Chu, T. M., and Murphy, G. P. (1974): The effects of aminoglutethimide on prostatic function. *Res. Commun. Chem. Pathol. Pharmacol.,* 9:561–574.
47. Voigt, W., and Hsia, S. L. (1973): The antiandrogenic action of 4-androsten-3-one-17β-carboxylic acid and its methyl ester on hamster flank organ. *Endocrinology,* 92:1216–1222.
48. Wagner, R. K., Schutze, K. H., and Jungblut, P. W. (1975): Estrogen and androgen receptors in human prostate and prostatic tumor tissue. *Acta Endocrinol.* [*Suppl. 193*] *(Kbh),* p. 52.
49. Westphal, V. (1971): Steroid-protein interactions. In: *Monographs on Endocrinology, Vol. 4,* edited by F. Gross, A. Labhart, T. Mann, L. T. Samuels, and J. Zander, p. 359. Springer-Verlag, Berlin.
50. Wilson, J. D. (1972): Recent studies on the mechanism of action of testosterone. *N. Engl. J. Med.,* 287:1284–1291.

Endocrine Control in Neoplasia, edited by
R. K. Sharma and W. E. Criss.
Raven Press, New York © 1978.

Regulation of Citrate-Related Metabolism in Normal and Neoplastic Prostate

L. C. Costello, G. K. Littleton, and R. B. Franklin

Department of Physiology and Biophysics, College of Medicine, Howard University, Washington, D.C. 20059

In humans, the prostate has a major physiological function of secreting citrate, which accounts for the characteristically high citrate content of semen. Correspondingly, tissue citrate content of human prostate is uniquely high as compared to that of other soft tissues and plasma. Metabolically, citrate usually functions as an oxidizable substrate providing a major source of energy and also a cytoplasmic source of acetyl coenzyme A (CoA) required for lipogenesis. Consequently, one must conclude that the prostate epithelial cell expends a tremendous potential energy source by accumulating and secreting high levels of citrate. Such conditions emphasize the important functional relationship of citrate production as a physiological characteristic of prostatic epithelium. However, the metabolic mechanism(s) responsible for this prostate function remains unresolved. Of additional importance is the expectation that alterations in citrate-related metabolism will be associated with prostate pathology.

Although this report will not deal with a review of the earlier literature on prostate metabolism and physiology, several excellent reviews have described the many outstanding contributions that should be recognized (15,18,19,25, 26,33). In this report we will review the recent studies and current status relating to the following aspects of prostatic citrate metabolism:

1. Citrate accumulation and related intermediary metabolism in normal prostate
2. Hormonal control of citrate production
3. Changes in citrate-related metabolism associated with hyperplasia and carcinoma.

CITRATE ACCUMULATION AND RELATED INTERMEDIARY METABOLISM IN NORMAL PROSTATE

The fundamental question regarding normal prostatic citrate physiology must be "What is the metabolic mechanism(s) responsible for the characteristically high citrate production?" Table 1 presents comparative data from rats that exemplify the unique citrate relationship of prostate. In rats, the ventral prostate

TABLE 1. *Comparison of citrate levels in prostate and other soft tissues from male rats*

Tissue	Citrate
Prostate	4,000 ± 380[a]
Plasma	140 ± 11
Liver	240 ± 22
Kidney	330 ± 28
Heart	290 ± 24

[a] Tissue values are micromoles per kilogram; plasma value is micromoles per liter. Values presented are mean ± SEM.

is physiologically or metabolically analagous (if not embryologically homologous) to the human prostate in that both are major citrate-producing accessory organs. Furthermore, the rat ventral prostate and human prostate are similar in that neither functions as a fructose-producing gland; therefore the metabolic machinery is not "complicated" by this specialized function. The high prostate citrate content must arise from one of two sources: diffusion or transport from extracellular fluid derived from blood; intracellular formation from precursors.

Regarding the former possibility, no information or studies exist. One could suggest that, consistent with its function, prostatic epithelium contains a unique transport mechanism existing at the basal membrane surface of the cell that permits a net uptake of citrate from plasma. Under such conditions, measurements of the citrate extraction coefficient of the prostate (arteriovenous difference) should reveal a large net removal of citrate from circulation. Since prostatic citrate levels greatly exceed circulating levels, the possibility exists that citrate diffuses into plasma. Under such conditions the prostatic venous circulation would contain a higher citrate level than arterial blood. This would not seem to be physiologically rational in that the prostatic epithelium would be sacrificing its secretory product and potential energy source to circulation. However, this important question of citrate uptake from circulation needs to be investigated in order to understand this aspect of prostate physiology.

In the absence of a currently demonstrable citrate transport mechanism, intracellular production of citrate seems more plausible. The relationship of citrate to prostate intermediary metabolism becomes a focal point. The results of numerous studies related to prostate metabolism are complicated and confused because of the use of tissue preparations of different species and different accessory organs, making interpretations most difficult. At present, we would emphasize that the unique citrate relationship is a function of the prostate epithelial cell and not stromal tissue. Table 2 demonstrates that stromal tissue contains very little citrate, whereas glandular tissue contains extraordinarily high levels of citrate. Furthermore, teased fragments of rat ventral prostate represent preparations with minimal nonepithelial tissue, and such preparations exhibit a high citrate level (13). With this in mind, relationships between citrate and intermedi-

TABLE 2. *Comparison of citrate contents of TUR chips from patients with BPH and carcinoma of the prostate*

Patient number	Diagnoses	Number of chips	Mean epithelium (%)	Mean[a] citrate (nmoles/g)	Citrate[b] normalized (nmoles/g)
6	Cancer	3	86	5,709	6,638
9	Cancer	3	66	1,281	1,940
11	Cancer	3	70	1,244	1,777
2	BPH	3	30	7,649	25,496
10	BPH	3	50	11,596	23,196
15	BPH	3	20	9,649	48,295
4	BPH[c]	3	5	484	9,680
1	Bladder (epi)[c]	3	80	116	145

[a]Epithelium content estimated from histological examination of chips.
[b]Citrate value normalized to 100% epithelium.
[c]These chips were taken from BPH patients, but these chips contained mainly prostate stroma or bladder epithelium.

ary metabolism must be coupled to metabolic machinery within the prostatic epithelial cell.

One may typically represent citrate-related intermediary metabolism by the glycolytic Krebs cycle (Fig. 1). A high citrate accumulation may result from a high rate of citrate formation and/or a low rate of citrate oxidation. Consequently, the first question to examine is "Does prostate possess an accelerated citrate production rate that in itself would permit accumulation of high citrate levels?" Discussion of this question for the moment assumes a "normal or typical" Krebs cycle activity for citrate oxidation. Since glucose generally serves as the carbon source of citrate (through pyruvate), this possibility will be examined first. Numerous studies strongly indicate that prostatic epithelium contains glycolytic machinery that permits the utilization of glucose. Early studies (1,28) indicated that anaerobic glycolysis was the major aspect of carbohydrate metabolism. Hexokinase activity in prostate has been described by several investigators (2,35,36). Farnsworth (8) demonstrated lactate production from glucose utilization by rat ventral prostate, and Muntzing et al. (29) reported a high dependency of human prostate on aerobic glycolysis. In addition, key glycolytic and HMP enzymes have been identified (35,37,38). The capability of prostate to utilize glucose has been demonstrated by the production of $^{14}CO_2$ from labeled glucose (8,16,21,34). From these studies and others one would suggest that prostate epithelium could utilize glucose via aerobic glycolysis as a carbon source for citrate production.

However, some serious questions must still be raised concerning this possibility. To date, no one has demonstrated experimentally that utilized glucose can maintain the characteristic high citrate levels of prostate. Prendergast et al. (32) reported that pyruvate was more efficient than glucose in increasing the

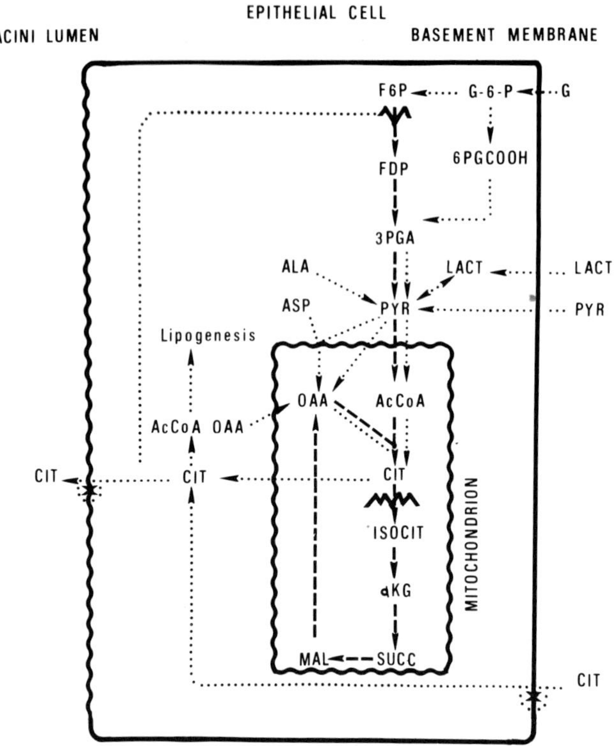

FIG. 1. Proposed scheme of citrate-related metabolism in the prostate epithelial cell. The steps indicated by dots are proposed as keys of citrate production and secretion in prostate.

citrate level of guinea pig seminal vesicle. In recent unpublished studies (Table 3) we observed that glucose did not maintain or increase citrate production of isolated ventral prostate fragments, although CO_2 production from glucose was evident. Farnsworth (8) demonstrated that lactate accumulated from aerobic utilization of glucose; unfortunately no stoichiometric studies relating glucose utilization to citrate production were reported. A major problem with virtually all of the aforementioned studies on glucose utilization arises from the absence of consideration of possible effects of the normally high prostate citrate level on glycolysis. One of the key regulating steps of glycolysis is PFK, and citrate along with ATP and AMP is a major regulator of PFK. In other tissues, citrate is a strong inhibitor of PFK and glycolysis, and the inhibition is potentiated by ATP (30,41). In the presence of the high citrate content of prostate, one might expect glycolysis to be inhibited. Unfortunately, none of the earlier studies employed conditions to study glucose utilization while maintaining high prostate citrate levels. Franklin et al. (13) demonstrated that prostate preparations *in vitro* will rapidly lose citrate to the medium unless the medium contains high citrate levels; consequently the intracellular citrate levels in such studies would

TABLE 3. *Production of citrate and CO_2 from glucose by ventral prostate in vitro*

Total citrate[a] (nmoles)				$^{14}CO_2$ production[b] (cpm/100 mg tissue)		
No glucose	Glucose 50 mg/dl	Glucose 100 mg/dl	Glucose 200 mg/dl	Glucose 18 mg/dl	Glucose 90 mg/dl	Glucose 180 mg/dl
403 ± 46	394 ± 21	352 ± 22	388 ± 5	3,149 ±352	12,263 ±1,615	27,406 ±3,251

[a] Total citrate is sum of tissue citrate and medium citrate.
[b] $^{14}CO_2$ production from ^{14}C-labeled glucose. All flasks contained 100 mg tissue. Values are mean ± SEM.

not represent the true *in vivo* situation. In view of this relationship, several considerations must be investigated. The high prostate citrate level may not be reflected as a high cytosol level. Farnsworth (8,10) suggested that the major citrate content of the prostate resides in the secretory extracellular space; consequently the intracellular citrate level is considerably lower. Whereas it may be likely that residual secretory product in prostate preparations would tend to increase the tissue citrate level, it is not plausible to presume that the intracellular citrate level is not uniquely high. Even pressed and washed prostate preparations contain much higher citrate levels than blood or other soft tissues (11,13), although such washings would cause removal of intracellular citrate (13). Furthermore, if citrate is formed intramitochondrially and secreted as high concentrations from the cell, the citrate must diffuse from the mitochondrial space to the cytosol. Consequently, we must presume that prostate epithelial cytosol does contain a high citrate concentration. It is possible that prostate PFK is uniquely different from other tissues in its substrate affinity properties and the inhibitory effects of citrate as a regulator. Since Franklin et al. (13) demonstrated that exogenous citrate will enter prostatic epithelium and accumulate without being oxidized, it should be possible to measure the glycolytic rate in the presence of high citrate levels. In the absence of such information, we must currently suggest that glycolysis in prostate epithelium would be reduced by a citrate inhibition of PFK. It would be tempting to suggest that this inhibition of glycolysis could be circumvented by the HMP pathway, resulting in 3-phosphoglyceraldehyde entry into glycolysis. Studies involving $^{14}CO_2$ production from 6-^{14}C glucose (8,16) cannot conclusively establish the major involvement of aerobic glycolysis. More meaningful and corroborating evidence must be obtained by other approaches such as 1-C/6-C CO_2 ratio from 1-^{14}C and 6-^{14}C glucose.

Although glucose utilization via glycolysis or HMP may provide some limited citrate production, the flux rate through these pathways could not account for the high concentration of citrate in prostate assuming "normal" Krebs cycle activity. An alternate carbon source for citrate might be derived from the uptake of circulating lactate or pyruvate. Prendergast et al. (32) reported that pyruvate increases citrate synthesis in guinea pig seminal vesicle (which also secretes citrate), and Farnsworth (8) observed that malate plus acetate can be converted to citrate, but the production level seems slow. It must be recognized that the high level of citrate accumulation and secretion characteristic of prostate necessitates a total six-carbon source, not the two-carbon source required to recycle citrate oxidation. Consequently a source of oxalacetate as well as acetyl CoA is required if prostate citrate production results from intracellular citrate synthesis as opposed to exogenous citrate uptake. No information exists concerning this question, but we might suggest that carboxylation of pyruvate or amino acid transamination and deamination might serve as sources of oxalacetate.

Attention will now be directed to the relationship of citrate oxidation to citrate accumulation in prostate. Generalized conclusions that prostate contains complete machinery for Krebs cycle oxidation have been made by several investigators (8,11,16,32). However, most of the information has been derived from whole homogenate or tissue preparations with very little direct study of Krebs cycle activity in mitochondrial preparations. The utilization of oxygen and production of CO_2 have been taken as indicators of Krebs cycle activity, but compared to other tissues these parameters are indicative of relatively low respiratory rates in prostate (1,5). The existence of a functional cytochrome system coupled to substrate oxidation has been identified (6). Citrate accumulation could result from a mitochondrial deficiency of isocitrate dehydrogenase; however, our recent studies (6) demonstrated the existence of an active NADP-IDH that is readily coupled to the cytochrome system. The suggestion (17) that IDH activity would be limited by accumulation of NADPH would not be applicable to prostate mitochondria. In addition, ventral prostate also contains an NAD-IDH that is activated by ADP (6) and that may be an important regulatory enzyme, as is the case in other tissues. In spite of the existence of significant mitochondrial IDH activity, citrate is not (or only slightly) oxidized by either mitochondrial preparations or teased fragments of ventral prostate (12,13), although isocitrate is readily utilized. Although teased ventral prostate will accumulate high citrate levels intracellularly, virtually none of the citrate is oxidized (13). In comparison, kidney preparations readily utilize citrate. Neither sonicated nor unsonicated mitochondria utilize or oxidize any appreciable amount of citrate; so permeability cannot be the limiting factor (5,6). A most significant relationship of ventral prostate is the unique citrate/isocitrate ratio of about 30/1, which compares with a 9/1 to 10/1 ratio in other soft tissues (13). It is of further importance to recall the findings (3,4) in which no α-ketoglutarate (α-KG) or succinate was detected in human prostate, although high levels of citrate and other Krebs cycle imtermediates were found. Our unpublished studies with ventral prostate also revealed a low α-KG content. These observations lead us to conclude that citrate oxidation is markedly impeded at the aconitase step. We suggest that prostate epithelium contains a unique aconitase in which the equilibrium is far to the citrate side.

$$\text{citrate} \longleftarrow \text{cis aconitate} \longleftarrow \text{isocitrate}$$

Under these conditions, complete oxidation via the Krebs cycle would be limited at aconitase to a slow flux. This is not typical of other tissues in which citrate oxidation to α-KG is not rate-limiting in an oxidizing system that prevents reduced nucleotide accumulation. One might alternatively suggest that a "typical" aconitase is absent or greatly reduced in prostate mitochondria, instead of indicating a "unique" aconitase. Whereas this may be the case, it will not explain the consistently high citrate/isocitrate ratio we have observed for prostate. Consequently, further studies of aconitase properties of prostate are urgently required.

In summary, the currently available information leads us to the following suggestions regarding prostate citrate production (Fig. 1):

1. Limited citrate oxidation is an important characteristic of prostate epithelium.
2. The rate-limiting reaction for citrate oxidation is the aconitase step.
3. Intramitochondrially formed citrate is at best only slightly oxidized, and the major portion of mitochondrial citrate effluxes to cytosol.
4. Cytosol citrate (a) is mainly secreted into the acini lumen, (b) inhibits glycolysis at the PFK step, and (c) may be utilized as a source of acetate (via citrate lyase) for lipogenesis.
5. Glucose may be utilized via glycolysis (if PFK is not significantly inhibited) or via HMP as a PFK bypass, resulting in a pyruvate source for citrate formation.
6. A more rapid source of pyruvate may be obtained from lactate or pyruvate uptake from circulation or from deamination of alanine.
7. Pyruvate enters mitochondria and gives rise to acetyl CoA for citrate synthesis.
8. Possible sources of oxaloacetic acid for synthesis of citrate are (a) carboxylation of pyruvate and (b) amino acid transamination.
9. Citrate may be extracted from circulation at the basement border and secreted at the luminal border.

HORMONAL CONTROL OF CITRATE PRODUCTION

Prostate citrate production and secretion evidently are regulated by androgenic control. Humphrey and Mann (20) demonstrated that seminal fluid content and tissue content of citrate were decreased by castration and restored by testosterone treatment. Several studies since have verified this relationship. Lostroh (23) demonstrated a marked increase in citrate content of mouse prostate caused by testosterone. Dondero et al. (7) reported that no correlation existed in rats between testosterone level of testicular venous plasma and citrate content of seminal vesicle. It is not clear why they would choose to measure seminal vesicle citrate rather than prostate citrate levels, since the former is not a major citrate-producing gland. Recent studies in our laboratory (Table 4) demonstrated that castration results in decreased citrate content of rat ventral prostate. Grayhack

TABLE 4. *Effect of castration (4 days) on ventral prostate citrate levels and citrate oxidation*

Group	Citrate content (nmoles/g tissue)	$^{14}CO_2$ production (cpm/150 mg tissue)
Control	2,558 ± 161	513 ± 28
Castrate	1,732 ± 137 (−36%)	705 ± 29 (+32%)

(14) and Walvoord et al. (42) reported that citrate content of rat lateral lobe was altered by testosterone, but this was evidently a growth response rather than a specified increased citrate production.

It is probable that the regulation of citrate production by testosterone is modulated by other hormonal influences. Prolactin and estradiol appear to exert a potentiating action on androgenic effects; however, neither directly stimulated citrate production in the absence of testosterone (9,14,24,42). Insulin also appears to potentiate testosterone stimulation of citrate production without having a direct effect (23). Consequently, at present the primary regulation of prostate citrate production appears to be mediated directly only by androgenic control.

The mechanism by which citrate production by prostate is stimulated by androgen is not known. Increased citrate formation from glucose may be suggested. Numerous studies have demonstrated that testosterone stimulates glucose utilization by prostate (8,16,34). The activities of several key enzymes of glycolysis and HMP pathway, as well as hexokinase, are stimulated by testosterone (31,35–37). Consequently, androgen stimulation of glucose utilization, presumably via accelerated glycolysis or HMP pathways, seems evident. Harkonen et al. (16) concluded that testosterone stimulated phosphorylation of glucose by ventral prostate and increased oxidation of glucose. Thomas et al. (40) had suggested that testosterone acted primarily by increasing glucose metabolism. As described earlier in this review, androgenic stimulation of complete oxidation of glucose to CO_2 would be inconsistent with androgen production of citrate. Increased glucose utilization by testosterone may provide a carbon source for the acetyl CoA moiety of citrate, but if complete oxidation occurs, no net production of citrate will be accomplished. Farnsworth (8,10) suggested that androgen stimulated the secretion of citrate from the prostate epithelial cell and thereby permitted accelerated conversion of glucose to citrate. However, the essential problem is not reconciled by such proposals without some additional androgen effects to permit elevated citrate production. Therefore we are still impressed with the possibility that androgen stimulation of citrate production in prostate is due principally to an effect on citrate oxidation more than on citrate formation. Unfortunately no direct studies of this aspect have been reported except for the very early reports of respiratory and total enzyme changes associated with androgen effects (1,45). We have recently demonstrated that citrate oxidation by rat ventral prostate was increased by castration, with a concomitant decrease in prostate citrate concentration (Table 4). From this and other preliminary unpublished information, we suggest that testosterone regulates mitochondrial citrate oxidation, possibly by regulating the unique aconitase activity described in the preceding section.

CHANGES IN CITRATE—REGULATED METABOLISM ASSOCIATED WITH PROSTATE CARCINOMA AND HYPERPLASIA

Citrate accumulation and secretion are evidently physiological functions of normal prostate epithelium. One might expect that neoplastic disease of prostate epithelium would be associated with alterations in citrate-related metabolism. Mann (26) recently reviewed some of these considerations. Marberger et al. (27) indicated that metastatic tissue derived from prostatic carcinoma contains little citrate. In contrast, elevated citrate content appeared to be associated with benign prostatic hypertrophy (BPH). Cooper and Farid (3,4) also observed low citrate levels in prostatic carcinoma. Recent studies in our laboratory (Table 2) confirmed these earlier studies. We have observed that extraordinarily high citrate levels exist in BPH epithelium, as contrasted with significantly lower citrate levels in epithelial carcinoma. Our findings also established that prostate stroma and adjacent bladder epithelium contain little citrate.

An evaluation of these pathological changes in prostatic citrate is not possible without the elucidation of the metabolic mechanisms responsible for normal citrate production in prostate. If limited citrate oxidation characterizes normal prostate epithelium, we would further suggest that the decreased citrate content of prostate carcinoma is due to increased citrate oxidation by the cancer cell. However, one could alternatively suggest that decreased citrate formation is characteristic of the cancer epithelial cell. In the case of BPH, elevated citrate might be the result of cellular and glandular enlargement, increased secretory activity, and a characteristic low citrate oxidation.

Warburg (43,44) has generalized that an increased glycolytic rate is characteristic of neoplasm. More specifically, Cooper and Farid (3) reported accumulation of lactate and pyruvate in untreated malignant prostate, thereby suggesting an increased glycolytic rate. Muntzing et al. (29) also suggested that increased glycolysis is characteristic of prostate carcinoma. Consequently, decreased citrate formation from glucose could not be reconciled in prostatic carcinoma, and the most plausible explanation for decreased citrate would be increased citrate oxidation in the cancer cell. Indeed, we would suggest that increased citrate oxidation accounting for decreased cellular citrate concentration would result in increased glycolysis by removal of citrate inhibition of PFK.

Since we have proposed that citrate oxidation in normal prostate is limited at the aconitase step, we would also suggest that this unique aconitase has been altered in the cancer cell, thereby permitting an increased rate of citrate oxidation. Admittedly, aconitase generally is not considered to be under regulatory control as are other enzymes (e.g., PFK, NAD-IDH, citrate synthase). However, the unique citrate-secreting function of the prostate is not evident in other tissues.

Obviously the normal prostate requires androgen for maintenance of growth and for production and secretion of citrate. Androgen is also required for the development and maintenance of the prostate cancer cell (22), which does not accumulate citrate. The role of androgen in stimulating growth and in stimulating citrate production apparently has been differentiated in the cancer cell. Consequently, the decrease in citrate observed in prostatic carcinoma is probably the result of specific alterations in the enzymatic machinery of the prostate epithelial cell independent of androgen regulation of growth. In contast, androgen stimulation of both growth and citrate production appears to be retained in BPH. Therefore, we suggest that aberrant alteration in the regulation of citrate production appears to be characteristic of the prostatic cancer cell. However, it is difficult to describe the pathological relationships of prostatic neoplasms without an understanding of the fundamental mechanisms of normal prostate citrate metabolism. It is hoped that this discussion has generated interest and ideas in the many unresolved aspects of physiological and pathological relationships of prostate citrate metabolism that must be studied.

ACKNOWLEDGMENT

Some of the studies reported were part of NIH research grant programs HD-08420 and CA-14718.

REFERENCES

1. Barron, E. S. G., and Huggins, C. (1944): The metabolism of isolated prostate tissue. *J. Urol.,* 51:630–634.
2. Bergamini, E., Bonbara, G., and Pellegrino, C. (1969): The effect of testosterone on glycogen metabolism in rat levator ani muscle. *Biochim. Biophys. Acta,* 177:220–234.
3. Cooper, J. E., and Farid, I. (1963): The role of citric acid in the physiology of the prostate. A chromatographic study of citric acid cycle intermediates in benign and malignant prostatic tissue. *J. Surg. Res.,* 3:112–121.
4. Cooper, J. F., and Farid, I. (1964): The role of citric acid in the physiology of the prostate. 3. Lactic/citrate ratios in benign and malignant prostatic homogenates as an index of prostatic malignancy. *J. Urol.,* 92:533–536.
5. Costello, L. C., Fadika, G., and Franklin, R. (1978): Citrate and isocitrate utilization by rat ventral prostate mitochondria. *Enzyme, (in press).*
6. Costello, L. C., Franklin, R., and Stacey, R. (1976): Mitochondrial isocitrate dehydrogenase and isocitrate oxidation of rat ventral prostate. *Enzyme,* 21:495–506.
7. Dondero, F., Sciara, F., and Isidori, A. (1972): Evaluation of relationship between plasma testosterone and human seminal citric acid. *Fertil. Steril.,* 23:168–171.
8. Farnsworth, W. E. (1966): Testosterone stimulation of citric acid synthesis in the rat prostate. *Biochim. Biophys. Acta,* 117:247–254.
9. Farnsworth, W. E. (1970): The normal prostate and its endocrine control. In: *Some Aspects of the Aetiology and Biochemistry of Prostatic Cancer, Proceedings 3rd Tenovus Workshop,* edited by K. Griffiths and C. G. Pierrepoint, pp. 3–15. Alpha Omega Alpha Publishing, Cardiff.
10. Farnsworth, W. E. (1972): The role of the steroid-sensitive cation-dependent ATPase in human prostatic tissue. *J. Endocrinol.,* 54:375–385.
11. Farnsworth, W. E., and Brown, J. R. (1961): Androgen on prostate biosynthetic reactions. *Endocrinology,* 68:978–986.

12. Franklin, R. B., and Costello, L. C. (1978): Isocitrate uptake and citrate production by rat ventral prostate fragments. *Invest. Urol. (in press).*
13. Franklin, R. B., Costello, L. C., and Littleton, G. K. (1977): Citrate uptake and oxidation by fragments of rat ventral prostate. *Enzyme,* 22:45–51.
14. Grayhack, J. T. (1965): Effect of testosterone-estradiol administration on citric acid and fructose content of the rat prostate. *Endocrinology,* 77:1068–1074.
15. Griffiths, K., and Pierrepoint, C. G. (editors) (1970): *Some Aspects of the Aetiology and Biochemistry of Prostatic Cancer, Proceedings 3rd Tenovus Workshop.* Alpha Omega Alpha Publishing, Cardiff.
16. Harkonen, P., Isoltald, A., and Santti, R. (1975): Studies on the mechanism of testosterone action on glucose metabolism in the rat ventral prostate. *J. Steroid Biochem.,* 6:1405–1413.
17. Harding, B. W., and Samuels, L. T. (1961): A tissue factionation study of rat ventral prostate: Subcellular distribution of nucleic acids, succinate oxidizing systems, cytochrome C reductase, cytochrome oxidase and acid phosphatase. *Biochim. Biophys. Acta,* 54:42.
18. Huggins, C. (1945): Physiology of the prostate gland. *Physiol. Rev.,* 25:281.
19. Huggins, C. (1947): The prostatic secretion. *Harvey Lect.,* 42:148–293.
20. Humphrey, G. F., and Mann, R. (1949): Studies on the metabolism of semen. 5. Citric acid in semen. *Biochem. J.,* 44:97–105.
21. Isotalo, A., and Santti, R. S. (1972): Effect of inhibitors of RNA and protein synthesis on the prostatic response to testosterone. *Biochim. Biophys. Acta,* 277:595–615.
22. Liavag, I. (1968): Atrophy and regeneration in the pathogenesis of prostatic carcinoma. *Acta Pathol. Microbiol. Scand.,* 73:338–350.
23. Lostroh, A. J. (1968): Regulation by testosterone and insulin of citrate secretion and protein synthesis in explanted mouse prostates. *Proc. Natl. Acad. Sci. U.S.A.,* 60:1312–1318.
24. Manandhar, M. S., and Thomas, J. A. (1976): Effect of prolactin on the metabolism of androgens by the rat ventral prostate gland in vitro. *Invest. Urol.,* 14:20–22.
25. Mann, R. (1964): *The Biochemistry of Semen and of the Male Reproductive Tract.* Metheun, London.
26. Mann, R. (1974): Secretory function of the prostate, seminal vesicle and other male accessory organs of reproduction. *J. Reprod. Fertil.,* 37:179–188.
27. Marberger, H., Marberger, E., Mann, R., and Lutwak-Mann, C. (1962): Citric acid in human prostatic secretion and metastasizing cancer of prostate gland. *Br. Med. J.,* 1:835.
28. McDonald, D. F., and Latta, M. J. (1954): Anaerobic glycolysis of human benign prostatic hypertrophy slices: Inhibition by testosterone. *J. Appl. Physiol.,* 7:325–328.
29. Muntzing, J., Varkarakis, M. J., Saroff, J., and Murphy, G. P. (1975): Comparison and significance of respiration and glycolysis of prostatic tissue from various species. *J. Med. Primatol.,* 4:245–251.
30. Newsholme, E. A. (1970): Theoretical and experimental considerations on the control of glycolysis in muscle. In: *Essays in Cell Metabolism,* edited by W. Bartley, H. L. Kornberg, and J. R. Quala, pp. 189–223. Wiley-Interscience, New York.
31. Ozols, R. F., and Hilf, R. (1973): Effect of androgen on glucose-6-phosphate dehydrogenase isoenzymes in rat ventral prostate and seminal vesicles. *Proc. Soc. Exp. Biol. Med.,* 144:73–77.
32. Prendergast, F., and Veneziale, D. (1975): Control of fructose and citrate synthesis in guinea pig seminal vesicle epithelium. *J. Biol. Chem.,* 250:1282–1289.
33. Price, D., and Williams-Ashman, H. G. (1961): The accessory reproductive glands of mammals. In: *Sex and Internal Secretions,* edited by W. D. Young, pp. 366–447. Williams & Wilkins, Baltimore.
34. Santti, R. S., and Johansson, R. (1973): Some biochemical effects of insulin and steroid hormones on the rat prostate in organ culture. *Exp. Cell Res.,* 77:111–120.
35. Santti, R. S., and Villee, C. A. (1971): Hormonal control of hexokinase in male sex accessory glands. *Endocrinology,* 89:1162–1170.
36. Singhal, R. L., and Ling, G. M. (1969): Metabolic control mechanisms in mammalian systems. II. Androgenic induction of hexokinase and glucose-6-phosphate dehydrogenase in rat seminal vesicles. *Can. J. Physiol. Pharmacol.,* 47:233–239.
37. Singhal, R. L., Parulekar, M. R., and Vijayvargiya (1971): Metabolic control mechanisms in mammalian systems. *Biochem. J.,* 125:329–342.
38. Singhal, R. L., and Valdares, J. R. E. (1968): Metabolic control mechanisms in mammalian systems. *Biochem. J.,* 110:703–711.

39. Szymik, N., and Buntner, B. (1975): Testosterone concentration in testicular venous blood of adult rats and seminal citric acid and fructose concentration as well as weight of accessory sex organs. *Endocrinology,* 64:304–310.
40. Thomas, J. A., Mawhinney, M. G., Smith, C. G., and Lee, T. J. (1971): The action of testosterone on the assimilation of nonmetabolizable hexoses by the prostate. *J. Pharmacol. Exp. Ther.,* 197:499–504.
41. Underwood, A., and Newsholme, E. (1967): Some properties of phosphofructokinase from kidney cortex and their relation to glucose metabolism. *Biochem. J.,* 104:296–299.
42. Walvoord, D. J., Resnick, M. I., and Grayhack, J. T. (1976): Effect of testosterone, dihydrotestosterone, estradiol, and prolactin on the weight and citric acid content of the lateral lobe of the rat prostate. *Invest. Urol.,* 14:60–65.
43. Warburg, O. (1930): *Metabolism of Tumors.* Arnold Constable, London.
44. Warburg, O. (1956): On the origin of cancer cells. *Science,* 123:309–314.
45. Williams-Ashman, H. G. (1954): Changes in the enzymatic constitution of the ventral prostate gland induced by androgenic hormones. *Endocrinology,* 45:121–129.

Endocrine Control in Neoplasia, edited by
R. K. Sharma and W. E. Criss.
Raven Press, New York © 1978.

Role of Steroid Hormones in Mammary Cancer

Suresh Mohla* and Winston A. Anderson†

Department of Oncology, Department of Zoology,† and Howard University Cancer Research Center, Howard University College of Medicine, Washington, D.C. 20059*

Breast cancer remains the cancer of highest incidence and causes the most deaths among American women. It also strikes men, but the rate among men is extremely low. One in 13 American women, or 7%, will develop breast cancer during her lifetime (81). It has been known for over a century that a relationship exists between mammary cancer and the endocrine glands (5,19,50,114). The endocrine cycles of the body modify the size, activity, and subjective quality of mammary tissue, and female breast tissue is 100 times more susceptible to neoplastic change than male tissue (6). Pilot studies have shown that after oophorectomy-induced regression, estrogen treatment may reactivate tumor growth (114). After hypophysectomy-induced regression, estrogens fail to reactivate the disease, which suggests that a pituitary factor is involved in the estrogenic stimulation of tumor growth (113). In addition to estrogens (31,45,58,82,91,94), progesterone (45,49,96), androgens (47,65,86,94,123), glucocorticoids (82,87, 93,124), prolactin (4,8,18,23,29,46,83,84,94,96–98,106–108,112,113,118,120, 126,128,129), insulin (44,47), and cyclic nucleotides (15,47,74) have been implicated in the regulation of breast cancer.

In recent years, significant advances have been made in at least three areas of investigation that may be particularly important in gaining an understanding of hormones and tumor development: (a) studies on intracellular macromolecules with high affinity and stereospecific affinity have revealed the existence of specific protein "receptors" in hormone-responsive tissues; (b) the presence of estrogenic substances in the urine of breast cancer patients after both ovaries and adrenals have been removed has led several investigators to search for the site(s) of production of these estrogens; (c) not least in importance is the substantial progress achieved in the last decade in understanding the relationship of estrogen and prolactin to tumorigenesis in the mammary gland.

Recent evidence suggests that mammary cancers that respond to hormone intervention are those that contain specific estrogen and progesterone receptors (31,49,58,82,91,94,96). Thus it appears that during neoplastic transformation, some breast cancers retain the hormone-dependent characteristic of normal mammary tissue, whereas other cancers somehow escape from this control. Although considerable progress has been made during the last decade, precise information concerning the molecular mechanisms of hormone dependency and regulation of growth, differentiation, and regression in breast cancer is lacking. Because of the inherent difficulties of conducting such experiments in humans, several experimental animal models have been employed, viz., the transplantable tumors (48,117) and chemically induced tumors (51,52,117). Both types are of interest in the study of hormone dependency. However, in this chapter only the rat mammary tumor induced by the carcinogen 7,12-dimethylbenz(*a*)anthracene (DMBA) will be considered. This model offers important advantages for study of the detailed interactions with hormones. In the first place, it provides both hormone-dependent and -independent forms that apparently are evoked from the same tissue, so that one can determine at what level(s) the hormone dependency exists. In addition, the hormone-responsive forms in the animal model and in human breast tumors respond to endocrine therapy.

The present discussion will be confined to the role of steroid hormones in mammary cancer; the roles of other hormones (prolactin and insulin) will be discussed by other investigators in this volume.

ESTROGENS

Of the various steroid hormones capable of inducing normal tissue growth and neoplasia, none has such diversified effects as the estrogens. If administration of an estrogen under appropriate circumstances can cause the development of a malignant tumor that otherwise would not have arisen, then estrogen can be classified as a carcinogen. Estrogens have long been implicated as primary agents in breast cancer. The incidence of breast cancer in men is approximately 1% of that in women (6). The beneficial effects of oophorectomy in advanced breast cancer were reported as early as 1896 by Beatson (5). Significant remissions were observed following treatment of breast cancer patients with synthetic estrogen (117). Thus both removing and administering estrogen have been used as approaches for inducing objective remissions in patients with breast cancer, which leads to a paradox: How can both removal and administration of estrogens cause tumor regression? (47).

Considerable information has been obtained regarding subcellular interactions of estrogen with both normal and cancerous target tissues. In this interaction pathway, which is derived essentially from studies with immature rat uterus (39,67), estrogen enters the cell, where it associates rapidly with extranuclear specific estrogen-binding protein, the estrogen receptor, in a very high affinity interaction. The association of estrogen with its specific receptor can be shown by sedimentation analysis to consist of a complex that moves with a characteristic mobility of 8S in low ionic media; it is dissociated in the presence of KC1 to a smaller core binding unit for the hormone sedimenting in the 4S region. The association of estrogen with its specific cytosol receptor unit endows the complex with a unique property: its ability to undergo temperature-dependent estrogen-requiring transformation of the receptor protein to a new form that, unlike its precursor, is able to permeate the nucleus and associate with the nuclear chromatin. Exposure of such treated nuclei or chromatin to buffered KCl solution extracts the intact complex from the DNA or chromatin; it is shown by sedimentation analysis to consist of the 5S complex. Although judicious use of sucrose gradient ultracentrifugation has provided valuable information about the estrogen receptor substance, including the cytosol and nuclear forms and hormone-induced receptor transformation, it must be emphasized that the complexes observed in sucrose gradients may not be indentical with those present in the cell (64). Unlike the case of immature rat or calf uterus, where the extranuclear estradiol-receptor complex sediments exclusively in the 8S region in low-salt sucrose gradients, the sedimentation patterns of cytosol complexes obtained from mature uterus (111,119), as well as from some breast cancers (94), show a significant amount of a more slowly sedimenting component (4S or 3S).

Estrogen dependency is well established in these DMBA-induced mammary tumors: the tumor regresses after ovariectomy; it grows, with marked increases in DNA synthesis and RNA syntheses, after estrogen therapy (3,41,46,78). By use of this model the first evidence was obtained for estrogen receptors in breast cancer (56,72,99). These hormone-dependent tumors resemble uterus and vagina in their affinity for estradiol, which is incorporated without chemical transformation, and in the sensitivity of this uptake to nafoxidine and similar binding inhibitors (56,59,60,72,78,99). Detailed study of the interaction of estradiol with these tumors has demonstrated that this is preceded by a two-step mechanism in which an 8S receptor protein in the cytosol (dissociable into 4S subunits) serves as the precursor of the 5S estradiol receptor complex extractable from the nucleus. However, one difference between tumor and uterus is that in tumor, a greater proportion (85 to 90%) of the estradiol incorporated is found in the nuclear fraction (78). Small fractions (10 to 20%) of these induced tumors appear to be independent in that they do not regress after ovariectomy; uptake of estradiol by these nonregressing tumors is considerably lower than uptake by the dependent ones (99). However, recent evidence indicates that certain DMBA-induced mammary tumors that continued to grow after ovariectomy of the host contained significant amounts of estradiol receptors in cytoplasm (3,7) as well as in the nucleus (7). The sedimentation properties of these components were indistinguishable from those of either hormone-dependent DMBA-induced tumors or rat uterus. The cytoplasmic binding components of both classes of tumors exhibited similar specificities for estrogens (7). In addition, it has been reported that essentially all DMBA-induced rat mammary tumors contained some specific estrogen receptor, which suggests that previous considerations of hormone dependence on the basis of the presence or absence of hormone receptors may be oversimplified (29). However, preovariectomy estradiol receptor levels of the hormone-dependent groups were significantly higher than estradiol receptor levels of the hormone-independent group. Ovariectomy decreased estradiol receptor levels only in the hormone-dependent group; as a consequence, postovariectomy levels were less suitable than preovariectomy levels to discriminate between hormone-dependent and hormone-independent tumors (75). A smaller number of hormone-dependent tumors showed low preovariectomy receptor values, indicating that there is no correlation between the estrogen-binding capacity of a tumor and its growth response to ovariectomy (7,75,100).

As methods to determine receptors have been made more sensitive, it has become evident that the numbers of human breast cancers that contain this protein are greater than was originally thought (79). However, it is also clear that mammary tumors with only small amounts of receptor rarely respond to endocrine therapy (66). Evidence has recently been presented suggesting that only one of the two forms of estrogen receptors observed in breast cancers may be important in predicting response to endocrine therapy. Objective remissions were reported only with tumors containing receptors that sedimented at 8S in sucrose gradients of low ionic strength; no remissions were seen when most or all of the receptor sedimented at 4S under the same conditions (130).

With the use of a human breast cancer cell line (MCF-7) in tissue culture, estrogen receptors in the nuclei of these cells have been observed even in the absence of estrogen in the culture medium (133). Recent data also indicate the presence of proteolytic activity in extracts from myofibrillar nuclear pellets of human breast tumors; this interferes with or prevents the measurement of estrogen receptor in the nucleus. This problem can be circumvented by using the hydroxyapatite assay, by which human breast cancers have been shown to contain both cytoplasmic and nuclear receptors. Furthermore, the nuclear receptor may be bound to estradiol or may be found in free form; the binding of free receptor in nuclei raises the possibility that unoccupied nuclear receptor may be able to stimulate cell replication even in the absence of estrogen (36).

Ovariectomy-induced depletion of estrogen receptors in DMBA-induced hormone-dependent regressing mammary tumors can be corrected by administration of estrogen and/or prolactin (4,83,127). In rat mammary tumors estrogen receptor levels (unfilled sites) are found to fluctuate in inverse relationship with plasma estrogen concentration (42). Such ovariectomy-induced regression of hormone-dependent mammary tumors is accompanied by decreases in the numbers of receptors for estrogen, progesterone, and prolactin (4,83,127); there are also transient increases in RNA synthesis (41) and tumor acid ribonuclease and cathepsin (14), as well as increased susceptibility of cytosol proteins to proteolytic digestion (116). Regression in estrone-induced mammary tumors in rats is accompanied by shrinkage of cells, decreased numbers of dividing cells, increased nuclear pyknosis, and increases in lysosomal enzymes, acid phosphatase, β-glucuronidase, and cathepsin (25,26).

Recent experiments using dibutyryl cyclic AMP indicated that treatment of DMBA-induced tumors with this cyclic nucleotide can mimic ovariectomy-induced tumor regression and, further, that a regression-associated nonhistone protein may be phosphorylated by a specific cyclic-AMP-dependent protein kinase of the tumor nucleus (15). These studies provided some of the first evidence for differential endogenous phosphorylatin of nuclear proteins during growth and regression of hormone-dependent mammary carcinoma. An aromatase inhibitor (4-hydroxy-4-androstene-3,17-dione) was recently shown to cause regression of estrogen-dependent DMBA-induced breast tumors, presumably by inhibiting the final step in estrogen biosynthesis, the aromatization of androgens to estrogens (9).

Although there is general agreement that most of the DMBA-induced tumors in the rat are hormone-dependent, there is considerable disagreement whether the necessary hormone is prolactin or estrogen (97,112,118,120,128). Synergism between estrogen and prolactin presumably regulates transformation of breast nodule to tumor and tumor maintenance; the relative roles of estrogen and prolactin in tumorigenesis and dependency have not yet been elucidated (8,23, 29,84,118,128). The ovarian hormones and prolactin, or at least their residual effects, are critical, perhaps essential, in the chemical transformation of the rat mammary gland epithelium; but pituitary hormones alone can promote the growth of these transformed cells, even in the absence of normal ovarian function (129). It is probable that growth dependency of carcinogen-induced rat mammary tumors on prolactin and ovarian hormones will vary from tumor to tumor (18,106). Although physiological doses of estrogen may enhance the action of prolactin, larger doses may inhibit the direct stimulatory effect of prolactin on normal and neoplastic mammary tissues (98,107,108). Recent evidence has also indicated that prolactin may increase the quantity of estrogen receptors in rats (4,83,126).

Since antiestrogens or estrogen antagonists have been shown to prevent the uterotrophic effect of estrogens (12,30,103,104), probably acting by preventing the association of estrogen with specific estrogen receptors (34,61,80,110), it is reasonable to assume that they could effectively counter any endogenous estrogenic stimulation of breast cancer growth. Antiestrogens have been shown to induce regression of DMBA-induced rat mammary carcinoma (13,28,70,125) and cause objective remissions in human mammary carcinoma (32,43,57, 122,127). Recent work in rat uterus and mammary tumors (17,34,76,125) indicates that antiestrogens can bind to receptor sites and translocate to the nucleus and that the processing step that removes receptor complex from the nucleus is somehow defective; this results in prolonged retention of the complex in the nucleus, a situation that may render the mammary tissue insensitive to the animal's own endogenous estrogens. In addition, antiestrogens may also partially counteract the estrogen-induced increase in prolactin levels (46), but not as efficiently as ergocryptine (inhibitor of prolactin secretion). Since the general effects of antiestrogen and prolactin inhibitor differ markedly, it is apparent that the antiestrogens cannot be acting simply as prolactin inhibitors, although reduction of an estrogen-induced increase in serum prolactin may contribute to the overall results seen when an antiestrogen is used *in vivo.*

Biochemical studies of rodent mammary tumors have provided knowledge about some properties of experimental tumors and their relationship to biological behavior of these lesions *in vivo.* The carcinogen-induced tumor has become a most valuable model for biochemical studies of the hormone dependence of breast cancer as applied to the disease in man. Early work demonstrated that estrogen-treated ovariectomized rats had high levels of uterine peroxidase and that this enzyme was within the endometrial epithelium (10,11,89,92,109). These studies were recently confirmed (1,16) when it was shown that estrogen-17β and the synthetic estrogen diethylstilbestrol administered to ovariectomized animals and to immature females play regulatory roles in inducing synthesis of endometrial peroxidase. At this point, it should be made clear that the enzyme is called a peroxidase because uterine peroxidase is a well-documented enzyme and because the histochemical medium employed in its localization is designed to reveal endogenous peroxidases in tissues (40). It is, of course, entirely possible that what is being revealed may be one or more heme proteins with peroxidatic activity; the biochemical characterization of this enzyme is still very limited. What appears clear is that endogenous peroxidase or heme proteins with peroxidatic activity are produced in the estrogen-stimulated uterus; it also appears that peroxidase activity is absent from endometrial cells of ovariectomized rats not receiving estrogen therapy and is present in uteri of rats only during proestrus, estrus, and constant estrus when the plasma levels of estrogen are high. Estrogen-induced peroxidase activity in the uterine mucosal cell has been shown to be a marker enzyme for tissues dependent on estrogen for growth. Competitive growth antagonists also induce synthesis of peroxidase in these cells. The partial antagonist effects of such antiestrogens suggest that the nonsteroidal agents also participate in estrogen-receptor-mediated gene activation in such tissues (1,16,69).

Like the uterus, hormone-dependent rat mammary tumor peroxidase is also estrogen-dependent, the intense peroxidase activity being located within the acinar cells (27). The enzyme reaction product is also relegated to perinuclear cisternae, granular endoplasmic reticulum, and Golgi apparatus and is secreted into the acinar lumen. The tumor regressing after ovariectomy loses its acinar cell peroxidase activity; however, when the tumor is again induced to grow in the ovariectomized animal by estrogen therapy, peroxidase activity reappears within the acinar cells (Figs. 1 and 2). Since estrogen induces synthesis of uterine peroxidase, it seems possible that estrogen may also play an inductive role in synthesis of mammary gland peroxidase in DMBA-induced breast tumors. There is no evidence whether estrogen directly or indirectly induces mammary tumor cell peroxidase synthesis, and one cannot discount an inductive role of prolactin. It is indeed pertinent to this subject that previous studies (46) have shown that administration of 2-Br-α-ergocryptine (CB-154), an inhibitor to prolactin secretion, and nafoxidine (estrogen antagonist) inhibits formation of preneoplastic nodules in DMBA-treated rats, blocks transformation of nodules to tumors, and blocks growth of established tumors. Administration of Parke-Davis CI-628 to intact animals induces rapid regression of DMBA-induced mammary

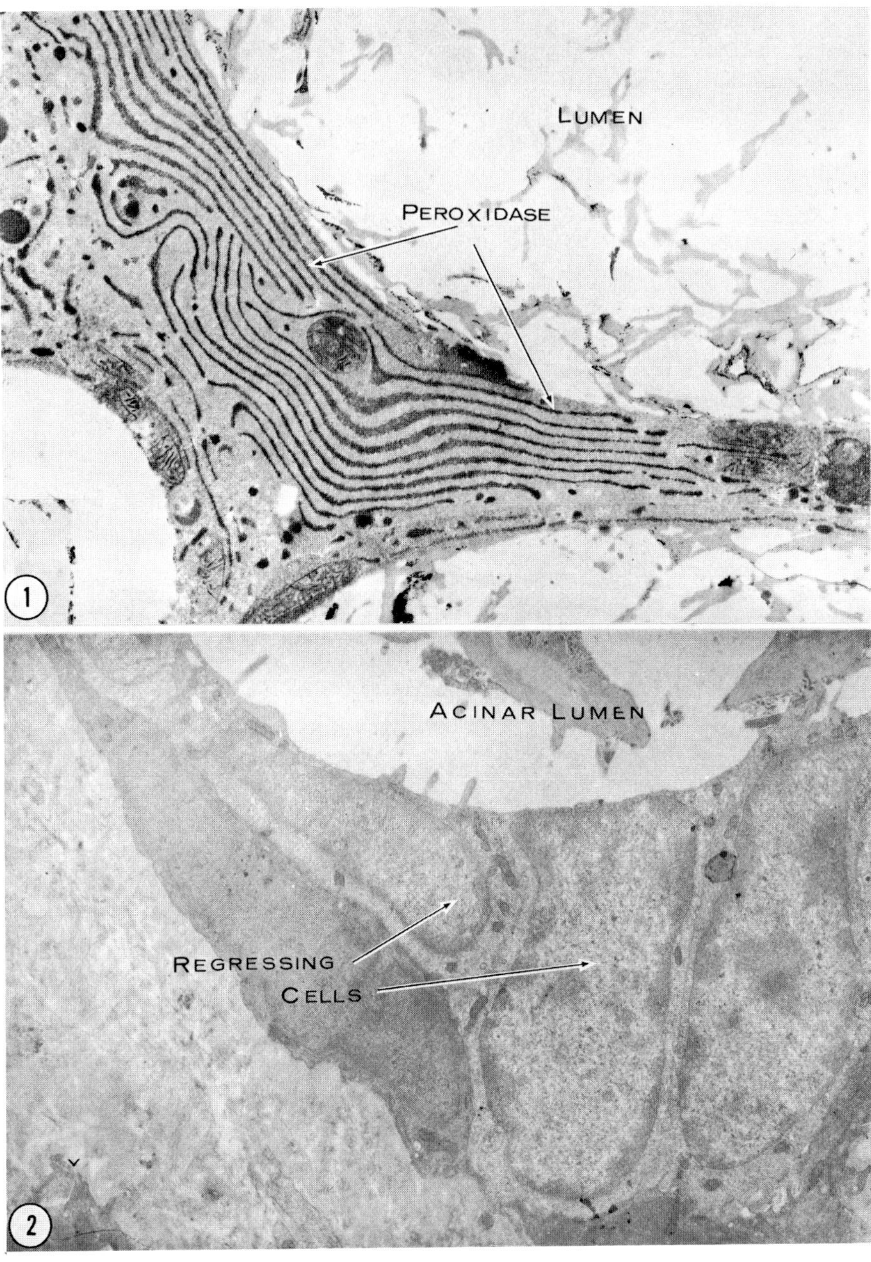

FIG. 1. Mammary tumor cells from hypophysectomized-ovariectomized female rat that received 3 daily doses of estrogen (0.1 μg diethylstilbestrol). Endogenous peroxidase is present within cisternae of granular endoplasmic reticulum. Epithelial cells remain relatively undeveloped in spite of marked development of protein synthetic apparatus.

FIG. 2. Acinar cells from mammary tumor of hypophysectomized-ovariectomized female rat. Low columnar and flattened epithelial cells have poorly developed granular endoplasmic reticulum system and no endogenous peroxidase staining.

tumors in rats (28). These results provided the first ultracytochemical criterion to allow differentiation of an estrogen-dependent mammary tumor, albeit in rodents (27). This ultracytochemical localization of endogenous peroxidase activity may provide a direct diagnostic device for detecting estrogen dependency, and it could supplement the radioactive estrogen-affinity binding procedures for the screening of estrogen-dependent tumors. Progesterone has been shown to block estrogen-induced peroxidase synthesis in the rat uterus (2). This antagonism to estrogen action does not result from blocks to entry of estrogen into target cells, estrogen binding to the receptor, temperature-dependent transformation of native (4S) to active (5S) complex, or entry into the binding of the active complex to chromatin in target cells (2). However, progesterone effects reduction in cytoplasmic receptor levels especially when administered along with estrogen; such reductions in the receptor are believed to explain, at least partially, the progesterone antagonism (2).

Recent studies (3) have shown that incubation of estradiol with tumor homogenates effects stimulation of RNA polymerase activity in nuclei of hormone-dependent tumors. This *in vitro* effect of estrogen is characteristic for the hormone-dependent tumor nuclei, but requires the presence of cytosol receptor and conditions that bring about nuclear localization of the receptor complex (3). Similar results have also been reported for *in vitro* stimulation of uterine nuclear RNA synthesis by estradiol receptor protein complexes (62–64,101,102). Experiments on hormone-dependent tumors have also revealed that lack of hormone dependence is accompanied by altered biochemical characteristics; anaerobic glycolysis and glucose-6-phosphate dehydrogenase (G6PD/2GPD) activity ratios are inversely related to hormone dependence, whereas capacity to bind hormones (estrogen and prolactin) decreases as hormone dependence decreases. There are indications that estrogens are capable of stimulating *de novo* synthesis of G6PD (47). Pharmacological doses of estrogen can also cause a lactation-like response, such as production of short-chain fatty acids, "milk proteins," and lactose; these estrogen-induced biochemical changes are accompanied by a decrease in growth rate, which suggests that secretory activities and function are not compatible with maximum tumor growth. Taken together, these observations suggest that hormone-directed substrate utilization leading to differentiated products competes with substrate utilization for cell growth and proliferation. This may help to explain the paradox of tumor growth inhibition resulting from estrogen removal or administration; the former response occurs because of metabolic embarrassment, and the latter occurs because of metabolism toward differentiation and nonusable product formation (47).

Glucose oxidation has recently been examined as a potential indicator for hormone dependency in responsive tissues; a correlation exists between the presence of estrogen and progesterone receptors in cytosols of human mammary tissue and the effect of those hormones on glucose oxidation by isolated tissue. These data suggest that glucose oxidation may serve as a metabolic marker for hormonal expression in isolated breast tumor tissue (85).

PROGESTERONE

Progesterone is one of the steroid hormones that influence differentiation, development, and functions of the mammary gland (35,68,77,90). However, considerably fewer studies exist regarding the effects of progesterone on breast cancer, perhaps because the major role of progesterone is to synergize or possibly antagonize the effects of estrogen (47). Results obtained on the inhibition of mammary cancer after administration of progesterone have been inconsistent. Recently the subject of progesterone and progesterone receptors has received a great deal of attention from both reproductive biologists and tumor biologists. Measurement of progesterone receptors in mammary cancers and other responsive tissues has been hampered by lack of suitable ligand. However, this problem may now be overcome by a new synthetic progestin that shows high affinity for progestin receptor, lack of tight plasma binding, slow dissociation rate of the complex, and negligible interference with other steroid receptors, thus permitting its successful use as a radioactive ligand for detection of progesterone receptor in target tissues, both normal and malignant (96). By use of this compound (R 5020; 17,21-dimethyl-19-nor-4,9-pregnadiene-3,20-dione) specific progesterone receptors have been demonstrated in normal and neoplastic tumors of rat, mouse, human breast, and normal human endometrium and in endometrial carcinoma (96).

In estrogen target tissues the synthesis of progesterone receptor depends on the action of estrogen (35). It has been suggested that the presence of progesterone receptor may indicate that the tumor is capable of synthesizing at least one end product under estrogenic regulation and that tumors remain endocrine-responsive (49). In DMBA-induced hormone-dependent tumors progesterone receptors decrease after ovariectomy and antiestrogen treatment (4,71,75), conditions that result in tumor regression. Estrogen treatment can reinitiate tumor growth in regressing animals, and progesterone receptors also increase in number. In mammary tumors the prolactin receptor is probably also implicated in the control of progesterone receptor, since the estrogen receptor seems to be dependent on prolactin (71).

Progesterone has been reported to be both stimulatory (44,53,54,71) and inhibitory (73) on the development of DMBA-induced mammary tumors. However, tumors growing under the stimulating effects of either estrogens or progesterone display totally different histological features (74). Estradiol-stimulated tumors closely resemble tumors growing in nonovariectomized untreated rats; their cells are actively proliferating and are round and closely packed over wide areas containing a fair number of alveolar structures. In sharp contrast, progesterone-stimulated tumors are made up of variably sized cavities surrounded by a regular wall, most often composed of a double layer of large cuboidal cells. It therefore appears that the usual structure of DMBA tumors in nonovariectomized rats is predominantly determined by estrogens, which are the main hormones produced by the ovaries of virgin rats. Large doses of progesterone in the absence of ovarian estrogens profoundly distort the architecture of the tumor tissue. This may result either from proliferation of distinct progesterone-dependent cell clones or from a special configuration of the tumor tissue induced by the differentiation effect of progesterone (74). These alternative hypotheses are worth further investigation. The ability of progesterone to enhance mammary tumorigenesis is not due to an effect of hormone on DNA synthesis (54,55). However, progesterone antagonizes the estrogen-induced peroxidase, and this antagonism could partly be due to reduction of estrogen receptors by progesterone (2).

ANDROGENS

Although the first regressions of breast cancer induced by administration of hormones were observed with the use of estrogens, a systematic search for active hormones was first carried out on androgenic compounds (20,24). The overall objective response was approximately 20%. Use of androgens to antagonize an obviously estrogen-related disease such as breast cancer was a direct outcome of early animal studies.

Pharmacological doses of androgens have been shown to induce regression of DMBA-induced mammary carcinomas of rat (131) as well as human mammary carcinomas (37,38,95). Regression is correlated with a dramatic decline in estrogen receptor of the cytosol in rat mammary tumors; testosterone affects the number of estrogen receptor binding sites and not the affinity of receptor for estrogen (132). Similar results have also been demonstrated in androgen-induced regression of human breast cancers (95). It is possible that the regression observed could be due to translocation of cytoplasmic estrogen receptor to inappropriate nuclear acceptor sites and then its elimination, leaving insufficient cytoplasmic estrogen receptor to carry out estrogen-mediated events required for growth of the tumor cell (132). The other possibility is that prolactin may be involved in this androgen-induced regression. Prolactin stimulates estrogen receptors in DMBA tumors (4,83,126), and prolactin receptors decrease after testosterone therapy; therefore, loss of prolactin receptors may at least partly explain the reduction of cytoplasmic estrogen receptor following androgen therapy (22). Furthermore, prolactin in large doses is also able to counteract androgen-induced tumor regression (115) and is capable of stimulating prolactin receptors (21); it is then conceivable that large doses of prolactin restore prolactin receptors in regressing tumors, which in turn help to restore cytoplasmic estrogen receptors sufficiently to achieve normal estrogen receptor translocation and resumption of tumor growth (132).

Biochemical studies on androgen-induced tumor regression indicate that androgens probably cause tumor inhibition by inhibiting carbohydrate metabolism and macromolecular synthesis (47). The exact mechanisms involved in these effects are not yet elucidated.

GLUCOCORTICOIDS

The role of glucocorticoids in breast cancer is far less clear. Considerably fewer studies exist regarding the effects of glucocorticoids on breast cancer. Pharmacological administration of glucocorticoids either is without effect or leads to tumor regression in 15% of cases of breast cancer (121). Glucocorticoids evoke strikingly diverse responses in different target tissues (80,87,88,105); these effects are probably mediated by a common mechanism involving steroid–cytoplasmic receptor interaction followed by translocation of the steroid complex to the nucleus, leading to accumulation of new mRNA species that code for proteins characteristic of the observed tissue-specific responses (33). Glucocorticoids have been shown to inhibit thymidine incorporation in human breast cancer cells in tissue culture; only cells that contain glucocorticoid receptor show this inhibitory response (87,88). These data indicate that glucocorticoids may directly inhibit the growth of some breast cancers, and it has been suggested that determination of glucocorticoid receptors in human breast cancer samples may help to identify patients who might benefit from glucocorticoid therapy (88).

CONCLUSIONS AND FUTURE RESEARCH

This overview of some recent work on DMBA-induced mammary tumors of rats indicates that this animal model is of value for improving our knowledge of the hormone dependence mechanisms of breast tumors; based on this improved knowledge, the model is useful in selecting and screening new compounds of potential value in the treatment of breast cancer. Regulatory proteins, the steroid hormone receptors, provide some of the most advanced models for rational physicochemical and physiological approaches to pharmalogical and therapeutic problems. Their purification and complete characterization will undoubtedly lead to even more progress in clinical medicine.

The DMBA-induced tumor responds to estrogen administration in a manner analogous to other estrogen-responsive tissues, such as uterus and mammary gland. The ability of estrogen to induce synthesis of specific proteins (peroxidase) supports the conclusion that the usual mechanisms attributed to hormonal control of enzyme synthesis are intact and function in the neoplasm. Furthermore, endogenous peroxidase may be a possible diagnostic protein for the detection of estrogen-dependent neoplasms, including breast cancer and uterine and cervical carcinomas. A suitable radioimmunoassay for detecting steroid receptors is the big attraction for the future.

There are several ways in which a mammary tumor containing abundant cytoplasmic estrogen receptors might not respond to endocrine therapy, including defective nuclear transfer of cytoplasmic receptor, heterogeneity of tumors, and defects in subsequent expression of the steroid effect at a point distal to chromatin activation. Many aspects of the relationship between hormones and the responses they evoke remain to be elucidated. Among these, the role of prolactin in breast cancer, the mechanisms of inhibitory effects of pharmacological concentrations of estrogens, androgens, and progestins, and the role of glucocorticoids in inhibition of tumor growth are particularly vexing problems. Finally, the data obtained in these animal tumors need confirmation in human breast cancer. Judicious use of information gained from the experimental models should lead to more successful treatment of the disease. At present, it is difficult to understand how simple carcinogenic agents (chemical or viral) can bring about the staggering number of changes found in tumor cells. The problem depends on the search for mechanisms that are central or basic to eukaryotic gene expression. How are genes or sets of genes regulated, and how can one alteration or a small number of alterations in regulatory agents result in such a dramatic change in the tumor cell phenotype? Can we discover which sets are involved, and can we then learn to predict the perturbations that will ensue? Can the key sets, if they exist, be turned off again? Further applications of the techniques of molecular biology for the study of gene expression should provide much needed insights into the nature of cancer and precancerous cells.

REFERENCES

1. Anderson, W. A., DeSombre, E. R., and Kang, Y. H. (1977): Estrogen-progesterone antagonism with respect to specific marker protein synthesis and growth by the uterine endometrium. *Biol. Reprod.,* 16:409–419.
2. Anderson, W. A., Kang, Y. H., and DeSombre, E. R. (1975): Endogenous peroxidase: Specific marker enzyme for tissues displaying growth-dependency on estrogen. *J. Cell Biol.,* 64:668–681.
3. Arbogast, L. Y., and DeSombre, E. R. (1975): Estrogen-dependent *in vitro* stimulation of RNA synthesis in hormone-dependent mammary tumors of the rat. *J. Natl. Cancer Inst.,* 54:483–485.
4. Asselin, J., Kelly, P. A., Caron, M. C., and Labrie, F. (1977): Control of hormone receptor levels and growth of 7,12-dimethylbenz*(a)*anthracene-induced mammary tumors by estrogens, progesterone and prolactin. *Endocrinology,* 101:666–671.
5. Beatson, G. T. (1896): On treatment of inoperable cases of carcinoma of mamma: Suggestion for new method of treatment with illustrative cases. *Lancet,* 2:104–107, 162–165.
6. Bernstein, T. C. (1977): What are my chances of getting breast cancer? *J.A.M.A.,* 238:345–346.
7. Boylan, E. S., and Witliff, J. L. (1975): Specific estrogen binding in rat mammary tumors induced by 7,12-dimethylbenz*(a)*anthracene. *Cancer Res.,* 36:506–511.
8. Bradley, C. J., Kledzik, G. S., and Meites, J. (1976): Prolactin and estrogen dependency of rat mammary cancers at early and late stages of development. *Cancer Res.,* 36:319–324.
9. Brodie, A. M. H., Schwarzel, W. C., Shaikh, A. A., and Brodie, H. J. (1977): The effect of an aromatase inhibitor, 4-hydroxy-4-androstene-3,17-dione, on estrogen-dependent processes in reproduction and breast cancer. *Endocrinology,* 100:1684–1695.
10. Brokelmann, J. (1969): Peroxidase-associated binding of estradiol by the rat uterus. *J. Histochem. Cytochem.,* 17:394–407.
11. Brokelmann, J., and Fawcett, D. W. (1969): The localization of endogenous peroxidase in the rat uterus and its induction by estradiol. *Biol. Reprod.,* 1:59–71.
12. Callentine, M. R., Humphrey, R. R., Lee, L. L., Windsor, B. L., Schottin, N. H., and O'Brien, O. P. (1966): Action of an estrogen antagonist on reproductive mechanism in the rat. *Endocrinology,* 79:153–167.

13. Chan, P. C., and Cohen, L. A. (1974): Effects of dietary fat, antiestrogen, and anti-prolactin on the development of mammary tumors in rats. *J. Natl. Cancer Inst.,* 52:25–30.
14. Cho-Chung, Y. S., and Gullino, P. M. (1973): Mammary tumor regression. V. Role of acid ribonuclease and cathepsin. *J. Biol. Chem.,* 248:4743–4749.
15. Cho-Chung, Y. S., and Redler, B. H. (1977): Dibutyryl cyclic AMP mimics ovariectomy: Nuclear protein phosphorylation in mammary tumor regression. *Science,* 197:272–274.
16. Churg, A., and Anderson, W. A. (1974): Induction of endometrial peroxidase synthesis and secretion by estrogen antagonist. *J. Cell Biol.,* 62:449–459.
17. Clark, J. H., Anderson, J. N., and Peck, E. J., Jr. (1973): Estrogen-receptor antiestrogen complex: Atypical binding by uterine nuclei and effects on uterine growth. *Steroids,* 22:707–718.
18. Clemens, J. A., Welsch, C. W., and Meites, J. (1968): Effect of hypothalamic lesions on incidence and growth of mammary tumors in carcinogen-treated rats. *Proc. Soc. Exp. Biol. Med.,* 127:969–972.
19. Cooper, A. P. (1836): *The Principles and Practice of Surgery: Founded on the Most Extensive Hospital and Private Practice, during a Period of Nearly 50 Years; with Numerous Plates, Illustrative Both of Healthy and Diseased Structures, Vol. 1,* p. 333. E. Cox, London.
20. Cooperative Breast Cancer Group (1961): Progress report: Results of studies by the Cooperative Breast Cancer Group 1956–60. *Cancer Chemother. Rep.,* 11:109–141.
21. Costlow, M. E., Buschow, R. A., and McGuire, W. L. (1975): Prolactin stimulation of prolactin receptors in rat liver. *Life Sci.,* 17:1457–1466.
22. Costlow, M. E., Buschow, R. A., and McGuire, W. L. (1976): Prolactin receptors and androgen-induced regression of 7,12-dimethylbenzanthracene-induced mammary carcinoma. *Cancer Res.,* 36:3324–3329.
23. Costlow, M. E., Buschow, R. A., and McGuire, W. L. (1976): Prolactin receptors in 7,12-dimethylbenz*(a)*anthracene-induced mammary tumors following endocrine ablation. *Cancer Res.,* 36:3941–3943.
24. Council on Drugs (1960): Androgens and estrogens in the treatment of disseminated mammary carcinoma. *J.A.M.A.,* 172:1271–1283.
25. Cutts, J. H. (1973): Enzyme activities in regressing estrone-induced mammary tumors of the rat. *Cancer Res.,* 33:1235–1237.
26. Cutts, J. H., and Froude, G. C. (1968): Regression of estrone-induced mammary tumors in the rat. *Cancer Res.,* 28:2413–2418.
27. DeSombre, E. R., Anderson, W. A., and Kang, Y. H. (1975): Identification, subcellular localization and estrogen regulation of peroxidase in 7,12-dimethylbenz*(a)*anthracene-induced rat mammary tumors. *Cancer Res.,* 35:172–179.
28. DeSombre, E. R., and Arbogast, L. Y. (1974): Effect of the antiestrogen CI628 on the growth of rat mammary tumors. *Cancer Res.,* 34:1971–1976.
29. DeSombre, E. R., Kledzik, G., Marshall, S., and Meites, J. (1976): Estrogen and prolactin receptor concentrations in rat mammary tumors and response to endocrine ablation. *Cancer Res.,* 36:354–358.
30. Duncan, G. W., Lyster, S. C., Clark, J. J., and Lednicer, D. (1963): Antifertility activities of two diphenyl-dihydro-naphthalene derivatives. *Proc. Soc. Exp. Biol. Med.,* 112:439–442.
31. Engelsman, E., Persijn, J. P., Korsten, C. B., and Cleton, F. J. (1973): Oestrogen receptor in human breast cancer tissue and response to endocrine therapy. *Br. Med. J.,* 2:750–752.
32. European Organization for Research on Treatment of Cancer. Breast Cancer Group (1972): Clinical trial of nafoxidine, an oestrogen antagonist in advanced breast cancer. *Eur. J. Cancer,* 8:387–389.
33. Feigelson, P., and Schutz, G. (1974): Studies in the control of the level of the messenger RNA for hepatic tryptophan oxygenase during hormonal induction of the enzyme. *J. Steroid Biochem.,* 5:356.
34. Ferguson, E. R., and Katzenellenbogen, B. S. (1977): A comparative study of antiestrogen action: Temporal patterns of antagonism of estrogen stimulated uterine growth and effects on estrogen receptor levels. *Endocrinology,* 100:1252–1259.
35. Friefeld, M. L., Feil, P. D., and Bardin, C. W. (1974): The *in vitro* regulation of progesterone receptor in guinea pig uterus: Dependence on estrogen and progesterone. *Steroids,* 23:93–103.
36. Garola, R. E., and McGuire, W. L. (1977): Estrogen receptor and proteolytic activity in human breast tumor nuclei. *Cancer Res.,* 37:3329–3332.

37. Goldenberg, I. S. (1964): Testosterone propionate therapy in breast cancer. *J.A.M.A.*, 188:1069–1072.
38. Goldenberg, I. S., Sedransk, N., Volk, H., Segaloff, A., Kelly, R. M., and Haines, C. R. (1975): Combined androgen and antimetabolite therapy of advanced female breast cancer. *Cancer,* 36:308–310.
39. Gorski, J., Toft, D., Shyamala, G., Smith, D., and Notides, A. (1968): Hormone receptors: Studies on the interaction of estrogen with uterus. *Recent Prog. Horm. Res.,* 24:45–80.
40. Graham, R. C., and Karnovsky, J. J. (1966): The early stages of the absorption of injected horseradish peroxidase in the proximal tubules of the mouse kidney; ultrastructural cytochemistry by a new technique. *J. Histochem. Cytochem.,* 14:291–302.
41. Gulliano, P. M., Cho-Chung, Y. S., Losanczy, I., and Grantham, F. H. (1974): Increase of RNA synthesis during mammary tumor regression. *Cancer Res.,* 34:751–757.
42. Hawkins, R. A., Hill, A., Freedman, B., Killern, E., Buchan, P., Miller, W. R., and Forrest, A. P. M. (1977): Oestrogen receptor activity and endocrine status in DMBA-induced rat mammary tumours. *Eur. J. Cancer,* 13:223–228.
43. Heuson, J. C., Coune, A., and Staquet, M. (1972): Clinical trial of nafoxidine, an estrogen antagonist in advanced breast cancer. *Eur. J. Cancer,* 8:387–389.
44. Heuson, J. C., Legros, N., Heuson-Stiennon, J. A., Leclercq, G., and Pasteels, J. L. (1976): Hormone dependency of rat mammary tumors. In: *Breast Cancer: Trends in Research and Treatment,* edited by J. C. Heuson, W. H. Mattheiem, and M. Rosencweig, pp. 81–93. Raven Press, New York.
45. Heuson, J. C., Mattheiem, W. H., and Rozencweig, M. (editors) (1976): *Breast Cancer: Trends in Research and Treatment.* Raven Press, New York.
46. Heuson, J. C., Waelbroeck, C., Legros, N., Gallez, G., Robyn, C., and L'Hermit, N. (1972): Inhibition of DMBA-induced mammary carcinogenesis in the rat by 2-Br-α-ergocryptine (CB154), an inhibitor of prolactin secretion, and by nafoxidine (U11100), an estrogen antagonist. *Gynecol. Invest.,* 2:130–137.
47. Hilf, R., Harmon, J. T., Matusik, R. J., and Ringler, M. B. (1976): Hormonal control of mammary cancer. In: *Control Mechanisms in Cancer,* edited by W. E. Criss, T. Ono, and J. R. Sabine, pp. 1–24. Raven Press, New York.
48. Hilf, R., Michel, I., Bell, C., Freeman, J. J., and Borman, A. (1965): Biochemical and morphological properties of a new lactating mammary tumor line in the rat. *Cancer Res.,* 25:286–299.
49. Horwitz, K. B., McGuire, W. L., Pearson, O. H., and Segaloff, A. (1975): Predicting response to endocrine therapy in human breast cancer: A hypothesis. *Science,* 189:726–727.
50. Huggins, C., and Bergenstal, D. M. (1952): Inhibition of human mammary and prostatic cancers by adrenalectomy. *Cancer Res.,* 12:134.
51. Huggins, C., Briziarelli, G., and Sutton, H., Jr. (1959): Rapid induction of mammary carcinoma in the rat and the influence of hormones on the tumors. *J. Exp. Med.,* 109:25–41.
52. Huggins, C., Grand, L. C., and Brillantes, F. P. (1961): Mammary cancer induced by a single feeding of polynuclear hydrocarbon and its suppression. *Nature,* 189:204–207.
53. Huggins, C., Moon, R. C., and Morh, S. (1962): Extinction of experimental mammary cancer. I. Estradiol and progesterone. *Proc. Natl. Acad. Sci. U.S.A.,* 48:379–386.
54. Jabara, A. G. (1967): Effects of progesterone on 9,10-dimethyl-1,2-benzanthracene-induced mammary tumors in Sprague-Dawley rats. *Br. J. Cancer,* 21:418–429.
55. Jabara, A. G., and Harcourt, A. G. (1971): Effect of progesterone, ovariectomy and adrenalectomy on mammary tumors induced by 7,12-dimethylbenz*(a)*anthracene in Sprague-Dawley rats. *Pathology,* 3:209–214.
56. Jensen, E. V. (1965): Mechanism of estrogen action in relation to carcinogenesis. *Proc. Canadian Cancer Res. Conf.,* 6:143–164.
57. Jensen, E. V., Block, G. E., Smith, S., and DeSombre, E. R. (1973): Hormonal dependency of breast cancer. In: *Breast Cancer: A Challenging Problem,* edited by M. L. Griem, E. V. Jensen, J. E. Ultmann, and R. W. Wisler, pp. 55–62. Springer-Verlag, Berlin.
58. Jensen, E. V., Block, G. E., Smith, S., Kyser, K., and DeSombre, E. R. (1971): Estrogen receptors and breast cancer response to adrenalectomy. *Natl. Cancer Inst. Monogr.,* 34:55–70.
59. Jensen, E. V., Block, G. E., Smith, S., Kyser, K., and DeSombre, E. R. (1972): Estrogen receptors and hormone dependency. In: *Estrogen Target Tissue and Neoplasia,* edited by T. L. Dao, pp. 23–57. University of Chicago Press, Chicago.

60. Jensen, E. V., DeSombre, E. R., and Jungblut, P. W. (1967): Estrogen receptors in hormone-responsive tissues and tumors. In: *Endogenous Factors Influencing Host-Tumor Balance,* edited by R. W. Wissler, T. L. Dao, and S. Wood, Jr., p. 15. University of Chicago Press, Chicago.
61. Jensen, E. V., Jacobson, H. I., Smith, S., Jungblut, P. W., and DeSombre, E. R. (1972): The use of estrogen antagonist in hormone receptor studies. *Gynecol. Invest.,* 3:108–122.
62. Jensen, E. V., Mohla, S., Brecher, P. I., and DeSombre, E. R. (1973): Estrogen receptor transformation and nuclear RNA synthesis. In: *Receptors for Reproductive Hormones,* edited by B. W. O'Malley and A. R. Means, pp. 60–79. Plenum Press, New York.
63. Jensen, E. V., Mohla, S., and DeSombre, E. R. (1974): Receptor transformation, a key step in estrogen action. In: *Lymphocyte Recognition and Effector Mechanisms,* edited by K. Lindahl-Kiessling and D. Osoba, p. 479. Academic Press, New York.
64. Jensen, E. V., Mohla, S., Gorell, T. A., and DeSombre, E. R. (1975): The role of estrophilin in estrogen action. *Vitam. Horm.,* 32:89–127.
65. Jensen, E. V., Polley, T. Z., Smith, S., Block, G. E., Ferguson, D. J., and DeSombre, E. R. (1975): Prediction of hormone dependency in human breast cancer. In: *Estrogen Receptors in Human Breast Cancer,* edited by W. L. McGuire, P. P. Carbone, and E. P. Vollmer, pp. 37–56. Raven Press, New York.
66. Jensen, E. V., Smith, S., and DeSombre, E. R. (1976): Hormone dependency in breast cancer. *J. Steroid Biochem.,* 7:911–917.
67. Jensen, E. V., Suzuki, J., Kawashima, T., Stump, W. E., Jungblut, P. W., and DeSombre, E. R. (1968): A two step mechanism for the interaction of estradiol with rat uterus. *Proc. Natl. Acad. Sci. U.S.A.,* 59:632–638.
68. Juergens, W. G., Stockdale, F. E., Topper, Y. J., and Elias, J. J. (1965): Hormone-dependent differentiation of mammary gland *in vitro. Proc. Natl. Acad. Sci. U.S.A.,* 54:629–634.
69. Kang, Y. H., Anderson, W. A., and DeSombre, E. R. (1975): Modulation of uterine morphology and growth by estradiol-17β and the estrogen antagonist Parke Davis, CI-628. *J. Cell Biol.,* 64:682–691.
70. Kelly, P. A., Asselin, J., Caron, M. G., Labrie, F., and Raynaud, J. P. (1977): Potent inhibitory effect of a new antiestrogen (RU16117) on the growth of 7,12-dimethylbenz*(a)*anthracene-induced rat mammary tumors. *J. Natl. Cancer Inst.,* 58:623–628.
71. Kelly, P. A., Asselin, J., Labrie, F., and Raynaud, J. P. (1977): Regulation of hormone receptor levels and growth of DMBA-induced mammary tumors by RU16117 and other steroids in the rat. In: *Progesterone Receptors in Normal and Neoplastic Tissues,* edited by W. L. McGuire, J. P. Raynaud, and E. E. Baulieu, pp. 85–101. Raven Press, New York.
72. King, R. J., Cowan, D. M., and Inman, D. R. (1965): The uptake of (6,7-^{3}H)oestradiol by dimethylbenzanthracene-induced rat mammary tumours. *J. Endocrinol.,* 32:83–90.
73. Kledzik, G. S., Bradley, C. J., and Meites, J. (1974): Reduction of carcinogen-induced mammary cancer incidence in rats by early treatment with hormones or drugs. *Cancer Res.,* 34:2953–2956.
74. Klein, D. M., and Loizzi, R. F. (1977): Enhancement of R3230AC rat mammary tumor growth and cellular differentiation by dibutyryl cyclic adenosine monophosphate. *J. Natl. Cancer Inst.,* 58:813–818.
75. Koenders, A. J. M., Moespot, A. G., Zolingen, S. J., and Benraad, T. J. (1977): Progesterone and estradiol receptors in DMBA-induced mammary tumors before and after ovariectomy and after subsequent estradiol administration. In: *Progesterone Receptors in Normal and Neoplastic Tissues,* edited by W. L. McGuire, J. P. Raynaud, and E. E. Baulieu, pp. 71–101. Raven Press, New York.
76. Koseki, Y., Zava, D. T., Chamness, G. C., and McGuire, W. L. (1977): Estrogen receptor translocation and replishment by the antiestrogen tamoxifen. *Endocrinology,* 101:1104–1110.
77. Kuhn, N. J. (1969): Progesterone withdrawal as a lactogenic trigger in the rat. *J. Endocrinol.,* 44:39–54.
78. Kyser, K. A. (1970): The tissue subcellular and molecular binding of estradiol to dimethylbenzanthracene-induced rat mammary tumors. Ph.D. dissertation, University of Chicago.
79. Leclercq, G., Heuson, J. C., Deboel, M. C., and Mattheiem, W. H. (1975): Oestrogen receptors in breast cancer: A changing concept. *Br. Med. J.,* 1:185–189.
80. Lee, K., and Kenny, F. T. (1971): Regulation of tyrosine-ketoglutarate transaminase in rat livers. *J. Biol. Chem.,* 246:7595–7601.
81. Leis, H. P., Jr. (1977): The diagnosis of breast cancer. *CA,* 27:209–232.
82. Leung, B. S., Fletcher, W. S., Lindell, T. D., Wood, D. C., and Krippaehne, W. W. (1973):

Predictability of response to endocrine ablation in advanced breast carcinoma. *Arch. Surg.*, 106:515–519.
83. Leung, B. S., and Sasaki, G. H. (1975): On the mechanism of prolactin and estrogen action in 7,12-dimethyl-benzanthracene-induced mammary carcinoma in the rat. II. *In vivo* tumor responses and estrogen receptor. *Endocrinology,* 97:654–572.
84. Leung, B. S., Sasaki, G. H., and Leung, J. S. (1975): Estrogen-prolactin dependency in 7,12-dimethylbenz*(a)*anthracene-induced tumors. *Cancer Res.*, 35:621–627.
85. Levy, J., and Glick, S. M. (1977): Estrogen and progesterone receptors and glucose oxidation in mammary tissue. In: *Progesterone Receptors in Normal and Neoplastic Tissues,* edited by W. L. McGuire, J. P. Raynaud, and E. E. Baulieu, pp. 211–225. Raven Press, New York.
86. Lippman, M. E., Bolan, G., and Huff, K. (1975): Androgen responsive human breast cancer in continuous tissue culture. *Nature,* 256:592–593.
87. Lippman, M. E., Bolan, G., and Huff, K. (1976): The effects of glucocorticoids and progesterone on hormone responsive human breast cancer in long term culture. *Cancer Res.,* 36:4610–4618.
88. Lippman, M. E., Osborne, C. K., Knazek, R., and Young, N. (1977): *In vitro* model systems for the study of hormone-dependent human breast cancer. *N. Engl. J. Med.,* 296:154–159.
89. Lucas, F. V., Neufeld, H. A., Utterback, J. G., Martin, A. P., and Stotz, E. (1955): The effect of estrogen on the production of a peroxidase in the uterus. *J. Biol. Chem.,* 214:775–780.
90. Lyons, W. R., Li, C. H., and Johnson, R. E. (1958): Hormonal control of mammary growth. *Recent Prog. Horm. Res.,* 14:219–254.
91. Maass, H., Engel, B., Hohmeister, H., Lehmann, F., and Trans, G. (1972): Estrogen receptors in human breast cancer tissue. *Am. J. Obstet. Gynecol.,* 113:377–382.
92. Martin, A. P., Neufeld, H. A., Lucas, F. V., and Stotz, E. (1958): Characterization of uterine peroxidase. *J. Biol. Chem.,* 233:206–208.
93. McGuire, W. L., Carbone, P. P., Sears, M. E., and Escher, G. C. (1975): Estrogen receptors in human breast cancer: An overview. In: *Estrogen Receptors in Human Breast Cancer,* edited by W. L. McGuire, P. P. Carbone, and E. P. Vollmer, pp. 1–7. Raven Press, New York.
94. McGuire, W. L., Carbone, P. P., and Vollmer, E. P. (editors) (1975): *Estrogen Receptors in Human Breast Cancer.* Raven Press, New York.
95. McGuire, W. L., Chamness, G. C., Costlow, M. E., and Horwitz, K. B. (1976): Hormone receptors in breast cancer. In: *Modern Pharmacology,* edited by G. S. Levy, pp. 265–299. Marcel Dekker, New York.
96. McGuire, W. L., Raynaud, J. P., and Baulieu, E. E. (editors) (1977): *Progesterone Receptors in Normal and Neoplastic Tissues.* Raven Press, New York.
97. Meites, J. (1972): The relation of estrogen and prolactin to mammary tumorigenesis in the rat. In: *Estrogen Target Tissue and Neoplasia,* edited by T. L. Dao, pp. 275–286. University of Chicago Press, Chicago.
98. Meites, J., Cassell, E., and Clark, J. (1971): Estrogen inhibition of mammary tumor growth in rats; counteraction by prolactin. *Proc. Soc. Exp. Biol. Med.,* 137:1225–1227.
99. Mobbs, B. G. (1966): The uptake of tritiated oestradiol by dimethylbenzanthracene-induced mammary tumours of the rat. *J. Endocrinol.,* 36:409–414.
100. Mobbs, B. G., and Johnson, I. E. (1974): Estrogen-binding *in vitro* by DMBA-induced rat mammary tumors: Its relationship to hormone responsiveness. *Eur. J. Cancer,* 10:757–763.
101. Mohla, S., DeSombre, E. R., and Jensen, E. V. (1972): Tissue specific stimulation of RNA synthesis by transformed estradiol-receptor complex. *Biochem. Biophys. Res. Commun.,* 46:661–667.
102. Mohla, S., DeSombre, E. R., and Jensen, E. V. (1975): Stimulation of RNA synthesis in uterine nuclei by estradiol-estrophilin complexes. *Fed. Proc.,* 34:320.
103. Mohla, S., and Prasad, M. R. N. (1968): Inhibition of oestrogen-induced glycogen synthesis in the rat by clomiphene. *Steroids,* 11:571.
104. Mohla, S., and Prasad, M. R. N. (1969): Estrogen-antiestrogen interaction. Effect of U11100A, MRL-41, and U1155A on estrogen-induced glycogen synthesis in the rat during delayed implantation. *Acta Endocrinol. (Kbh),* 62:489–497.
105. Munck, A. (1971): Glucocorticoid inhibition of glucose uptake by peripheral tissues: Old and new evidence, molecular mechanisms, and physiological significance. *Perspect. Biol. Med.,* 14:265–289.
106. Nagasawa, H., Chen, C., and Meites, J. (1973): Relation between growth of carcinogen-induced

mammary cancers and serum prolactin values in rats. *Proc. Soc. Exp. Biol. Med.*, 142:625–627.
107. Nagasawa, H., and Yanai, R. (1971): Reduction by pituitary isograft of inhibitory effect of large doses of estrogen on incidence of mammary tumors induced by carcinogen in ovariectomized rats. *Int. J. Cancer,* 8:463–467.
108. Nagasawa, H., and Yanai, R. (1974): Effects of estrogen and/or pituitary isograft on nucleic acid synthesis of carcinogen-induced mammary tumors in rats. *J. Natl. Cancer Inst.*, 52:1219–1222.
109. Neufeld, H. A., Levan, A. N., Lucas, F. V., Martin, A. P., and Stotz, E. (1958): Peroxidase and cytochrome oxidase in rat tissues. *J. Biol. Chem.*, 233:209–211.
110. Nicholson, R. I., Davies, P., and Griffiths, K. (1977): Effects of oestradiol-17β and tamoxifen on nuclear oestradiol-17β receptors in DMBA-induced rat mammary tumours. *Eur. J. Cancer,* 13:201–208.
111. Notides, A. C., Hamilton, D. E., and Rudolph, J. H. (1973): The action of a human uterine protease on the estrogen receptor. *Endocrinology,* 93:210–216.
112. Pearson, O. H., Molina, A., Butler, T. P., Uerena, L., and Nasr, H. (1972): Estrogens and prolactin in mammary cancer. In: *Estrogen Target Tissue and Neoplasia,* edited by T. L. Dao, pp. 287–305. University of Chicago Press, Chicago.
113. Pearson, O. H., and Ray, B. S. (1959): Results of hypophysectomy in the treatment of metastatic mammary carcinoma. *Cancer,* 12:85.
114. Pearson, O. H., West, C. D., Hollander, V., and Treves, N. L. (1954): Evaluation of endocrine therapy for advanced breast cancer. *J.A.M.A.*, 154:234.
115. Quadri, S. K., Kledzik, G. S., and Meites, J. (1974): Counteraction by prolactin of androgen-induced inhibition of mammary tumor growth in rats. *J. Natl. Cancer Inst.*, 52:875–878.
116. Rouleau, M., and Gullino, P. M. (1977): Increased susceptibility of cytosol proteins to proteolytic digestion during regression of a hormone-dependent mammary tumor. *Cancer Res.*, 37:670–677.
117. Segaloff, A. (1966): Hormones and breast cancer. *Recent Prog. Horm. Res.*, 22:351–379.
118. Sinha, D., Cooper, D., and Dao, T. L. (1973): The nature of estrogen and prolactin effect on mammary tumorigenesis. *Cancer Res.*, 33:411–414.
119. Steggles, A. W., and King, R. J. B. (1970): The use of protamine to study (6,7-^{3}H) oestradiol-17β binding in rat uterus. *Biochem. J.*, 118:695–701.
120. Sterental, A., Dominguez, J. M., Weismann, C., and Pearson, O. H. (1963): Pituitary role in the estrogen dependency of experimental mammary cancer. *Cancer Res.*, 23:481–484.
121. Stoll, B. A. (1972): Androgen, corticosteroid and progestin therapy. In: *Endocrine Therapy of Malignant Disease,* edited by B. A. Stoll, pp. 176–182. W. B. Saunders, Philadelphia.
122. Tagnon, H. J. (1976): Antiestrogens. In: *Breast Cancer: A Report to the Profession,* p. 62. Sponsored by The White House, The National Cancer Institute, and the American Cancer Society, Nov. 22–23. Washington, D.C.
123. Tagnon, H. J. (1976): Role of hormones in the modern treatment of advanced breast cancer. In: *Breast Cancer: Trends in Research and Treatment,* edited by J. C. Heuson, W. H. Mattheiem, and M. Rozencweig, pp. 187–192. Raven Press, New York.
124. Teulings, F. A. G., Treurniet, R. E., and Van Gilse, H. A. (1976): Glucocorticoid receptors in human breast carcinomas. In: *Proceedings of Fifth International Congress of Endocrinology,* abstract #136:55, Hamburg, Germany.
125. Tsai, T. L. S., and Katzenellenbogen, B. (1977): Antagonism of development and growth of 7,12-dimethylbenz*(a)*anthracene-induced rat mammary tumors by the antiestrogen U23,469 and effects on estrogen and progesterone receptors. *Cancer Res.,* 37:1537–1543.
126. Vignon, F., and Rochefort, H. (1976): Regulation of estrogen receptors in ovarian-dependent rat mammary tumors. I. Effects of castration and prolactin. *Endocrinology,* 98:722–729.
127. Ward, H. W. C. (1973): Anti-estrogen therapy for breast cancer. A trial of tamoxifen at two dose levels. *Br. Med. J.*, 1:13–14.
128. Welsch, C. W. (1972): Effect of brain lesions on mammary tumorigenesis. In: *Estrogen Target Tissue and Neoplasia,* edited by T. L. Dao, pp. 317–331. University of Chicago Press, Chicago.
129. Welsch, C. W., and Nagasawa, H. (1977): Prolactin and murine mammary tumorigenesis: A review. *Cancer Res.*, 37:951–963.
130. Witliff, J. L., Beatty, B. W., Savlov, E. D., Patterson, W. B., and Cooper, R. A., Jr. (1976): Estrogen receptors and hormone dependency in human breast cancer. Recent results. *Cancer Res.*, 57:59–77.

131. Young, S., Baker, R. A., and Helfenstein, J. E. (1965): The effects of androgens on induced mammary tumors in rats. *Br. J. Cancer,* 19:155–159.
132. Zava, D. T., and McGuire, W. L. (1977): Estrogen receptors in androgen-induced breast tumor regression. *Cancer Res.,* 37:1608–1610.
133. Zava, D. T., and McGuire, W. L. (1977): Estrogen receptor: Unoccupied sites in nuclei of a breast tumor cell line. *J. Biol. Chem.,* 252:3703–3708.

CYCLIC NUCLEOTIDES

Endocrine Control in Neoplasia, edited by
R. K. Sharma and W. E. Criss.
Raven Press, New York © 1978.

Interaction of Cyclic AMP and Estrogen in Tumor Growth Control

Yoon Sang Cho-Chung

Laboratory of Pathophysiology, National Cancer Institute, National Institutes of Health, Bethesda, Maryland 20014

The roles of cyclic nucleotides in the control of tumor growth *in vivo* have been discussed in a recent review (9). The purpose of this chapter is threefold: (a) to describe the reciprocal relationship between cyclic adenosine 3′,5′-monophosphate (cyclic AMP) and estrogen in growth control of a hormone-dependent mammary tumor; (b) to show how cyclic AMP might counteract estrogen effects during regression of mammary tumors; (c) to introduce the concept that intracellular availability of estrogen may selectively regulate cyclic nucleotide participation in modulating mammary tumor growth.

ARREST OF MAMMARY TUMOR GROWTH *IN VIVO*

Effects of Cyclic Nucleotides

Sapag-Hagar and Greenbaum (53) reported that the tissue content of cyclic AMP in rat mammary gland rises continuously during gestation and then falls progressively to its lowest level by the 16th day of lactation. The transition at parturition coincides in time with the increased metabolic activity of the gland due to the initiation of lactation. A reverse pattern is seen for cyclic guanosine 3′,5′-monophosphate (cyclic GMP) during the various stages of the cycle. These observations suggest an involvement of cyclic nucleotides in the growth and development of the mammary gland.

Studies by Klein and Loizzi (35) provided an example of the effect of cyclic AMP on cell differentiation and growth in the hormone-responsive R323OAC rat mammary adenocarcinoma. Following daily subcutaneous injections of $N^6,O^{2'}$-dibutyryl cyclic AMP (dibutyryl cyclic AMP) beginning on day 1 after tumor implantation, the growth rate increased appreciably. R323OAC tumor is composed primarily of epithelial cells with a histologic organization resembling mammary gland alveoli (26,62). The ultrastructure of cells treated with dibutyryl cyclic AMP showed a rough endoplasmic reticulum in short dilated segments, proliferation of the Golgi complex with extensive membrane, dilated cisternae, and numerous vesicles of various sizes containing fine granular material indicative of cell differentiation. With these data Klein and Loizzi suggested that the increase in tumor size after dibutyryl cyclic AMP treatment is attributable to an increase in cell size rather than an increase in cell number. These *in vivo* studies are compatible with *in vitro* studies in which changes in morphology, synthesis of specialized cell products, and cell differentiation are often associated with cyclic-AMP-induced inhibition of cell proliferation (31,51).

Growth inhibition of R323OAC tumors by cyclic nucleotides has also been observed. Bogden and associates *(personal communication)* compared the growth curves of R323OAC and 13762 mammary adenocarcinomas following daily intraperitoneal injections of dibutyryl cyclic AMP (20 mg/kg) for 22 days after tumor implantation and found appreciable inhibition of only the R323OAC tumor. The studies of Cho-Chung et al. (8,19,20) have shown growth-inhibiting effects on a variety of established rat mammary tumors. Dibutyryl cyclic AMP treatment (8 mg/day/200-g rat s.c.) of rats bearing R323OAC tumors produced growth arrest of some tumors but had no effect on others. The same treatment of hormone-independent Walker 256 (W256) mammary carcinoma produced regression in only a fraction of the transplants, thus suggesting a mixed cell population with different degrees of susceptibility to the nucleotide. When rats bearing hormone-dependent tumors, primary 7,12-dimethylbenz(α)anthracene-(DMBA)-induced tumors, and transplantable MTW9 tumors were injected similarly with dibutyryl cyclic AMP, 8-thiomethyl cyclic AMP, and 8-bromo cyclic AMP, respectively, tumor growth was arrested, and this inhibition was reversible only on cessation of the treatment. However, the same nucleotides had less inhibitory effect on the growth of primary nitrosomethylurea-(NMU)-induced mammary carcinoma. Thus it appears that exogenous cyclic nucleotides can inhibit mammary tumor growth, but the inhibition varies with tumor cell populations.

Effects of Hormones

Mammary tumors can be classified into three types: (a) hormone-dependent tumors, which grow only in the presence of hormone and regress either in the absence of hormone or with pharmacological doses of hormone; (b) hormone-responsive tumors, which do not require hormone for growth but whose growth is retarded by pharmacological doses of hormone; (c) hormone-independent tumors, which grow in the absence and presence of hormone and may or may not regress with pharmacologic doses of hormone. These models have been empirically defined on the basis of their responses to hormonal manipulation of the host, although in any single tumor all types of cells may coexist, and thus partial responses have been most often observed.

It has long been assumed that estrogens may be essential for the growth of mammary carcinomas. Evidence for the beneficial effects of ovariectomy in some, but not all, advanced breast cancers was obtained by Beatson (1), Schinzinger (54), and Huggins and Bergenstal (27). Later reports demonstrated the efficacy of treating breast cancer with synthetic estrogens (25) and nonsteroidal agents with antiestrogenic activity (7,40). These findings have since been repeatedly examined and confirmed (55). Thus deprivation, administration, and antagonization of estrogens all produced remission in certain mammary carcinomas.

The hormone dependency of mammary tumors was subsequently shown to correlate with certain biochemical properties of the tumors. Of particular importance were the findings that the majority of hormone-dependent tumors specifically incorporate [^{3}H]estradiol (30,32,47,52,61) and that tumor cytosol and nuclei contain specific estrogen-binding proteins (34,39,45), just as do estrogen-responsive normal tissues (29,33,41,50,63). It has therefore become possible to predict the hormone dependency of tumors by determining the estrogen receptor proteins in biopsy specimens. However, the presence of estrogen receptors per se is not an absolute indication of hormone dependency (5), as revealed by clinical studies in which only 50% of those patients whose tumors contained estrogen receptors showed a favorable response to hormone therapy (44). Thus it appears that estrogen may promote the growth of certain mammary tumors, but estrogen deprivation may or may not produce regression.

DIBUTYRYL CYCLIC AMP MIMICS OVARIECTOMY

Data described in the preceding section showed clearly that the growth of mammary tumors can be influenced by either cyclic nucleotide treatment or hormonal manipulation. For example, hormone-dependent DMBA-induced mammary carcinoma undergoes growth arrest following either ovariectomy or dibutyryl cyclic AMP treatment of the host (8). Recently Cho-Chung et al. (3,4,11,12,21) obtained evidence that regulation of hormone-dependent tumor growth may depend on an antagonistic action between cyclic AMP and estrogen. The observations supporting this relationship are described below.

Cyclic AMP Level

Ovariectomy and dibutyryl cyclic AMP treatment of respective DMBA-tumor-bearing hosts resulted in an immediate increase in cyclic AMP content of the tumors (3,4,11,12). The time course of change of cyclic AMP content in these tumors is shown in Fig. 1. A peak level (~ threefold that of the growing tumor) was reached 1 day after dibutyryl cyclic AMP treatment and 2 days after ovariectomy. The increase in cyclic AMP content of the tumors followed a sharp increase in adenylate cyclase activity (4,12). Three days after both treatments, the cyclic AMP content decreased simultaneously with the increased cyclic AMP phosphodiesterase activity (4,12). The increases in cyclic AMP level and adenylate cyclase and phosphodiesterase activities subsided in those tumors resuming growth following the injection of estradiol valerate or cessation of dibutyryl cyclic AMP treatment (Fig. 1).

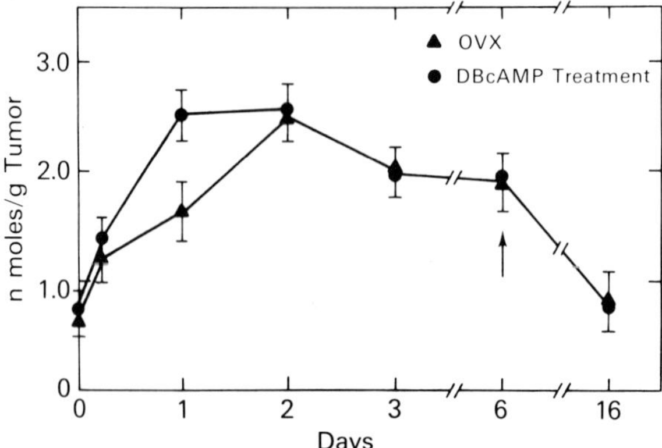

FIG. 1. Cyclic AMP content of DMBA-induced mammary tumors during ovariectomy or dibutyryl cyclic AMP treatment. Arrow indicates start of estradiol valerate injection (8) or cessation of dibutyryl cyclic AMP treatment (8). Cyclic AMP levels in tumors were measured by Gilman's competitive protein binding method as previously described (8). Values are means of 10 tumors ± S.E.

Cyclic-AMP- and Estrogen-binding Activities

Changes in the specific binding of estrogen and cyclic AMP to proteins of DMBA tumors were produced by both dibutyryl cyclic AMP treatment and ovariectomy (3,4,11,12) (Fig. 2). Three days after either ovariectomy or dibutyryl cyclic AMP treatment, cyclic AMP binding increased fivefold and twofold in the tumor nuclei and cytosols, respectively, whereas nuclear and cyto-plasmic estrogen binding decreased by 70% and 25%, respectively. Cyclic AMP binding increased first in the cytosol, and when the nuclei-associated cyclic AMP binding reached a peak activity, the cytosol binding decreased. Conversely, estrogen binding decreased first in the nuclei, followed by a decrease of cytoplasmic estrogen binding. These reciprocal changes in cyclic-AMP- and estrogen-binding activities were detectable within 1 day after either ovariectomy or dibutyryl cyclic AMP treatment, when there was no appreciable change in tumor size. The changes were reversed, however, when tumor growth was resumed following the injection of estradiol valerate or cessation of dibutyryl cyclic AMP treatment.

Concomitant with the increase in cyclic-AMP-binding activity in the regressing tumors was an increase in protein kinase activity. The identity between cyclic-AMP-dependent protein kinase and cyclic-AMP-binding protein (12), as found in DEAE cellulose column chromatography profiles and sucrose density-gradient sedimentation patterns, suggested a similar relationship between these proteins in DMBA tumors as shown in other tissues (36,38). The increased activities of both cyclic AMP binding and protein kinase due to ovariectomy could be attributed to new protein synthesis, since cycloheximide was found to block these activities.

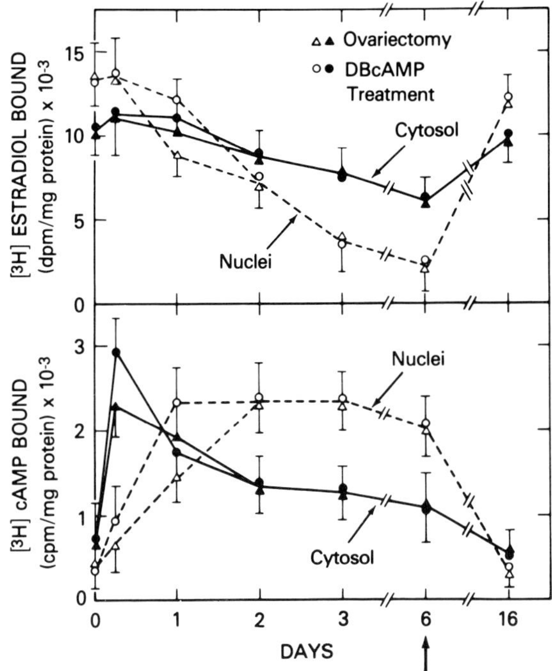

FIG. 2. Estrogen- and cyclic AMP-binding activities in cytosol and nuclei of DMBA-induced mammary tumors during ovariectomy or dibutyryl cAMP treatment. Vertical arrow indicates start of estradiol valerate injection (8) or cessation of dibutyryl cyclic AMP treatment (8). Tumors growing and regressing (at times indicated following ovariectomy or dibutyryl cyclic AMP treatment), respectively, were removed and homogenized, and cytosols and nuclear extracts were prepared by a method (14) previously described. Cyclic AMP- and estrogen-binding activities in the extracts were assayed by methods previously described (3,16). Values represent means of 10 tumors ± S.E.

Nuclear Protein Phosphorylation

A change in protein-kinase-dependent phosphate incorporation in isolated nuclei of DMBA tumors was also observed (21) following either ovariectomy or dibutyryl cyclic AMP treatment. As shown in Fig. 3, protein species IV was found to be the major endogenous substrate for nuclei-associated protein kinase in growing tumors (Fig. 3A), whereas in nuclei of regressing tumors (Figs. 3B and 3C) the radioactivity peaks associated with protein species IV decreased by approximately 40%, and new radioactivity peaks coincident with protein species I appeared. Phosphorylation of this regression-associated protein (RAP) began within 1 day after either ovariectomy or dibutyryl cyclic AMP treatment and stopped when tumor growth was resumed following the injection of estradiol valerate or cessation of dibutyryl cyclic AMP treatment.

Whether phosphorylation of RAP is, indeed, related to the effect of cyclic AMP was examined under more clearly defined conditions *in vitro*. As shown

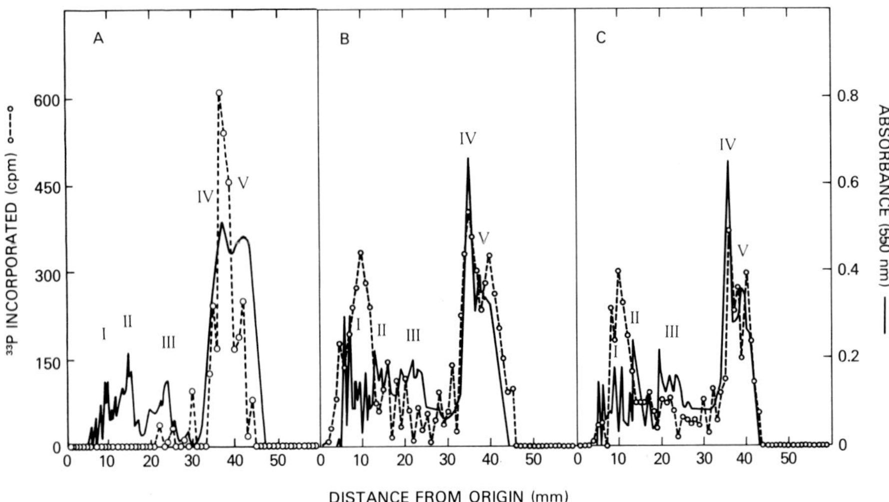

FIG. 3. SDS polyacrylamide gel electrophoresis of phosphorylated nuclear proteins from growing, regressing, and growth-arrested DMBA tumors. **A:** Growing tumors. **B:** Growth-arrested tumors 3 days after dibutyryl cyclic AMP treatment (8). **C:** Regressing tumors (regressed by 20% of original size) 3 days after ovariectomy. Isolated nuclei from each tumor were incubated with [γ-^{33}P]ATP to phosphorylate the nuclear proteins via intrinsic protein kinase; nuclear proteins were then treated with 1% SDS and 1% mercaptoethanol and subjected to electrophoresis. (From Cho-Chung and Redler, ref. 21, with permission.)

in Fig. 4, slices from growing DMBA tumors preincubated with cyclic AMP alone induced phosphorylation of RAP, whereas in the simultaneous presence of 17β-estradiol, phosphorylation by cyclic AMP was inhibited (Fig. 4, top). The phosphorylation patterns of nuclei isolated from hormone-independent mammary tumors (DMBA #1) did not respond to either cyclic AMP and/or estrogen preincubation (Fig. 4, bottom). Thus phosphorylation of RAP appears to be related to the specific action of cyclic AMP that counteracts the effect of estrogen in the nuclei of hormone-dependent mammary tumors.

Acid Ribonuclease and Glucose-6-phosphate Dehydrogenase

One of the earliest signs of regression of hormone-dependent rat mammary tumors following either dibutyryl cyclic AMP treatment or ovariectomy is the increase in activity and quantity of acid RNase that occurs within 6 hr after either treatment (8,17–19). Precipitation of prelabeled acid RNase with monospecific antiacid RNase antiserum showed that the increase in enzyme quantity was due to new synthesis (18,19).

On the other hand, a decrease in glucose-6-phosphate dehydrogenase (G6PD), particularly that found in the microsomal cell fraction, is observed within a few days after either treatment, followed by its reappearance when tumor growth is resumed either by injection of estradiol valerate or cessation of dibutytryl

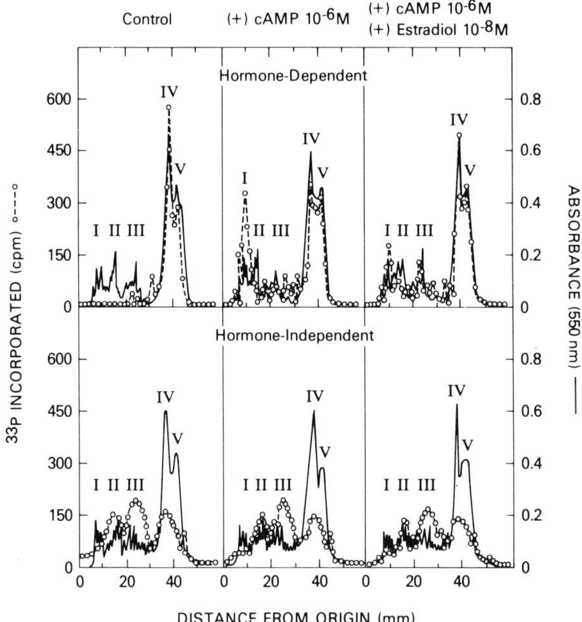

FIG. 4. Effects of cyclic AMP and 17β-estradiol on endogenous nuclear protein phosphorylation of hormone-dependent and -independent mammary tumor slices *in vitro.* Tumor slices (0.2 g) were incubated in 5 volumes of Tris-HCl (10 mM, pH 7.5) in the absence or presence of cyclic AMP (10^{-6} M) ± 17β-estradiol (10^{-8} M) at 30°C. Incubations were stopped by diluting the medium 2.5-fold with cold Tris-HCl after 30 min. Tumor slices were collected by immediate centrifugation and washed once with cold Tris-HCl; then nuclei were isolated, and nuclear protein phosphorylation by intrinsic protein kinase was measured (see legend for Fig. 3). Hormone-dependent, DMBA; hormone-independent, DMBA #1 (tumor received from Dr. W. F. Dunning in 1967 and carried on in the laboratory of pathophysiology by subcutaneous transplantation for 172 generations, then stored at −80°C).

cyclic AMP treatment (2,10). Thus the increase in acid RNase and the decrease in G6PD appear to be associated with the regression of hormone-dependent mammary tumors following ovariectomy or dibutyryl cyclic AMP treatment.

MECHANISM OF HORMONE-DEPENDENT MAMMARY TUMOR REGRESSION

The widely accepted hyothesis that the interaction of estrogen with its cellular receptors determines the hormone dependency of mammary tumors should now be challenged on the basis of the following observations: (a) Several autonomous tumors (those not regressing after hormonal deprivation) occurring in both experimental animals and humans contain significant amounts of estrogen receptors (5,44). (b) Tumors regrowing after complete or partial regression as a result of endocrine ablation are considered to be autonomous (57) but have been found to retain estrogen receptors (49). (c) Administration of a pharmacological dose of estrogen to an intact or ovariectomized host causes tumor regression instead of growth promotion (24,25,59,60). These findings suggest that estrogen receptors may not be the sole determinant of hormone dependency of mammary tumors.

Attempts to define the role of cyclic AMP as the mediator of estrogen action have resulted in conflicting conclusions that may well be due to differences in experimental conditions, especially with respect to the effective dose of estrogen used to stimulate target tissues. In ovariectomized rats, cyclic AMP levels were increased in the uterus within 30 sec following intravenous injection of 17 β-estradiol at a dose of 1 μg/100 g (58) and within 5 min after subcutaneous injection of 17β-estradiol benzoate at a high dose of 10 μg/day/100 g (23). However, other investigators found decreases in uterine cyclic AMP in similar animals, either with injection of a low dose of 17β-estradiol (1 μg/day/250 g i.p.) or with measurement during proestrus when the plasma estrogen level was maximal (37). In regressing DMBA tumors, as opposed to growing tumors, an increase in the cyclic AMP level follows a high dose of estrogen administration (Y. S. Cho-Chung et al., *unpublished observation*), ovariectomy (11,12,43), and dibutyryl cyclic AMP treatment (4). Thus it appears that cyclic AMP levels are low in estrogen target tissues that are under a physiological concentration of estrogen and high under supraphysiological or subphysiological concentrations of estrogen. Increased levels of cyclic AMP have also been found in DMBA tumors regressing due to inhibition of prolactin secretion or insulin deficiency (43). Since it has been suggested that insulin acts by lowering cyclic AMP (6,28), prolactin and estrogen may act accordingly, so that removal of these hormones may result in elevation of the cyclic AMP level. Thus tumor regression may be produced by elevated cyclic AMP in counteraction with estrogen or prolactin, just as with the countereffects of cyclic AMP and insulin that have been described in a plasma cell tumor in culture (48). However, arrest of tumor growth may not occur solely by increasing cellular cyclic AMP levels. Whereas elevated cyclic AMP levels have been found in some tumors (46,56), and an increase in cyclic AMP concentration has been produced in W256 mammary carcinomas after dibutyryl cyclic AMP treatment, tumor regression has occurred in only a fraction of the transplants (8).

The inverse relationship between cyclic-AMP- and estrogen-binding activities found during growth and regression of DMBA tumors (3,4,11,12) suggests that these binding proteins may interact in the growth control of this tumor. A possible counteraction between cyclic AMP and estrogen at the nuclear level has been indicated by the observation that cyclic-AMP-binding proteins accumulate into the nuclei of regressing tumors in a similar manner as estrogen receptors translocate into growing tumor nuclei. The stimulation and prevention of endogenous phosphorylation of nuclear proteins, RAP (regression-associated protein), as demonstrated by cyclic AMP and estrogen, respectively, in both *in vivo* and *in vitro* experiments, further indicate an interrelationship between cyclic AMP and estrogen at the nuclear level. However, these results do not exclude a possible interaction of cyclic AMP and estrogen in the cytoplasm. In fact, Liu and Greengard (42) reported opposing actions of cyclic AMP and steroid hormones in endogenous phosphorylation of a specific cytosol protein, SCARP, in several target tissues. The new synthesis of acid RNase found during the regression of hormone-dependent mammary tumors (8,17–19) also suggests a reciprocal relationship between cyclic AMP and estrogen. Furthermore, Wu (64) reported that when ornithine aminotransferase was induced in normal kidneys of old female rats injected with cyclic AMP, estrogen binding in the kidney cytosol was markedly decreased.

It is important to stress that the inverse relationship between cyclic-AMP- and estrogen-binding activities is closely related to the hormone dependency of tumor growth. DMBA tumors that continue to grow and fail to regress after hormonal deprivation possess a wide range of estrogen- and cyclic-AMP-binding activities that do not change after ovariectomy or dibutyryl cyclic AMP treatment. These findings suggest that integrity in both cyclic-AMP-binding proteins and estrogen receptors is probably essential for the control of hormone-dependent mammary tumor growth. Estrogen receptors may promote growth, whereas cyclic-AMP-binding proteins may play a role in the regression phase of these tumors similar to the pivotal role of cyclic-AMP-binding proteins in the growth arrest of other tumor models (13–16,22). Further investigations on the phosphorylation of nuclear proteins in conjunction with cyclic AMP binding and estrogen binding in the nuclei would help to elucidate the mechanism of hormone-dependent mammary tumor growth and regression.

SUMMARY

Evidence has been presented to show that (a) the intracellular concentration of estrogen may selectively regulate cyclic nucleotide participation in modulating growth of mammary tumors, (b) cyclic AMP and estrogen appear to be interrelated in the growth control of hormone-dependent mammary tumors, (c) integrity of both estrogen receptors and cyclic-AMP-binding proteins may be required for the interaction between estrogen and cyclic AMP, and (d) a counteraction between cyclic AMP and estrogen at the nuclear level is possible since cyclic-AMP- and estrogen-induced phosphorylations of nuclear proteins are demonstrable in both *in vivo* and *in vitro* experiments.

It seems probable that estrogen and cyclic AMP exert opposing actions on the growth-control mechanism of hormone-dependent mammary tumors: estrogen may promote growth, whereas cyclic AMP may be involved in the regression process.

REFERENCES

1. Beatson, G. T. (1896): On the treatment of inoperable cases of carcinoma of the mamma: Suggestions for a new method of treatment, with illustrative cases. *Lancet,* 2:104–107, 162–165.

2. Bodwin, J. S., and Cho-Chung, Y. S. (1975): Glucose 6-phosphate dehydrogenase isozymes in growing and regressing MTW9 rat mammary carcinomas. *Proc. Am. Assoc. Cancer Res.,* 16:89.
3. Bodwin, J. S., and Cho-Chung, Y. S. (1977): Decreased estrogen binding in hormone dependent mammary carcinoma following ovariectomy or dibutyryl cyclic AMP treatment. *Cancer Letters,* 3:289–294.
4. Bodwin, J. S., Clair, T., and Cho-Chung, Y. S. (1977): Role of estrogen receptor and cyclic AMP-binding protein in the growth control of hormone-dependent mammary carcinoma. *Proc. Am. Assoc. Cancer Res.,* 18:117.
5. Boylan, E. S., and Wittliff, J. L. (1975). Specific estrogen binding in rat mammary tumors induced by 7,12-dimethylbenz(α)anthracene. *Cancer Res.,* 35:506–511.
6. Butcher, R. W., Sneyd, J. G. T., Park, C. R., and Sutherland, E. W., Jr. (1966): Effect of insulin on adenosine 3′,5′-monophosphate in the rat epididymal fat pad. *J. Biol. Chem.,* 241:1651–1653.
7. Callentine, M. R. (1967): Nonsteroidal estrogen antagonists. *Clin. Obstet. Gynecol.,* 10:74–87.
8. Cho-Chung, Y. S. (1974): *In vivo* inhibition of tumor growth by cyclic adenosine 3′,5′-monophosphate derivatives. *Cancer Res.,* 34:3492–3496.
9. Cho-Chung, Y. S. (1978): Cyclic AMP and tumor growth *in vivo.* In: *Influence of Hormones on Tumor Development,* edited by J. A. Kellen. CRC Press, Cleveland. *(In press).*
10. Cho-Chung, Y. S., and Berghoffer, B. (1974): The role of cyclic AMP in neoplastic cell growth and regression. II. Growth arrest and glucose-6-phosphate dehydrogenase isozyme shift by dibutyryl cyclic AMP. *Biochem. Biophys. Res. Commun.,* 60:528–534.
11. Cho-Chung, Y. S., Bodwin, J. S., and Clair, T. (1978): Cyclic AMP-binding protein: Role in ovariectomy-induced regression of a hormone-dependent mammary tumor. *J. Natl. Cancer Inst., (in press).*
12. Cho-Chung, Y. S., Bodwin, J. S., and Clair, T. (1978): Cyclic AMP-binding protein: inverse relationship with estrogen-receptors in hormone-dependent mammary tumor regression. *(In press).*
13. Cho-Chung, Y. S., and Clair, T. (1977): Altered cyclic AMP-binding and db cyclic AMP-unresponsiveness *in vivo. Nature,* 265:452–454.
14. Cho-Chung, Y. S., Clair, T., and Huffman, P. (1977): Loss of nuclear cyclic AMP-binding in cyclic AMP-unresponsive Walker 256 mammary carcinoma. *J. Biol. Chem.,* 252:6349–6355.
15. Cho-Chung, Y. S., Clair, T., and Porper, R. (1977): Cyclic AMP-binding proteins and protein kinase during regression of Walker 256 mammary carcinoma. *J. Biol. Chem.,* 252:6342–6348.
16. Cho-Chung, Y. S., Clair, T., Yi, P. N., and Parkison, C. (1977): Comparative studies on cyclic AMP binding and protein kinase in cyclic AMP-responsive and -unresponsive Walker 256 mammary carcinomas. *J. Biol. Chem.,* 252:6335–6341.
17. Cho-Chung, Y. S., and Gullino, P. M. (1973): Mammary tumor regression. V. Role of acid ribonuclease and cathepsin. *J. Biol. Chem.,* 248:4743–4749.
18. Cho-Chung, Y. S., and Gullino, P. M. (1973): Mammary tumor regression. VI. Synthesis and degradation of acid ribonuclease. *J. Biol. Chem.,* 248:4750–4755.
19. Cho-Chung, Y. S., and Gullino, P. M. (1974): *In vivo* inhibition of growth of two hormone-dependent mammary tumors by dibutyryl cyclic AMP. *Science,* 183:87–88.
20. Cho-Chung, Y. S., and Gullino, P. M. (1974): Effect of dibutyryl cyclic adenosine 3′,5′-monophosphate on *in vivo* growth of Walker 256 carcinoma: isolation of responsive and unresponsive cell population. *J. Natl. Cancer Inst.,* 52:995–996.
21. Cho-Chung, Y. S., and Redler, B. H. (1977): Dibutyryl cyclic AMP mimics ovariectomy: nuclear protein phosphorylation in mammary tumor regression. *Science,* 197:272–275.
22. Coffino, P., and Yamamoto, K. R. (1976): Somatic genetic studies of steroid and cyclic AMP receptors. In: *Control Mechanisms in Cancer,* edited by W. E. Criss, T. Ono, and J. R. Sabin, pp. 57–66. Raven Press, New York.
23. Dupont-Mairesse, N., Van Sande, J., Rooryck, J., Fastrez-Boute, A., and Galand, P. (1974): Mechanism of estrogen action. Independence of several responses of the rat uterus from the early increase in adenosine 3′,5′-cyclic monophosphate. *J. Steroid Biochem.,* 5:173–178.
24. Griswold, D. P., Skipper, H. E., Laster, W. R., Wilcox, W. S., and Schabel, F. M., Jr. (1966): Induced mammary carcinoma in the female rat as a drug evaluation system. *Cancer Res.,* 26:2169–2180.
25. Haddow, A., Watkinson, J. M., Paterson, E., and Koller, P. C. (1944): Influence of synthetic oestrogens upon advanced malignant disease. *Br. Med. J.,* 2:393–398.

26. Hilf, R., Inge, M., and Carlton, B. (1965): Biochemical and morphologic properties of a new lactating mammary tumor line in the rat. *Cancer Res.,* 25:286–297.
27. Huggins, C., and Bergenstal, D. M. (1952): Inhibition of human mammary and prostatic cancers by adrenalectomy. *Cancer Res.,* 12:134–141.
28. Jefferson, L. S., Exton, J. H., Butcher, R. W., Sutherland, E. W., and Park, C. R. (1968): Role of adenosine 3′,5′-monophosphate in the effects of insulin and anti-insulin serum on liver metabolism. *J. Biol. Chem.,* 243:1031–1038.
29. Jensen, E. V., and DeSombre, E. R. (1972): Mechanism of action of the female sex hormones. *Annu. Rev. Biochem.,* 789:203–230.
30. Jensen, E. V., DeSombre, E. R., and Jungblut, P. W. (1967): Estrogen receptors in hormone-responsive tissues and tumors. In: *Endogenous Factors Influencing Host-Tumor Balance,* edited by R. W. Wissler, T. L. Dao, and S. Wood, pp. 15–30. University of Chicago Press, Chicago.
31. Johnson, G. S., and Pastan, I. (1972): $N^6,0^{2'}$-dibutyryl adenosine 3′,5′-monophosphate induces pigment production in melanoma cells. *Nature* [*New Biol.*], 237:267–268.
32. King, R. J. B., Cowan, D. M., and Inman, D. R. (1965): The uptake of (6,7-^{3}H) oestradiol by dimethylbenz-anthracene-induced rat mammary tumors. *J. Endocrinol.,* 32:83–90.
33. King, R. J. B., and Mainwaring, W. I. P. (1974): V. Glucocorticoid. VI. Mineralicorticoids. III. Estrogens. VIII. Progesterone. In: *Steroid Cell Interactions,* edited by R. J. B. King, pp. 102–287. University Park Press, Baltimore.
34. King, R. J. B., Smith, J. A., and Steggles, A. W. (1970): Oestrogen-binding and the hormone responsiveness of tumors. *Steroidologia,* 1:73–88.
35. Klein, D. M., and Loizzi, R. F. (1977): Enhancement of R3230AC rat mammary tumor growth and cellular differentiation by dibutyryl cyclic adenosine monophosphate. *J. Natl. Cancer Inst.,* 58:813–818.
36. Krebs, E. G. (1972): Protein kinase. *Curr. Top. Cell. Regul.,* 5:99–133.
37. Kuehl, F. A., Jr., Ham, E. A., Zanetti, M. E., Sanford, C. H., Nicol, S. E., and Goldberg, N. D. (1974): Estrogen-related increases in uterine guanosine 3′:5′-cyclic monophosphate levels. *Proc. Natl. Acad. Sci. U.S.A.,* 71:1866–1870.
38. Kuo, J. F., and Greengard, P. (1969): Cyclic nucleotide-dependent protein kinase. IV. Widespread occurrence of adenosine 3′,5′-monophosphate-dependent protein kinase in various tissues and phyla of the animal kingdom. *Proc. Natl. Acad. Sci. U.S.A.,* 64:1349–1355.
39. Kyser, K. A. (1970): The tissue, subcellular and molecular binding of estradiol to dimethylbenz-anthracene-induced rat mammary tumors. Ph.D. dissertation, University of Chicago.
40. Lerner, L. J., Holthaus, F. J., Jr., and Thompsen, C. R. (1958): A non-steroidal estrogen antagonist 1-(*p*-2-diethylaminoethoxyphenyl)-1-phenyl-2-*p*-methoxyphenyl ethanol. *Endocrinology,* 63:295–318.
41. Liao, S. (1975): Cellular receptors and mechanism of action of steroid hormones. *Int. Rev. Cytol.* 41:87–172.
42. Liu, A. Y. C., and Greengard, P. (1976): Regulation by steroid hormones of phosphorylation of specific protein common to several target organs. *Proc. Natl. Acad. Sci. U.S.A.,* 73:568–572.
43. Matusik, R. J., and Hilf, R. (1976): Relationship of adenosine 3′,5′-cyclic monophosphate and guanosine 3′,5′-cyclic monophosphate to growth of dimethylbenz[α]anthracene-induced mammary tumors in rats. *J. Natl. Cancer Inst.,* 56:659–661.
44. McGuire, W. L. (1975): Current status of estrogen receptors in human breast cancer. *Cancer,* 36:638–644.
45. McGuire, W. L., and Julian, J. (1971): Comparison of macromolecular binding of estradiol in hormone-dependent and hormone-independent rat mammary carcinoma. *Cancer Res.,* 31:1440–1445.
46. Minton, J. P., Matthews, R. H., and Wisenbaugh, T. W. (1976): Elevated adenosine 3′,5′-cyclic monophosphate levels in human and animal tumors *in vivo. J. Natl. Cancer Inst.,* 57:39–41.
47. Mobbs, B. G. (1966): The uptake of tritiated oestradiol by dimethyl-benzanthracene-induced mammary tumors of rat. *J. Endocrinol.,* 36:409–414.
48. Naseem, S. M., and Hollander, V. P. (1973): Insulin reversal of growth inhibition of plasma cell tumor by prostaglandin or adenosine 3′,5′-monophosphate. *Cancer Res.,* 33:2909–2912.
49. Nomura, Y., Abe, Y., Yamagata, J., and Takenaka, K. (1976): Possible retention of the estrogen-binding capacity after endocrine-ablation therapy in the rat and human breast cancer. *Gann,* 67:101–104.

50. O'Malley, B. W., and Means, A. R. (1974): Female steroid hormones and target cell nuclei. The effects of steroid hormones on target cell nuclei are of major importance in the interaction of new cell functions. *Science,* 183:610–620.
51. Prasad, K., and Vernadakis, A. (1972): Morphological and biochemical study in X-ray and dibutyryl cyclic AMP-induced differentiated neuroblastoma cells. *Exp. Cell Res.,* 70:27–32.
52. Sander, S. (1969): *In vitro* uptake of oestradiol in DMBA induced breast tumor of the rat. *Acta Pathol. Microbiol. Scand.,* 75:520–526.
53. Sapag-Hagar, M., and Greenbaum, A. L. (1974): The role of cyclic nucleotides in the development and function of rat mammary tissue. *F.E.B.S. Lett.,* 46:180–183.
54. Schinzinger, A. (1889): Über Carcinoma mammae. *Verh. Dtsch. Ges. Chir.,* 18:28–29.
55. Segaloff, A (1966): Hormones and breast cancer. *Recent Prog. Horm. Res.,* 22:351–379.
56. Singer, A. L., Sherwin, R. P., Dunn, A. S., and Appleman, M. M. (1976): Cyclic nucleotide phosphodiesterase in neoplastic and non-neoplastic human mammary tissue. *Cancer Res.,* 36:60–66.
57. Stoll, B. A. (1972): The basis of endocrine therapy. In: *Endocrine Therapy in Malignant Disease,* edited by B. A. Stoll, pp. 111–114. W. B. Saunders, Philadelphia.
58. Szego, C. M., and Davis, J. S. (1967): Adenosine 3′,5′-monophosphate in rat uterus: Acute elevation by estrogen. *Proc. Natl. Acad. Sci. U.S.A.,* 58:1711–1718.
59. Teller, M. N., Kaufman, R. J., Stock, C. C., and Bowie, M. (1968): Criteria for evaluating hormones in the 7,12-dimethylbenz[α]anthracene-induced mammary tumor-rat experimental chemotherapy system. *Cancer Res.,* 28:368–371.
60. Teller, M. N., Stock, C. C., Stohr, G., Merker, P. C., Kaufman, R. J., Escher, G. C., and Bowie, M. (1966): Biologic characteristics and chemotherapy of 7,12-dimethylbenz-[α]anthracene-induced tumors in rats. *Cancer Res.,* 26:245–252.
61. Terenius, L. (1968): Selective retention of estrogen isomers in estrogen-dependent breast tumors of rat demonstrated by *in vitro* methods. *Cancer Res.,* 28:328–337.
62. Turkington, R. W. (1970): Homogeneity of differentiated function in mammary carcinoma cell populations. *Cancer Res.,* 30:1841–1845.
63. Wittliff, J. L. (1975): Steroid binding proteins in normal and neoplastic mammary cells. *Methods Cancer Res.,* 11:293–354.
64. Wu, C. (1976): Hormonal regulation of glutamine synthetase and ornithine aminotransferase in normal and neoplastic rat tissues. In: *Control Mechanisms in Cancer,* edited by W. E. Criss, T. Ono, and J. R. Sabine, pp. 125–138. Raven Press, New York.

CIRCULATING HORMONES

Endocrine Control in Neoplasia, edited by
R. K. Sharma and W. E. Criss.
Raven Press, New York © 1978.

Plasma Hormone Concentrations in Human Breast and Prostate Cancer

Barnett Zumoff

Clinical Research Center, Institute for Steroid Research, and Department of Oncology, Montefiore Hospital and Medical Center, Bronx, New York 10467

Cancer of the breast and prostate are described as hormone-dependent on the basis of two findings: (a) they arise from tissues that are normally responsive to endogenous hormones and (b) their courses can often be influenced, favorably or unfavorably, by administration of hormones or removal of hormones (by surgical or radiation ablation of endocrine glands or by administration of antihormones). Because of the therapeutic effects of iatrogenic alterations in the hormonal environment, considerable interest has developed in the possibility that the spontaneous endogenous hormonal environment is related either to the induction of these cancers or to the untreated clinical courses of these cancers.

In the absence of data concerning the concentration of a hormone at its intracellular effector site the next best parameter of its biological impact is probably its plasma concentration. Although this concept has been clear for some time, it has been only recently, with the advent of satisfactory radioimmunoassay methods, that several studies of plasma hormone concentrations in breast cancer and a smaller number of studies in prostate cancer have been carried out. The total number of such studies to date is surprisingly small, and their results are often in conflict with one another. This review will describe in some detail the data that have been published by other workers and will examine possible limitations and sources of error in their studies; finally, it will describe unpublished data that have been obtained in our laboratory.[1]

There are three major sources of error in nearly all of the published studies:

1. Plasma hormone concentrations have been determined on the basis of a single "spot" sample, usually an early morning sample. Studies from our laboratory and other laboratories (13–15,31,43,52,84,94,95,99) have clearly established that the plasma concentrations of many hormones fluctuate markedly during a 24-hr cycle, so that spot values can be unrepresentative and therefore misleading. This is particularly a problem with cortisol, follicle-stimulating hormone (FSH), luteinizing hormone (LH), and prolactin, all of which are secreted even more actively during the nocturnal sleep period than during the day. Given these facts, we have concluded that a critical evaluation of plasma hormone concentrations in various disease states can best be carried out by taking blood

[1] These studies have been carried out in collaboration with David K. Fukushima, Jack Fishman, Robert S. Rosenfeld, Jacob Kream, Joseph Levin, John O'Connor, and Leon Hellman.

samples at very frequent intervals (every 20 min) throughout the 24 hr and analyzing a pool made from aliquots of each of the 72 samples, thereby obtaining a 24-hr mean value. Virtually no such data from cancer patients have been published; only the abstract by Malarkey et al. (59) reported 24-hr mean values, whereas the article by McFadyen et al. (60) reported partial profiles, i.e., samples at 15-min intervals for 8 hr (9 A.M. to 5 P.M.). All the data from our laboratory that will be described later in this review represent 24-hr mean values for plasma hormone concentrations.

2. The groups of patients reported in most studies have been heterogeneous, complicated by other diseases and/or medications, and poorly or not at all characterized. We have studied only well-characterized, rigidly selected, "clean" patients; any patient fulfilling any of the following criteria has been excluded from study:

a. Any significant (i.e., nontrivial) current disease.

b. History of any major chronic disease (e.g., cardiac, renal, pulmonary, metabolic, rheumatic, neurological, psychiatric, etc.).

c. Abnormal thyroid, kidney, or liver function.

d. Current regular ingestion of any medication (except sporadic minor analgesics, laxatives, etc.) and past history of ingestion of any thyroid preparation at any time, oral contraceptives within a year, any drug capable of causing intrahepatic cholestasis (e.g., phenothiazines) within 6 months, and any other medication within 3 months.

e. Any previous endocrine or antiendocrine therapy or endocrine ablation at any time.

f. Any previous cancer chemotherapy at any time.

3. The relationship between age and plasma hormone concentrations often is ignored or considered only grossly (e.g., premenopausal versus postmenopausal). We have found that nearly all hormones show a clear-cut ontogeny, i.e., predictable secular changes with age; therefore it becomes necessary to plot the patients' values against age and compare the graph with a similar plot for normal controls, rather than compare patients as a group with controls as a group.

With these points in mind, let us consider the reports that have been published to date.

BREAST CANCER[2]

Cortisol

Deshpande et al. (25) reported that plasma 17-hydroxycorticosteroid concentrations (determined colorimetrically) were elevated in metastatic breast cancer

---

[2] Only female breast cancer is reviewed in this chapter. Just one article (19) has been published concerning plasma hormone concentrations in male breast cancer; this study found elevated levels of estradiol, estrone, and estriol and normal levels of androstenedione and testosterone.

but not in early localized disease; these workers used early morning "spot" samples.[3] Brownsey et al. (17), using a fluorimetric method, failed to find elevated concentrations. McFadyen et al. (60) studied "partial plasma profiles" (i.e., every 15 min from 8 A.M. to 5 P.M.) in 6 postmenopausal women and found no abnormalities. Smethurst et al. (80), using a fluorimetric method, reported that the concentration of cortisol in early breast cancer was lower than that seen in other cancers; true normal controls were not studied. Rose et al. (71) studied plasma cortisol concentrations in 73 women with primary operable, locally recurrent, or metastatic disease, some of whom had previously received cancer chemotherapy; the three groups did not differ from each other or from normal controls. Borkowski et al. (12) found normal cortisol levels in patients with early breast cancer and in those with advanced breast cancer. Jones et al. (48) found normal cortisol levels after mastectomy in postmenopausal patients with early breast cancer.

We have found that 24-hr mean plasma cortisol concentrations show no age trend in women between the ages of 22 and 75, so that comparison of cancer patients as a group with normals as a group is permissible. Using this approach, we have found no difference between 15 normal women and 30 women with breast cancer; it made no difference whether the cancer was localized and operable, localized and inoperable, or metastatic.

Summarizing, the weight of evidence appears to indicate that plasma cortisol concentrations are normal in women with breast cancer.

Testosterone

Wang et al. (89) studied plasma testosterone concentrations in 19 normal women and 24 women with primary operable breast cancer. They used "spot" samples drawn in the early afternoon from the normals and in the morning from the patients, stating that testosterone showed no diurnal variations. [We have found that there is considerable fluctuation of plasma testosterone concentration in men (15) but much less in women (B. Zumoff, *unpublished data*)]. They also studied the correlation of testosterone concentration with age and found age invariance in both normals and patients. Their final conclusion was that testosterone concentrations were the same in controls and breast cancer patients, but their values (average of 120 ng/dl for both groups) were unacceptably high by current standards. Horn and Gordan (44) studied 13 women with metastatic breast cancer (4 of whom had had either surgical or radiation castration) and 10 normal controls; their values were in an acceptable range and they observed no difference between controls and breast cancer patients. McFadyen et al. (60), studying the same group of 6 postmenopausal women mentioned

[3] All studies reviewed in this chapter employed morning spot samples, except the "partial profiles" reported by McFadyen et al. (60), the 24-hr mean concentrations reported by Malarkey et al. (19), and our own studies.

previously, reported a significant difference between the mean value of 31 ng/dl in patients and the mean value of 18 ng/dl in controls.

Our own 24-hr mean values were just under 30 ng/dl in both normals and cancer patients, with no significant difference between the two groups. The very low values for normals reported by McFadyen et al. are puzzling and unexplained. Malarkey et al. (59) reported in abstract that the 24-hr mean concentration of testosterone was normal in women with breast cancer. The most recent study, by Borkowski et al. (12), reported normal testosterone levels in women with breast cancer, early or advanced.

Summarizing, the weight of evidence appears to indicate that plasma testosterone concentration is normal in women with breast cancer.

Dihydrotestosterone

Dihydrotestosterone, an immediate metabolite of testosterone, is of great interest because it is biologically active as an androgen (56) and because receptors for it have been described in breast cancer tissue (57). Despite this, there appears to have been only one study of its plasma concentration in breast cancer, an article in Russian by Vitola and Zeikate (86), who reported a tendency toward elevated dihydrotestosterone concentrations in breast cancer. Because of a very wide range of values, the elevation was not statistically significant. In our own studies we found that the 24-hr mean plasma concentration of dihydrostestosterone was age-invariant in women between 22 and 75 years of age. Breast cancer patients showed a small but statistically significant elevation, 58 ng/dl versus 42 ng/dl in normal controls. This interesting finding obviously requires further exploration.

Dehydroisoandrosterone and Dehydroisoandrosterone Sulfate

These two hormones are the major secreted "adrenal androgens" and are quantitatively the major sources of urinary 17-ketosteroids, specifically androsterone, etiocholanolone, and dehydroisoandrosterone. Since it has been claimed (2,3,18,49,53) and also denied (1,7,61,87,96) that some women with breast cancer have subnormal urinary excretion of 17-ketosteroids that is correlated with poor prognosis and poor response to endocrine ablation, considerable interest attaches to the determination of plasma concentrations of the major precursors of these urinary steroids.

Brownsey et al. (17) reported slightly decreased levels of dehydroisoandrosterone sulfate (DS) in advanced breast cancer but not in localized cancer. The control subjects were women with benign breast disease rather than normals. The authors did not relate the values obtained to age, although it was stated that the mean ages of the groups were the same. (It has repeatedly been shown, and our own data confirm it, that plasma concentrations of DS decrease with age.) No description was given of the clinical state of the advanced cancer patients, and no comment was made concerning any current or previous therapy. Wang (90) initially reported that women with breast cancer did not differ from controls with respect to plasma DS concentration. However, in a later publication, Wang et al. (90) reported normal DS concentrations in early localized cancer but subnormal concentrations in advanced cancer; age was taken into account. No description was given of the clinical state of the advanced cancer patients, and no comment was made concerning any current or previous therapy. Rose et al. (71) found, as did others, that plasma DS concentration decreased with age; they reported that DS levels were subnormal in all stages of breast cancer, early or late. Some of their patients had received previous cancer chemotherapy; since only regression lines, rather than individual values, were reported, it is not possible to determine what effect this factor may have had on the results. Plasma levels of "dehydroisoandrosterone" were studied by Šonká et al. (81). Their method appears to have determined free plus esterified dehydroisoandrosterone (i.e., DHA + DHAS). Since the latter is present at hundreds of times the concentration of the former, their study represents essentially a measurement of DHAS levels. They found subnormal levels of DHAS nonspecifically in various types of cancer, including breast cancer. Few clinical data were provided.

Our studies of 24-hr mean concentrations of DS have shown a linear negative correlation of the logarithm of plasma DS concentration with age in both normal individuals and cancer patients. The semilog plots of DS concentration versus age in these two groups are superimposable, indicating that there is no difference between normals and cancer patients with respect to plasma DS concentration. The reasons for the discrepancy between our data and those of other workers remain to be clarified.

The only published study of plasma free dehydroisoandrosterone (DHA) appears to be that of Thomas et al. (85). These workers plotted DHA concentration versus age in normal women and women with early or advanced breast cancer and reported that the cancer patients showed lower values. However, inspection of the graphs in their article leaves considerable doubt that this is so. Our own results, handled as with the DS data, show that the semilog plots of plasma DHA concentration versus age in normals and breast cancer patients are superimposable, indicating no difference between these two groups.

Androsterone and Androsterone Sulfate

These two weak androgens are major metabolites of DHA and DHAS. Wang et al. appear to be the only authors who have published data concerning the plasma levels of androsterone sulfate (AS) in breast cancer. Initially, Wang reported (90) that AS levels were normal in breast cancer. In a later publication, however, Wang et al. (91) reported normal AS concentrations in early localized cancer but subnormal concentrations in advanced cancer; age was taken into account, since they found that AS levels declined with age in normal individuals.

No data have been published concerning plasma levels of free androsterone in breast cancer.

Our studies have shown a slight downward trend of AS with age in normal subjects and no differences between cancer patients and normals. We have found the levels of free androsterone to be age-invariant in women between 22 and 75 years of age, with no difference in concentration between cancer patients and normals.

Androstenedione

This steroid is a weak androgen secreted by the adrenal. There have been two reports concerning its plasma concentration in breast cancer: Wang et al. (93) and Rose et al. (71) both reported normal levels in cancer patients. We have not studied the plasma concentration of this steroid.

Progesterone

There have been three published reports concerning plasma progesterone in breast cancer: Smethurst et al. (80) found that patients with early breast cancer had lower values than other cancer patients; true normal controls were not studied. Malarkey et al. (59) published an abstract reporting that the 24-hr mean concentrations of this steroid were normal in both premenopausal and postmenopausal cancer patients. Jones et al. (48) found normal levels after mastectomy in postmenopausal women with early breast cancer. We have not studied the plasma concentration of this steroid.

Estrone and Estradiol

Because of the fluctuations of these steroids during the menstrual cycle, comparison of normals with cancer patients is very difficult in the premenopausal group. Indeed, it is virtually essential to compare data from entire menstrual cycles to make appropriate comparisons. Skinner et al. (79) published an abstract describing just such studies, and they reported that patients with breast cancer showed no significant divergence from normal with respect to plasma estradiol concentration; estrone concentrations were not measured. In a later article (29), the same group of authors stated that plasma estradiol levels were normal in postmenopausal women with breast cancer but were slightly elevated in premenopausal cancer patients. Inspection of the graphic presentation of the premenopausal data makes it difficult to accept this conclusion. McFadyen et al. (60) reported "partial profiles" of estradiol in postmenopausal cancer patients; they found no significant difference from normal values. Malarkey et al. (59) measured the 24-hr mean concentration of estradiol during the follicular and luteal phases in premenopausal women with breast cancer; they found no abnormalities in these patients; estrone was not measured. Borkowski et al. (12) measured the plasma concentrations of both estradiol and estrone in postmenopausal women with breast cancer; no abnormalities were found. Jones et al. (48) measured the concentration of estradiol in postmenopausal patients with primary breast cancer, after mastectomy, and observed no difference from normal; estrone was not studied. We have studied 24-hr mean concentrations in postmenopausal women with breast cancer but have not yet completed the analysis of our data. Our preliminary impression is that the cancer patients do not differ significantly from normal.

LH and FSH

Plasma FSH concentrations have been measured in postmenopausal women with breast cancer by three groups: Wang et al. (92) reported slightly subnormal values, but commented that "the difference is probably due to the hormonal treatment that most of these patients were receiving." McFadyen et al. (60) found normal levels. Malarkey et al. (59) reported normal 24-hr mean concentrations in both postmenopausal and premenopausal breast cancer patients. Our studies have also shown normal 24-hr mean concentrations in both premenopausal and postmenopausal patients.

LH concentrations were found to be normal in postmenopausal cancer patients by the same three groups of workers (59,60,92), and Malarkey et al. (59) reported normal LH concentrations in premenopausal patients also. Our studies have found normal 24-hr mean LH concentrations in postmenopausal cancer patients, but significantly *subnormal* concentrations in premenopausal patients, averaging 7.5 mIU/ml compared with 13.5 mIU/ml in normal controls. This finding is particularly interesting in view of the epidemiological finding that women with frequent anovulatory cycles are at increased risk for development of breast cancer (38,76).

Prolactin

Thirteen studies of plasma prolactin in breast cancer have been published, more than for any other hormone. The first of these studies (8) used a bioassay (all subsequent studies have employed radioimmunoassay) and reported only that more cancer patients than normal controls had "measurable levels" of prolactin, implying that prolactin concentrations were higher in the cancer patients; this was true in all age ranges. Boyns et al. (16) studied premenopausal and postmenopausal patients, using a heterologous radioimmunoassay, and found normal values in both groups. Wilson et al. (98), the same group, but now using a homologous radioimmunoassay, reported normal levels in both primary and metastatic cancer; the ages of patients and controls were not specified. Franks et al. (33) found normal values in premenopausal and postmenopausal patients. Mittra et al. (63) studied basal and TRH-stimulated prolactin levels in age-matched cancer patients and controls (age not specified); basal levels were normal in the patients, and stimulated levels showed a significant but slight elevation (about 20%) in the patients. Kwa et al. (54) studied cancer patients and age-matched controls and found no difference between the groups. Sheth et al. (77) measured prolactin levels in premenopausal and postmenopausal cancer patients and found no abnormalities in either group. Ohgo et al. (65) measured basal and TRH-stimulated plasma prolactin in 34 patients with primary breast cancer (equally divided between premenopausal and postmenopausal); 29 patients (85%) showed values in the normal range, whereas 5 patients (3 of them postmenopausal) showed slight to marked elevations; prolactin-elevating drugs were excluded as an explanation for these results. McFadyen et al. (60) reported slight elevation of prolactin in 5 patients with breast cancer, but the difference was not statistically significant. Malarkey et al. (59) reported normal 24-hr mean prolactin levels in premenopausal cancer patients, but significantly *subnormal* levels in postmenopausal patients. Golder et al. (35) studied prolactin levels in menopausal or oophorectomized breast cancer patients; the results were in the normal range. Cole et al. (22) studied prolactin levels in premenopausal cancer patients *after* mastectomy; this design differs from that of all other studies of prolactin except that of Jones et al. (48). They found slight elevations of prolactin in the patients during the follicular phase only. A puzzling feature of their data is their finding that prolactin levels in normal women rose somewhat with increasing age, a finding in contrast with that of other workers and ourselves that prolactin concentration decreases with age. Jones et al. (48) measured prolactin levels after mastectomy in premenopausal and postmenopausal women with primary cancer and reported that the values did not differ from normal.

Our own studies have shown a clear-cut continuous linear decrease of 24-hr mean prolactin levels with age in normal women; there was no discontinuity at or around the menopause. Accordingly, dividing patients and controls grossly into premenopausal and postmenopausal groups is oversimplified and misleading; detailed age versus concentration plots for patients and controls should be compared. When we did this in a group of 27 breast cancer patients, we found 2 younger women (in their thirties) with moderate elevations and 2 older women (about 60) with slight elevations; prolactin concentrations were within the normal range in the remaining 23 patients (i.e., 85% of the group). Thus our results were very similar to those of Ohgo et al. (65).

It appears, therefore, that prolactin concentrations are normal in the great majority of breast cancer patients. There is no obvious explanation for the elevations seen in a small percentage of patients, nor is there a clear-cut correlation of this finding with the stage of disease or the clinical course.

Thyroid Hormones

There is a considerable literature, going at least as far back as 1952 (69), suggesting on epidemiological grounds that breast cancer is associated with abnormalities of thyroid function. Most frequently it has been suggested that the association is with hypothyroidism, e.g., that the incidence of breast cancer parallels that of endemic goiter due to iodine deficiency (27,82), that the incidence of breast cancer is decreased in hyperthyroid patients (32,45), and that the incidence of cancer is increased in women who are receiving thyroid therapy for the treatment of hypothyroidism (50). An occasional report (88) described an association between *hyperthyroidism* and increased incidence of breast cancer. A careful study by Schottenfeld (73) of his own patients (including measurement of PBI levels) and of the literature up to that time (1968) failed to confirm a relationship between hypothyroidism and breast cancer. The American Thyroid Association has recently resummarized and commented on the evidence in two editorial statements (36,37) and has also found it unconvincing.

Only a few studies of thyroid function in breast cancer patients have been carried out. Most have used the uptake and/or conversion of radioactive iodide as criteria: the first was by Edelstyn et al. (28), who concluded that thyroid function was decreased; Reeve et al. (67) found normal function; Lencioni et al. (55) found slightly subnormal function; Stoll (83) found normal function; Bignazzi et al. (10) found values compatible with *hyperthyroidism,* although there were no corresponding clinical signs. Mittra and Hayward (62), using the indirect approach of measuring thyroid-stimulating hormone (TSH) levels, found slightly increased basal and thyrotropin-releasing hormone (TRH)-stimulated levels of TSH in breast cancer patients, which they interpreted as indicating "the presence of relatively low levels of circulating thyroid hormones in breast cancer." Unaccountably, they did not report the levels of the plasma thyroid hormones themselves in their patients, though these might have confirmed their hypothesis. It is of considerable interest, in interpreting the data of Mittra and Hayward, that elevated plasma TSH levels have been found occasionally in *hyperthyroidism;* in such cases (30,40) they have turned out to be due to TSH-secreting pituitary adenomas.

There have been only six reports of actual plasma concentrations of thyroid hormones in breast cancer. All of them were reports of PBI concentration, and all were published more than 10 years ago. There have been no published reports of concentrations of thyroxine or triiodothyronine. Carter et al. (20) reported a statistically significant elevation of PBI in breast cancer patients; the values in the patients did not exceed the upper limit of normal but were apparently clustered in the upper part of the normal range. Dargent et al. (24) also reported significantly elevated mean levels; some of the values were well above the normal range. Lencioni et al. (55) reported normal levels. Myhill et al. (64) reported elevated levels in metastatic cancer but not in localized disease. Schottenfeld (73) repooted normal levels. Sicher and Waterhouse (78) also reported normal levels. We have studied 24-hr mean concentrations of both triiodothyronine and thyroxine. T3 levels were normal. T4 levels were significantly elevated, by an average of about 48%, with some values in a clearly hyperthyroid range.

Thus the majority of studies that have investigated serum thyroid hormone concentrations have found a tendency toward elevation of thyroxine levels in cancer patients. The fact that T3 levels are not elevated, according to our studies, makes these elevated T4 values hard to interpret. There are two possible explanations for these results:

1. The elevated T4 values may represent elevated levels of thyroxine-binding globulin, giving increased total T4 levels but normal free T4 levels, and consequently euthyroidism.

2. The elevated T4 levels may indeed represent real hyperthyroidism, and the absence of elevated T3 levels may be due to the simultaneous presence, as a consequence of the patients' illness, of the "low-T3 syndrome" (9,21,68) in which peripheral conversion of T4 to T3 is diminished (72). There have been several case reports (47) of what has been called "T4 thyrotoxicosis" in which the authors have invoked just such a mechanism as I postulate, namely, the simultaneous presence of thyrotoxicosis plus the low-T3 syndrome. That breast cancer patients may indeed be slightly hyperthyroid as a group is suggested by our recent observation (101) that these patients have slightly increased cortisol production, a known physiological consequence of hyperthyroidism (42).

This interesting problem clearly requires further investigation.

Summary of Breast Cancer Findings

1. There is evidence for elevated plasma levels of dihydrotestosterone in this group of patients.

2. The findings with respect to plasma levels of dehydroisoandrosterone, dehydroisoandrosterone sulfate, and androsterone sulfate in breast cancer patients are controversial: some workers find subnormal levels, but our laboratory finds all three normal.

3. There is no consistent abnormality of plasma prolactin concentration in these patients; a small proportion of them (about 15%) may show elevated levels, but there are no clear-cut correlations of such findings with the stage or course of the disease.

4. The plasma levels of LH appear to be subnormal in premenopausal women with breast cancer. This may be related to the epidemiological fact that women with frequent anovulatory cycles are at increased risk for breast cancer.

5. The weight of evidence, including our own findings, is that women with breast cancer have modestly elevated plasma levels of thyroxine; this may or may not represent mild hyperthyroidism.

PROSTATE CANCER

Cortisol

Doe et al. (26) reported elevated plasma levels of non-protein-bound cortisol. Blackard et al., using both colorimetric determination of 17-hydroxycorticosteroids and competitive protein-binding determination of cortisol, again reported elevated levels 16 years later (11); with the colorimetric method the difference from normal was not statistically significant, but with the more accurate protein-binding method it was. These authors also found that the higher the plasma level of cortisol the poorer the prognosis for survival. Our studies have also shown a statistically significant elevation of plasma cortisol concentration in cancer patients, by about 40%. We have not followed the patients long enough to make a correlation with prognosis, but we have found that they show a statistically significant inverse relationship between plasma cortisol concentration and age (as opposed to age invariance of cortisol levels in normal men); since younger patients generally have a better survival prognosis than older ones (4), our data would suggest the opposite of the conclusion of Blackard et al., i.e., that higher cortisol levels are associated with *better* survival prognosis. Blackard et al. did not correlate age with cortisol concentration in their patients.

Testosterone

There have been 12 published studies in which the plasma testosterone concentration of prostate cancer patients has been compared with that of normal controls. Despite this large number, the results are still somewhat inconsistent. Isurugi (46), using the double-isotope derivative method, studied 5 patients and found that their plasma testosterone values tended to be somewhat lower than those of age-matched controls. Young and Kent (100), using the same method, found normal testosterone values in stage C prostate cancer patients and definitely subnormal values in stage D patients; they also found equally subnormal values in patients with other cancers and other chronic illnesses; no comment was made about any treatment the patients were receiving or had received. Robinson and Thomas (70), also using the double-isotope derivative method, found normal testosterone levels in patients with metastases (stage D). Mackler et al. (58), using a competitive protein-binding method, found that most of the stage C and D patients they studied had normal concentrations; about 25% of them had markedly subnormal levels, which they attributed to "debility" in these patients. No mention was made of the ages of the patients or controls. Sciarra et al. (74), using the same method, reported normal values in all of their patients (stage C) except one, who had a subnormal value. Shearer et al. (75) and all subsequent workers determined testosterone by radioimmunoassay; this group found normal levels in stage B patients and somewhat decreased levels in stage C and stage D patients. Kent et al. (51) reported normal testosterone values in both stage C and stage D patients, contrary to this group's previous report (100). Harper et al. (41) found that levels in cancer patients were the same as those in normal controls. Bartsch et al. reported normal values in patients with prostate cancer in one article (5) and subnormal values in another article (6). Habib et al. (39) reported that patients with prostate cancer did not differ in testosterone concentration, on the average, from patients with prostatic hypertrophy; they did not comment on the fact, which is apparent in Fig. 3 of their article, that testosterone levels *fell* with age in benign prostatic hypertrophy but tended to *rise* slightly with age in cancer patients to apparently supranormal levels in the oldest patients, a fact that is pertinent in the light of our own studies. We have found that normal individuals show a continuous fall in 24-hr mean testosterone concentration between ages 22 and 88, whereas prostate cancer patients show a *rise* between ages 55 (the youngest we studied) and 80 (the oldest we studied). The oldest cancer patients had values well above the normal range for age-matched controls, although not higher than those of younger controls (i.e., in their forties). This result may be pertinent to an understanding of the relationship of age to the response of prostate cancer patients to orchiectomy or antiandrogen therapy: we have observed a considerably higher remission rate in response to these measures in older patients (>65 years) than in younger patients (<65 years), a phenomenon that does not seem to have been recorded in the literature so far as we can determine.

Dihydrotestosterone

Despite the fact that dihydrotestosterone is the active tissue androgen in the prostate (97), there have been only three published studies concerning its plasma concentration in patients with prostate cancer. Habib et al. (39) reported normal levels in such patients. Bartsch et al. concurred with this finding in one article (5) but reported slightly subnormal levels in patients in a second article (6). Our studies have found normal dihydrotestosterone levels in prostate cancer.

Dehydroisoandrosterone, Dehydroisoandrosterone Sulfate, Androsterone, and Androsterone Sulfate

As far as I can determine, there have been no published studies of the plasma concentrations of these androgens in patients with prostate cancer. Our studies have found normal values for all four steroids in cancer patients.

Androstenedione

Gandy and Peterson (34) measured this steroid by a double-isotope derivative method and found higher values in cancer patients than in normal controls. Their method gave values that are unacceptably high by comparison with the values obtained by all subsequent workers, using radioimmunoassay methods, and are therefore hard to interpret. Sciarra et al. (74) found normal values in about 85% of cancer patients and slightly increased values in the others. Cowley et al. (23) found no difference between cancer patients and normal controls; the same conclusion was stated in another article from the same group (41).

Habib et al. also found normal levels in cancer patients (39). We have not studied the plasma levels of this steroid in prostate cancer.

Estradiol and Estrone

There appear to have been only three published reports of plasma estradiol concentrations in prostate cancer and only two concerning estrone levels. Harper et al. (41) reported normal levels of estradiol. Bartsch et al. reported normal levels in one article (5) and slightly subnormal levels in another (6). Our own studies of plasma estradiol levels in prostate cancer have not yet been completely analyzed. The two papers on estrone levels are both by Bartsch et al. These workers reported normal estrone levels in one article (5) and slightly subnormal levels in another (6). We have found significant elevation of this steroid in cancer patients, by about 50%. Furthermore, we have found a positive linear correlation between the plasma concentration of cortisol and that of estrone, suggesting that the "excess" estrone in cancer patients may be coming from the adrenal cortex, in response to the same stimulus that produces the hypercortisolemia in these patients.

LH and FSH

There has been only one published study comparing LH and FSH levels of prostate cancer patients with those of normals. Harper et al. (41) found no differences between these groups. We, too, have found no difference in LH and FSH levels between normals and cancer patients.

Prolactin

There have been three published reports comparing plasma prolactin levels in prostate cancer patients with those in normal controls. Harper et al. (41) and Bartsch et al. (5,6) reported no difference between these two groups. Our studies have also found no difference.

Thyroid Hormones

As far as I can ascertain, there have been no published studies comparing the plasma levels of triiodothyronine or thyroxine in prostate cancer patients as a group with those of normal controls. Some of the papers concerning the so-called low-T3 syndrome (9,21,68) have included some prostate cancer patients among the miscellaneous group of ill patients who show nonspecific depression of plasma T3 levels. Our studies of 15 patients with prostate cancer have shown 2 patients with abnormally low T3 levels; the others have all been in the normal range. We have found normal T4 levels in prostate cancer patients.

Summary of Prostate Cancer Findings

1. We and others have found definite elevations of plasma cortisol in this group of patients. This is not a "nonspecific" finding in cancer patients, since it has not been observed in women with breast cancer.

2. We have found elevated estrone levels in these patients; the only other group to study estrone found either normal or slightly subnormal levels in prostate cancer. In our patients there was a positive linear correlation between the plasma levels of estrone and cortisol.

3. The findings concerning testosterone are highly problematical. Several groups have found subnormal plasma levels in patients with metastatic prostate cancer, apparently those with advanced disease and considerable "debility." We have observed a unique feature in the ontogeny of plasma testosterone concentrations in prostate cancer patients: a rise with age instead of the normal fall with age; one other group has reported data somewhat suggestive of a similar phenomenon. This relationship of age to plasma testosterone concentration in prostate cancer patients may be pertinent to the findings with respect to the relationship of age to response to orchiectomy or antiandrogen therapy in these patients.

4. Plasma levels of dihydrotestosterone, dehydroisoandrosterone, dehydroisoandrosterone sulfate, androsterone, androsterone sulfate, androstenedione, estradiol, LH, FSH, prolactin, T3, and T4 appear to be normal in prostate cancer.

CONCLUSIONS

Several abnormalities in plasma hormone concentration have been found in women with breast cancer and several others in men with prostate cancer. Hormonal aberrations in cancer patients may be related to the cancer in one of two ways: (a) they may antedate the onset of the cancer, in which case it is not unreasonable to postulate that they may constitute one of the components of a "fertile soil" that favors the initiation and/or progression of the cancer; (b) they may appear after (thus presumably as a result of) the onset of cancer. In the latter case, it is, of course, possible that a hormonal aberration may be only an incidental occurrence with no biological implications; however, a more interesting possibility is that a hormonal aberration may secondarily favor the progression of the cancer, thus participating in a positive-feedback cycle in which the onset of cancer produces hormonal aberrations, which favors the progression of the cancer, which increases the hormonal aberrations, etc. Thus the question of whether observed hormonal abnormalities in cancer antedate or follow the onset of the cancer is not necessarily critical; one can envision ways in which the abnormalities might favor the progression of the cancer in either circumstance. It certainly seems an appropriate endeavor, therefore, to seek out and critically document hormonal abnormalities in breast and prostate cancer with a view to finding ways of normalizing them in the hope that such an approach may constitute a new and promising therapeutic avenue.

ACKNOWLEDGMENTS

These studies were supported in part by grants CA-07304 from the National Cancer Institute and RR-53 from the General Clinical Research Centers Branch, National Institutes of Health, Bethesda, Md.

REFERENCES

1. Ahlquist, K. A., Jackson, A. W., and Stewart, J. G. (1968): Urinary steroid values as a guide to prognosis in breast cancer. *Br. Med. J.,* 1:217.
2. Allen, B. J., Hayward, J. L., and Merrivale, W. H. H. (1957): The excretion of 17-ketosteroids in the urine of patients with generalized carcinomatosis secondary to carcinoma of the breast. *Lancet,* 1:496.
3. Atkins, H. J. B., Bulbrook, R. D., Falconer, M. A., Hayward, J. L., MacLean, K. S., and Schuir, P. H. (1968): Ten years' experience of steroid assays in the management of breast cancer. A review. *Lancet,* 2:1255.
4. Axtell, L. M., Asire, A. J., and Myers, M. H. (editors) (1976): Cancer Patients Survival, Report Number 5, p. 196. DHEW Publication No. (NIH) 77–992, Bethesda, Md.
5. Bartsch, W., Horst, H.-J., Becker, H., and Nehse, G. (1977): Sex hormone binding globulin-binding capacity, testosterone, 5α-dihydrotestosterone, oestradiol, and prolactin in plasma of patients with prostate carcinoma under various types of hormonal treatment. *Acta Endocrinol. (Kbh),* 85:650.
6. Bartsch, W., Steins, P., and Becker, H. (1977): Hormone blood levels in patients with prostatic carcinoma and their relation to the type of carcinoma growth differentiation. *Eur. Urol.,* 3:47.
7. Beck, J. C., Blair, A. J., Griffiths, M. M., Rosenfeld, M. W., and McGarry, E. E. (1966): In search of hormonal factors as an aid in predicting the outcome of breast carcinoma. *Can. Cancer Conf.,* 6:3.
8. Berle, P., and Voigt, K. D. (1972): Evidence of plasma prolactin levels in patients with breast cancer. *Am. J. Obstet. Gynecol.,* 114:1101.
9. Bermudez, F., Surks, M. I., and Oppenheimer, J. H. (1975): High incidence of decreased serum triiodothyronine concentration in patients with nonthyroidal disease. *J. Clin. Endocrinol. Metab.,* 41:27.
10. Bignazzi, A., d'Amico, P., and Veronesi, U. (1965): La funzionalitá tiroidea nelle pazienti affette da carcinoma mammaria (Thyroid function in patients with breast cancer). *Tumori,* 51:199.
11. Blackard, C. E., Byar, D. P., Seal, U. S., Doe, R. P., and V. A. Cooperative Urological Research Group (1975): Correlation of pre-treatment serum 17-hydroxycorticosteroid values with survival in patients with prostate cancer. *J. Urol.,* 113:517.
12. Borkowski, A., L'Hermite, M., Dor, P., Longeral, E., Rozencweig, M., Muquardt, C., and Van Canter, F. (1977): Steroid sex hormones and prolactin in postmenopausal women with generalized mammary carcinoma during prolonged dexamethasone treatment. *J. Endocrinol.,* 73:235.
13. Boyar, R. M., Finkelstein, J. W., David, R., Roffwarg, H., Kapen, S., Weitzman, E. D., and Hellman, L. (1973): Twenty-four hour patterns of plasma luteinizing hormone and follicle-stimulating hormone in sexual precocity. *N. Engl. J. Med.,* 289:282.
14. Boyar, R. M., Kapen, S., Finkelstein, J. W., Perlow, M., Sassin, J. F., Fukushima, D. K., Weitzman, E. D., and Hellman, L. (1974): Hypothalamic-pituitary function in diverse hyperprolactinemic states. *J. Clin. Invest.,* 53:1588.
15. Boyar, R. M., Rosenfeld, R. S., Kapen, S., Finkelstein, J. W., Roffwarg, H., Weitzman, E. D., and Hellman, L. (1974): Human puberty: Simultaneous augmented secretion of luteinizing hormone and testosterone during sleep. *J. Clin. Invest.,* 54:609.
16. Boyns, A. R., Cole, E. N., Griffiths, K., Roberts, M. M., Buchan, R., Wilson, R. G., and Forrest, A. P. M. (1973): Plasma prolactin in breast cancer. *Eur. J. Cancer,* 9:99.
17. Brownsey, G., Cameron, E. H. D., Griffiths, K., Gleave, E. N., Forrest, A. P. M., and Campbell, H. (1972): Plasma dehydroepiandrosterone sulphate levels in patients with benign and malignant breast disease. *Eur. J. Cancer,* 8:131.

18. Bulbrook, R. D., Greenwood, F. C., and Hayward, J. L. (1960): Selection of breast-cancer patients for adrenalectomy or hypophysectomy by determination of urinary 17-hydroxycorticosteroids and aetiocholanolone. *Lancet,* 1:1154.
19. Calabresi, E., DiGiuli, G., Becciolini, A., Giannoti, P., Lombardi, G., and Serio, M. (1976): Plasma estrogens and androgens in male breast cancer. *J. Steroid Biochem.,* 7:605.
20. Carter, A., Feldman, E. B., and Schwartz, H. L. (1960): Level of serum protein-bound iodine in patients with metastatic carcinoma of the breast. *J. Clin. Endocrinol. Metab.,* 20:477.
21. Chopra, I. J., Solomon, D. H., Chopra, V., Young, R. T., and Chua Teco, G. N. (1974): Alterations in circulating thyroid hormones and thyrotropin in hepatic cirrhosis: Evidence for euthyroidism despite subnormal serum triiodothyronine. *J. Clin. Endocrinol. Metab.,* 39:501.
22. Cole, E. N., England, P. C., Sellwood, R. A., and Griffiths, K. (1977): Serum prolactin concentrations throughout the menstrual cycle of normal women and patients with recent breast cancer. *Eur. J. Cancer,* 13:677.
23. Cowley, T. H., Brownsey, B. G., Harper, M. E., Peeling, W. B., and Griffiths, K. (1976): The effect of ACTH on plasma testosterone and androstenedione concentrations in patients with prostatic carcinoma. *Acta Endocrinol. (Kbh),* 81:310.
24. Dargent, M., Berger, M., and Lahneche, B. (1962): La fonction thyroïdienne chez les malades atteintes de cancer du sein (Thyroid function in patients with breast cancer). *Acta Unio Internationalis contra Cancrum,* 18:915.
25. Deshpande, N., Hayward, J. L., and Bulbrook, R. D. (1965): Plasma 17-hydroxycorticosteroids and 17-oxosteroids in patients with breast cancer and in normal women. *J. Endocrinol.,* 32:167.
26. Doe, R. P., Dickinson, P., Linneman, H. H., and Seal, U. S. (1959): Elevated nonprotein-bound cortisol (NPC) in pregnancy, during estrogen administration and in carcinoma of the prostate. *J. Clin. Endocrinol. Metab.,* 29:757.
27. Doll, R. (1969): The geographical distribution of cancer. *Br. J. Cancer,* 23:1.
28. Edelstyn, G. A., Lyons, A. R., and Welbaum, R. B. (1958): Thyroid function in patients with mammary cancer. *Lancet,* 1:670.
29. England, P. C., Skinner, L. G., Cottrell, K. M., and Sellwood, R. A. (1974): Serum oestradiol-17β in women with benign and malignant breast disease. *Br. J. Cancer.,* 30:571.
30. Fagalia, G., Ferrari, C., Neri, V., Beck-Peccoz, P., Ambrosi, B., and Valentini, F. (1972): High plasma thyrotrophin levels in two patients with pituitary tumour. *Acta Endocrinol. (Kbh),* 69:649.
31. Finkelstein, J. W., Boyar, R. M., Roffwarg, H. P., Kream, J., Fukushima, D. K., Gallagher, T. F., and Hellman, L. (1973): Growth hormone secretion in congenital adrenal hyperplasia. *J. Clin. Endocrinol. Metab.,* 36:121.
32. Finley, J. W., Bogardus, G. M. (1960): Breast cancer and thyroid disease. *Quart. Rev. Surg. Obstet. Gynecol.,* 17:139.
33. Franks, S., Ralphs, D. N. L., Seagroatt, V., and Jacobs, H. S. (1974): Prolactin concentrations in patients with breast cancer. *Br. Med. J.,* 4:320.
34. Gandy, H. M., and Peterson, R. E. (1968): Measurement of testosterone and 17-ketosteroids in plasma by the double isotope dilution derivative technique. *J. Clin. Endocrinol. Metab.,* 28:949.
35. Golder, M. P., Phillips, M. E. A., Fahmy, D. R., Preece, P. E., Jones, V., Henk, J. M., and Griffiths, K. (1976): Plasma hormones in patients with advanced breast cancer treated with tamoxifen. *Eur. J. Cancer,* 12:719.
36. Gorman, C. A., Becker, D. V., Greenspan, F. S., Lang, R. P., Oppenheimer, J. H., Rivlin, R. S., Robbins, J., and Vanderloan, W. P. (1977): Breast cancer and thyroid therapy: Statement by the American Thyroid Association. *J.A.M.A.,* 237:1459.
37. Gorman, C. A., Becker, D. V., Greenspan, F. S., Lang, R. P., Oppenheimer, J. H., Rivlin, R. S., Robbins, J., and Vanderloan, W. P. (1977): American Thyroid Association Statement: Breast cancer and thyroid hormone therapy. *Ann. Intern Med.,* 86:502.
38. Grattarola, R. (1964): The premenstrual endometrial pattern of women with breast cancer. *Cancer,* 17:1119.
39. Habib, F. K., Lee, I. R., Stitch, S. R., and Smith, P. H. (1976): Androgen levels in the plasma and prostatic tissues of patients with benign hypertrophy and carcinoma of the prostate. *J. Endocrinol.,* 71:99.
40. Hamilton, C. R., Jr., Adams, L. C., and Maloof, F. (1970): Hyperthyroidism due to thyrotrophin-producing chromophobe adenoma. *N. Engl. J. Med.,* 283:1077.

41. Harper, M. E., Peeling, W. B., Cowley, T., Brownsey, B. G., Phillips, M. E. A., Groom, G., Fahmy, D. R., and Griffiths, K. (1976): Plasma steroid and protein hormone concentration in patients with prostatic carcinoma, before and during estrogen therapy. *Acta Endocrinol. (Kbh),* 81:409.
42. Hellman, L., Bradlow, H. L., Zumoff, B., and Gallagher, T. F. (1961): The influence of thyroid hormone on hydrocortisone production and metabolism. *J. Clin. Endocrinol. Metab.,* 21:1231.
43. Hellman, L., Nakada, F., Curti, J., Weitzman, E. D., Kream, J., Roffwarg, H., Ellman, S., Fukushima, D. K., and Gallagher, T. F. (1970): Cortisol is secreted episodically by normal man. *J. Clin. Endocrinol. Metab.,* 30:411.
44. Horn, H. and Gordan, G. S. (1974): Plasma testosterone in advanced brest cancer. *Oncology,* 30:147.
45. Humphrey, L. J., and Swerdlow,, M. (1964): The relationship of breast disease to thyroid disease. *Cancer,* 17:1170.
46. Isurugi, K. (1967): Plasma testosterone production rates in patients with prostatic cancer and benign prostatic hypertrophy. *J. Urol.,* 97:903.
47. Joasoo, A. (1975): T3 thyrotoxicosis with normal or low serum T4 concentration. *Aust. N.Z. J. Med.,* 5:432.
48. Jones, M. K., Ramsay, I. D., Booth, M., and Collins, W. P. (1977): Hormone concentrations in postmenopausal patients with breast cancer. *Clin. Oncol.,* 3:177.
49. Juret, P., Hayem, M., and Flaisler, A. J. (1964): À propos de 150 implantations d'yttrium radio-actif intra-hypophysaires dans le traitement de cancer du sein à un stade avancé. Technique; Bilan clinique; Indications. (A report on 150 intrahypophysial implantations of radioactive yttrium in the treatment of advanced cancer of the breast. Technique; clinical findings; indications.) *J. Chir.,* 87:409.
50. Kapdi, C. C., and Wolfe, J. N. (1976): Breast cancer: Relationship to thyroid supplements for hypothyroidism. *J.A.M.A.,* 236:1124.
51. Kent, J. R., Bischoff, A. J., Arduino, L. J., Mellinger, G. T., Byar, D. P., Hill, M., and Kozbur, X. (1973): Estrogen dosage and suppression of testosterone levels in patients with prostatic carcinoma. *J. Urol.,* 109:858.
52. Krieger, D. T., and Glick, S. (1971): Absent sleep peak of growth hormone release in blind subjects: Correlation with sleep EEG stages. *J. Clin. Endocrinol. Metab.,* 33:847.
53. Kumaoka, S., Sakauchi, N., Abe, O., Kusama, M., and Takatani, O. (1968): Urinary 17-ketosteroid excretion of women with advanced breast cancer. *J. Clin. Endocrinol. Metab.,* 28:667.
54. Kwa, H. G., Engelsman, E., DeJong-Bakker, M., and Cleton, F. J. (1974): Plasma prolactin in human breast cancer. *Lancet,* 1:433.
55. Lencioni, L. J., Richiger de Arranz, E., Davidovich, D., and Staffieri, J. J. (1962): Exploración funcional tiroidea en pacientes con cancer mamario (A study of thyroid function in patients with breast cancer). *Medicina,* 22:215.
56. Liang, T., Tymoczko, J. L., Chan, K. M. B., Hung, S. C., and Liao, S. (1977): Androgen action: Receptors and rapid responses. In: *Androgens and Antiandrogens,* edited by L. Martini and M. Motta, p. 77. Raven Press, New York.
57. Lippman, M. E. (1976): Hormone-dependent human breast cancer in long-term tissue culture. In: *Hormones and Cancer,* edited by K. N. Charyulu and A. Sudarsanam, p. 219. Stratton Intercontinental, New York.
58. Mackler, M. A., Liberti, J. P., Vernon Smith, M. J., Koontz, W. W., Jr., and Prout, G. R., Jr. (1972): The effect of orchiectomy and various doses of stilbestrol on plasma testosterone levels in patients with carcinoma of the prostate. *Invest. Urol.,* 9:423.
59. Malarkey, W. B., Schroeder, L. L., James, A. G., Pipers, F. S., and Stevens, V. C. (1976): Twenty-four hour concentrations of various pituitary and steroid hormones in women with breast cancer. In: *Endocrine Society Proceedings* (abstract 416).
60. McFadyen, I. J., Prescott, R. J., Groom, G. V., Forrest, A. P. M., Golder, M. P., Fahmy, D. R., and Griffiths, K. (1976): Circulating hormone concentrations in women with breast cancer. *Lancet,* 1:1100.
61. Miller, H., and Durant, J. A. (1968): The value of urine steroid hormone assays in breast cancer. *Clin. Biochem.,* 1:287.
62. Mittra, I., and Hayward, J. L. (1974): Hypothalamic-pituitary-thyroid axis in breast cancer. *Lancet,* 1:885.

63. Mittra, I., Hayward, J. L., and McNeilly, A. S. (1974): Hypothalamic-pituitary-prolactin axis in breast cancer. *Lancet,* 1:889.
64. Myhill, J., Reeve, T. S., and Hales, I. B. (1966): Thyroid function in breast cancer. *Acta Endocrinol. (Kbh),* 51:290.
65. Ohgo, S., Kato, Y., Chihara, K., and Imura, H. (1976): Plasma prolactin responses to thyrotropin-releasing hormone in patients with breast cancer. *Cancer,* 37:1412.
66. Portnay, G. I., O'Brian, J. T., Bush, J., Vogenakis, A. G., Azizi, F., Arky, R. A., Ingbar, S. H., and Braverman, L. E. (1974): The effect of starvation on the concentration and binding of thyroxine and triiodothyronine in serum and on the response to TRH. *J. Clin. Endocrinol. Metab.,* 39:191.
67. Reeve, T. S., Hales, I. B., Rundle, F. F., Myhill, J., and Groydon, M. (1961): Thyroid function in the presence of breast cancer. *Lancet,* 1:632.
68. Reichlin, S., Bollinger, J., Nijad, I., and Sullivan, P. (1973): Tissue thyroid hormone concentration of rat and man determined by radioimmunoassay: Biologic significance. *Mt. Sinai Hosp. J.,* 40:503.
69. Repert, R. W. (1952): Breast carcinoma study: Relation of thyroid disease and diabetes. *J. Mich. St. Med. Soc.,* 51:1315.
70. Robinson, M. R. G., and Thomas, B. S. (1971): Effect of hormonal therapy on plasma testosterone levels in prostatic carcinoma. *Br. Med. J.,* 4:391.
71. Rose, D. P., Stauber, P., Thiel, A., Crowley, J. J., and Milbrath, J. R. (1977): Plasma dehydroepiandrosterone sulfate, androstenedione and cortisol, and urinary free cortisol excretion in breast cancer. *Eur. J. Cancer,* 13:43.
72. Schimmel, M., and Utiger, R. (1977): Thyroidal and peripheral production of thyroid hormones. Review of recent findings and their clinical implication. *Ann. Intern Med.,* 87:760.
73. Schottenfeld, D. (1968): The relationship of breast cancer to thyroid disease. *J. Chronic Dis.,* 21:203.
74. Sciarra, F., Sorcini, G., DiSilverio, F., and Galliardi, V. (1973): Plasma testosterone and androstenedione after orchiectomy in prostatic adenocarcinoma. *Clin. Endocrinol.,* 2:101.
75. Shearer, R. J., Hendry, W. F., Sommerville, I. F., and Fergusson, J. D. (1973): Plasma testosterone: An accurate monitor of hormone treatment in prostatic cancer. *Br. J. Urol.,* 45:668.
76. Sherman, B. M., and Korenman, S. G. (1974): Inadequate corpus luteum function: A pathophysiological interpretation of human breast cancer epidemiology. *Cancer,* 33:1306.
77. Sheth, N. A., Ranadine, K. J., Suraiya, J. N., and Sheth, A. R. (1975): Circulating levels of prolactin in human breast cancer. *Br. J. Cancer,* 32:160.
78. Sicher, K., and Waterhouse, J. A. H. (1967): Thyroid activity in relation to prognosis in mammary cancer. *Br. J. Cancer,* 21:512.
79. Skinner, L. G., England, P. C., Cottrell, K. M., and Selwood, R. A. (1974): Serum oestradiol-17β in normal premenopausal women and in patients with benign and malignant breast disease. *Br. J. Cancer,* 30:176.
80. Smethurst, M., Basu, T. K., and Williams, D. C. (1975): Levels of cholesterol, 11-hydroxycorticosteroids and progesterone in plasma from postmenopausal women with breast cancer. *Eur. J. Cancer,* 11:751.
81. Šonká, J., Vitková, M., Gregorová, I., Tomsová, Z., Hilgertová, J., and Staś, J. (1973): Plasma and urinary dehydroepiandrosterone in cancer. *Endokrinologie,* 62:51.
82. Stadel, B. V. (1976): Dietary iodine and risk of breast, endometrial and ovarian cancer. *Lancet,* 1:890.
83. Stoll, B. A. (1965): Breast cancer and hypothyroidism. *Cancer,* 18:1431.
84. Takahashi, Y. D., Kipnis, D. M., and Daughaday, W. H. (1968): Growth hormone secretion during sleep. *J. Clin. Invest.,* 47:2079.
85. Thomas, B. S., Kirby, P., Symes, E. K., and Wang, D. Y. (1976): Plasma dehydroepiandrosterone concentration in normal women and in patients with benign and malignant breast disease. *Eur. J. Cancer,* 12:405.
86. Vitola, G. Y., and Zeikate, G. A. (1976): The concentration of testosterone and dihydrotestosterone in blood plasma in patients with breast cancer. *Vopr. Onkol.,* 22:26.
87. Wade, A. P., Tweedie, M. C. K., Davis, J. C., Clarke, C. A., and Haggart, B. (1969): The discriminant function in early carcinoma of the breast. *Lancet,* 1:853.
88. Wanebo, H. J., Benna, R. J., and Rawson, R. W. (1966): Neoplastic disease and thyrotoxicosis. *Cancer,* 19:1523.

89. Wang, D. Y., Hayward, J. L., and Bulbrook, R. D. (1966): Testosterone levels in the plasma of normal women and patients with benign breast disease or with breast cancer. *Eur. J. Cancer,* 2:373.
90. Wang, D. Y. (1969): Plasma androgens in breast cancer. In: *The Human Adrenal Gland and Its Relation to Breast Cancer,* edited by K. Griffiths and E. H. D. Cameron, p. 71. First Tenovus Workshop, Alpha Omega Alpha, Cardiff, Wales.
91. Wang, D. Y., Bulbrook, R. D., Herian, M., and Hayward, J. L. (1974): Studies on the sulphate esters of dehydroepiandrosterone and androsterone in the blood of women with breast cancer. *Eur. J. Cancer,* 10:477.
92. Wang, D. Y., Goodwin, P. R., Bulbrook, R. D., and Hayward, J. L. (1976): Plasma FSH and LH in post-menopausal women with breast cancer. *Eur. J. Cancer,* 12:305.
93. Wang, D. Y., Bulbrook, R. D., and Hayward, J. L. (1977): Plasma androstenedione levels in women with breast cancer. *Eur. J. Cancer,* 13:187.
94. Weitzman, E. D. Schaumberg, H., and Fishbein, W. (1966): Plasma 17-hydroxycorticosteroid levels during sleep in man. *J. Clin. Endocrinol. Metab.,* 26:121.
95. West, C. D., Mahajan, D. K., Chavre, V. J., Nabors, C. J., and Tyler, F. H. (1973): Simultaneous measurement of multiple plasma steroids by radioimmunoassay demonstrating episodic secretion. *J. Clin. Endocrinol. Metab.,* 36:1230.
96. Wilson, R. E., Crocker, D. W., Fairgrieve, J., Bartholomay, A. F., Emerson, K., Jr., and Moore, F. D. (1967): Adrenal structure and function in advanced carcinoma of the breast. II. The relation of description of a new discriminant function. *J.A.M.A.,* 199:474.
97. Wilson, J. D., and Walker, J. D. (1969): The conversion of testosterone to 5α-androstene-17β-ol-3-one. *J. Clin. Invest.,* 48:371.
98. Wilson, R. G., Buchan, R., Roberts, M. M., Forrest, A. P. M., Boyns, A. R., Cole, E. N., and Griffiths, K. (1974): Plasma prolactin and breast cancer. *Cancer,* 33:1325.
99. Yen, S. S. C., Tsai, C. C., Naftolin, F., Vanderberg, G., and Ajabor, L. (1972): Pulsatile patterns of gonadotropin release in subjects with and without ovarian function. *J. Clin. Endocrinol. Metab.,* 34:671.
100. Young, H. H., II, and Kent, J. R. (1968): Plasma testosterone levels in patients with prostatic carcinoma before and after treatment. *J. Urol.,* 99:788.

Subject Index